C000264093

"Many parents and professionals have noted the co[...] children with ASD and music and some have incorp[...] their homes or school programs. Up until now, ho[...] a rigorous or comprehensive statement about the practice, its scope, and its possibilities. This new book is most welcome and long overdue. Its scholarly treatment of all aspects of musical approaches and therapy with young children with ASD promises to be an important contribution to the field.

The best thing about this book is that it has something to offer to everyone. For the practicing therapist it explains some of the rigors of scientific approaches and nicely illustrates how musical interventions fit into the prevailing practices in the field for young children. For the scientist, it offers a comprehensive description of research, evidence-based practice, and field studies and the scientific relevance and possibilities related to the work. And for the many parents and professionals who have noticed that music and ASD often have some connection in young children, it broadens their understanding of the current scope and future possibilities. We all owe a huge debt of gratitude to the authors for finally giving this field the kind of recognition that it deserves."

—*Gary B. Mesibov, Ph.D., Professor Emeritus,*
The University of North Carolina at Chapel Hill

"The editors of this book are highly distinguished in the use of music therapy with persons with autism spectrum disorders and have compiled an outstanding compendium of information in a much needed clinical specialty area. They cover all aspects of clinical music therapy treatment from identifying and defining the problem to assessment and multiple methods of intervention and evaluation. It is a comprehensive volume that will be invaluable to clinicians and educators and is a welcome addition to the field."

—*Jayne Standley, Ph.D., MT-BC, Ella Scoble Opperman and Robert O. Lawton,*
Distinguished Professor of Music Therapy, The Florida State University

"Petra Kern and Marcia Humpal have edited a remarkable book on children with autism spectrum disorders that includes a wide range of topics and approaches focusing on the use of music in therapy. The information is presented in reader-friendly terms and includes supporting research, case examples, and practical ideas. Contributions from seasoned researchers in the field make this book an incredible evidence-based resource for professionals, students, and parents."

—*Blythe LaGasse, Ph.D., MT-BC, Assistant Professor*
of Music Therapy, Colorado State University

"Music therapy potentially has practices to offer the professionals working with children with autism; those practices, however, must be evaluated experimentally to be of use. This book makes a significant contribution toward providing the field with the experimental methods for such evaluations."
—*Mark Wolery, Ph.D., Professor of Special Education, Vanderbilt University*

Early Childhood Music Therapy and Autism Spectrum Disorders

of related interest

Music Therapy in Schools
Working with Children of All Ages in Mainstream and Special Education
Edited by Jo Tomlinson, Philippa Derrington and Amelia Oldfield
Foreword by Dr. Frankie Williams
ISBN 978 1 84905 000 5
eISBN 978 0 85700 474 1

Developmental Speech-Language Training through Music
for Children with Autism Spectrum Disorders
Theory and Clinical Application
Hayoung A. Lim
Foreword by Karen Miller
ISBN 978 1 84905 849 0
eISBN 978 0 85700 415 4

Music for Special Kids
Musical Activities, Songs, Instruments and Resources
Pamela Ott
ISBN 978 1 84905 858 2
eISBN 978 0 85700 426 0

Music Therapy with Children and their Families
Edited by Amelia Oldfield and Claire Flower
Foreword by Vince Hesketh
ISBN 978 1 84310 581 7
eISBN 978 1 84642 801 2

Let's All Listen
Songs for Group Work in Settings that Include Students
with Learning Difficulties and Autism
Pat Lloyd
Foreword by Adam Ockelford
With CD
ISBN 978 1 84310 583 1
eISBN 978 1 84642 724 4

Fuzzy Buzzy Groups for Children with Developmental
and Sensory Processing Difficulties
A Step-by-Step Resource
Fiona Brownlee and Lindsay Munro
Illustrated by Aisling Nolan
ISBN 978 1 84310 966 2
eISBN 978 0 85700 194 8

Music Therapy, Sensory Integration and the Autistic Child
Dorita S. Berger
Foreword by Donna Williams
ISBN 978 1 84310 700 2
eISBN 978 1 84642 712 1

Early Childhood Music Therapy and Autism Spectrum Disorders

Developing Potential in Young Children and their Families

Edited by Petra Kern and Marcia Humpal
Foreword by David Aldridge

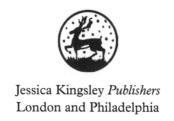

Jessica Kingsley *Publishers*
London and Philadelphia

Releases have kindly been provided for all photographs in the book.
Table 2.2, on pp. 49–50, has been reprinted with kind permission from The National Professional Development Center (NPDC) on ASD.
Figure 10.1, on pp. 92–3, has been reprinted with kind permission from De La Vista Publisher.
Table 12.4, on pp. 226–7, from Wakeford 2010 has been reprinted with permission.
The interviews in Chapter 14 have been reproduced with kind permission from the music therapists.

First published in 2012
by Jessica Kingsley Publishers
73 Collier Street
London N1 9BE, UK
and
400 Market Street, Suite 400
Philadelphia, PA 19106, USA

www.jkp.com

Copyright © Petra Kern and Marcia Humpal 2013
Foreword copyright © David Aldridge 2013

Printed digitally since 2015

Library of Congress Cataloging-in-Publication Data
Early childhood music therapy and autism spectrum disorders : developing potential in young children and their families / Petra Kern and Marcia Humpal ; foreword by David Aldridge.
pages cm
Includes bibliographical references and index.
ISBN 978-1-84905-241-2 (pbk. format : alk. paper) -- ISBN 978-0-85700-485-7 (electronic format) 1. Music therapy for children. 2. Music therapy--Instruction and study. 3. Autistic children--Education--Music. 4. Children with disabilities--Education--Music. 5. Special education--Music. 6. Autism in children. I. Kern, Petra. II. Humpal, Marcia Earl.
ML3920.E23 2012
618.92'89165154--dc23
2012015211

British Library Cataloguing in Publication Data
A CIP catalogue record for this book is available from the British Library

ISBN 978 1 84905 241 2
eISBN 978 0 85700 485 7

We dedicate this book to the children with autism spectrum disorders and their families who enriched our lives.

Contents

Part 3: Treatment Approaches

Part 4: Collaboration and Consultation

Part 5: Selected Resources

Foreword

David Aldridge

The body of the speaker dances in time with his speech.
Further, the body of the listener dances in
rhythm with that of the speaker!
(Condon and Ogston, 1966, p. 338)

I met Sidney over 30 years ago in a pediatric assessment unit. He was four years old. His mother was concerned about his delayed development. The unit pediatrician and teacher had tentatively diagnosed him as autistic. Sidney often walked on his tiptoes, flapped his hands, avoided eye contact, and was reluctant to play with other children. He refused to eat properly, his language skills were rudimentary, and he often repeated the same phrase, "Not 'day." meaning "Not today." Everything pointed to a diagnosis of early childhood autism. I was sent to interview his family after being advised by the pediatrician that Sidney's mother probably was emotionally detached (referred to in those days as a "refrigerator" mother).

In the past, myths were mixed with facts and there was no spectrum of disorder. You were either autistic or not. You were viewed by the myths that surrounded you, not as a person first. In this book, we see how things have changed, how each person with autism spectrum disorders (ASD) should be viewed as an individual with unique needs, and that assessment, diagnosis, and treatment are based on evidence.

At that first visit with Sidney, I rolled a toy car to him and he rolled it back. That is, he began to play. When sitting on a swing, he responded to "Sid" on the outward swing and "'Ney" on the return swing. When I sang his name, and then suspended the swing until he spoke his name, he then started to sing his name. Rhythm and playfulness were the cues for communication; that is why music therapy made so much sense to me when I first encountered it.

Later it became evident that Sidney had what we now know as tactile and oral defensiveness; his lips were extremely sensitive. This helped explain his eating issues. Sidney's mother was not a difficult mother, nor he a difficult child. Both were challenged by his compromised neurologic status. The important thing here is that parents usually know that something is not quite right with their child. It is challenging enough for them without being blamed for their child's difficulties. In terms of assessment and then intervention, it is important to accept the child as he is, starting with what he can do, and then treating him as a child, not a syndrome. In the pages that follow, you will find numerous examples that support these points.

These principles guided my earlier research with children with developmental delays (Aldridge, 1991; Aldridge, Gustorff, and Neugebauer, 1995). For instance, mutual listening is a prerequisite of effective mutual communication and dialogue; and hand–eye coordination, dependent on wider body awareness, appears to be a vital component in developmental change. Additionally, hand movements and gestures seem to play an important role in non-verbal communication and for the subtle aspects of emotional expression. Therefore, the active playing of a drum demands that the child listen to the therapist, who in turn is listening to, and playing for her. This coherence of the cognitive, gestural, emotional, and relational may be the strength of active music therapy for children who are developmentally challenged.

More recent studies have shown that the importance of this central coherence (i.e., a propensity to form meaningful links over a wide range of stimuli) may be compromised in children with ASD (Aljunied and Frederickson, 2011). Furthermore, addressing motor development is often highly indicated in early intervention (Lloyd, Macdonald, and Lord, 2011). Music therapy addresses these issues of coherence and motor skills by the very activity of performance.

Performance, the integration of coherence and timing, establishes our emotional being both biologically and socially (Aldridge, 2012). Studies have shown that individuals with ASD may have a different rhythm in their body response to sound that indicates their hearing is delayed (Aldridge, 1996; Condon, 1974, 1975; Condon and Sander, 1974) resulting in an interactional synchrony that may be compromised and thereby disrupting communication. It is this synchrony that may provide the awareness of our social relationship. When this is disturbed from birth, we often see the phenomena of social anxiety and communication difficulties in children with ASD. It is this very synchrony, based on mutual timing, which may be disordered; that may be the basis for both a central sense of coherence within ourselves (for the functioning of our own neural integrity), and with others. Therefore, a compromised neural development may be the basis for the coordination of interaction between child and caregiver in terms of facial expression and emotion (Camras and Shutter, 2010; Lopata et al., 2009).

Emotional development is individual and social, dependent upon a functioning neural substrate that is synchronized with another person. If this substrate is disturbed, then the child does not achieve the systemic regulators, internal and external, necessary for development. All of this discussion leads us back to the infant–mother interaction. If mothers do not receive the feedback that they expect, they know that something is not quite right.

We know that early behavioral intervention (Kovshoff, Hastings, and Remington, 2011) is important, and the upcoming chapters demonstrate that music therapy can be a valuable treatment option. Assessment is the key to an early diagnosis and potential intervention. While successful treatment is also dependent upon the level of the child's ability (Stahmer, Akshoomoff, and Cunningham, 2011), parents can play an important role in their child's program. As we saw with Sidney, his parents were concerned. We know now that parents require support (Ludlow, Skelly, and Rohleder, 2011) and also parents can initiate those early diagnoses, and thereby implementation of integrated treatments can be achieved in the preschool years (Lindsay, 2011).

Thirty years is a long time and the assessment and treatment of young children with ASD has moved forward by leaps and bounds. After finding a way to play with Sidney and alter the communicative environment in the unit, where he was always seen as a charming little boy, his behavioral difficulties receded. Playing with the charming child that was Sidney and simply singing with him opened up a world of communication and set me upon a research path that brought me into the world of music therapy.

We see in the following pages how that world has moved on. This book provides a resource of music therapy interventions firmly based in evidence from both research and practice. We now have a platform from which we can all develop further. The myths have been demolished. Music therapists continue to develop knowledge-based content that provides a resource for other professionals working in the field of early childhood and autism spectrum disorders.

References

Aldridge, D. (1991). Physiological change, communication and the playing of improvised music. *Arts in Psychotherapy, 18*, 59–64.

Aldridge, D. (1996). *Music Therapy Research and Practice in Medicine: From Out of the Silence.* London and Philadelphia: Jessica Kingsley Publishers.

Aldridge, D. (2012). Coherence and timing. In D. Aldridge and J. Fachner (Eds.) *Music Therapy and Addictions.* London and Philadelphia: Jessica Kingsley Publishers.

Aldridge, D., Gustorff, D., and Neugebauer, L. (1995). A pilot study of music therapy in the treatment of children with developmental delay. *Complementary Therapies in Medicine, 3*, 197–205.

Aljunied, M., and Frederickson, N. (2011). Does central coherence relate to the cognitive performance of children with autism in dynamic assessments? *Autism, 29* June, 1–16.

Camras, L.A., and Shutter, J.M. (2010). Emotional facial expressions in infancy. *Emotion Review, 2(2)*, 120–129.

Condon, W.S. (1974). Synchrony demonstrated between movements of the neonate and adult speech. *Child Development, 45*, 456–462.

Condon, W.S. (1975). Multiple response to sound in dysfunctional children. *Journal of Autism and Childhood Schizophrenia, 5*, 37–56.

Condon, W., and Ogston, W. (1966). Sound film analysis of normal and pathological behaviour patterns. *The Journal of Nervous and Mental Diseases, 143*, 338-347.

Condon, W.S., and Sander, L.W. (1974). Neonate movement is synchronised with adult speech: Interactional participation. *Science, 103*, 99–101.

Kovshoff, H., Hastings, R.P., and Remington, B. (2011). Two-year outcomes for children with autism after the cessation of early intensive behavioral intervention. *Behavior Modification, 35(5)*, 427–450.

Lindsay, G. (2011). The collection and analysis of data on children with speech, language and communication needs: The challenge to education and health services. *Child Language Teaching and Therapy*. Advanced online publication. doi:10.1177/0265659010396608.

Lloyd, M., Macdonald, M., and Lord, C. (2011). Motor skills of toddlers with autism spectrum disorders. *Autism*. Advanced online publication. doi:10.1177/1362361311402230.

Lopata, C., Smith, D.A., Thomeer, M.L., and Volker, M.A. (2009). Facial encoding of children with high-functioning autism spectrum disorders. *Focus on Autism and Other Developmental Disabilities, 24(4)*, 195–204.

Ludlow, A., Skelly, C., and Rohleder, P. (2011). Challenges faced by parents of children diagnosed with autism spectrum disorder. *Journal of Health Psychology*. Advanced online publication. doi:10.1177/1359105311422955.

Stahmer, A.C., Akshoomoff, N., and Cunningham, A.B. (2011). Inclusion for toddlers with autism spectrum disorders: The first ten years of a community program. *Autism: The International Journal of Research and Practice, 15(5)*, 625–641.

Acknowledgments

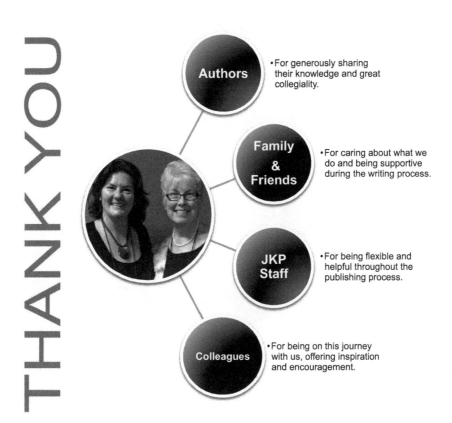

THANK YOU

Authors • For generously sharing their knowledge and great collegiality.

Family & Friends • For caring about what we do and being supportive during the writing process.

JKP Staff • For being flexible and helpful throughout the publishing process.

Colleagues • For being on this journey with us, offering inspiration and encouragement.

Preface

Petra Kern and Marcia Humpal

The increasing numbers of young children identified with autism spectrum disorders (ASD) calls for more evidence-based services and supports. Music therapists have a long tradition of serving individuals with ASD and their families. However, to offer effective services it is crucial to stay informed about the latest research and clinical practice in music therapy and related fields. Diagnostic criteria, theories about the causes, interventions and strategies, and application of the latest technology for young learners on the autism spectrum constantly change; new information and applications continue to rapidly evolve. Therefore, we recognized the need to bring together renowned researchers and practitioners from music therapy and related disciplines to provide a comprehensive perspective on existing knowledge and music therapy practice with young children with ASD and their families.

Starting with an ASD primer, Kern describes the core characteristics of ASD, early warning signs, current prevalence rates, research and theories about the causes, screening and diagnostic evaluation, as well as focused intervention practices and comprehensive treatment models. In Chapter 2, Humpal and Kern address evidence-based practice, its specific considerations for ASD, and implications for music therapy practice to identify the best available interventions, strategies, and supports for young children with ASD and their families. Whipple unveils her most recently conducted meta-analysis, published for the first time in Chapter 3 of this book. She reviews the current music therapy research literature and provides evidence that music therapy is an effective treatment option for developing communication, interpersonal, personal responsibility, and play skills in young children with ASD.

The rationale for conducting assessments, the role of the music therapist in the assessment process, and an overview of various approaches to music therapy assessment are highlighted by Martin, Snell, Walworth, and Humpal in Chapter 4. The authors feature the Four-Step Assessment Model to determine eligibility, the Music Therapy–Music Related Behavior assessment to gather information, and the SCERTS® Model to generate treatment goals.

The next five chapters focus on ASD-specific treatment approaches and strategies as applied in music therapy. Martin introduces four major principles of Applied Behavior Analysis (ABA), highlights three common treatment modalities widely utilized with young children with ASD, and discusses their relevance and application to music therapy practice. Brownell provides guidance for constructing Social Stories™ and gives examples that describe setting them to music for behavior modification of children with ASD. In a clinical vignette and research snapshot, Guerrero and Turry introduce the principles of Nordoff-Robbins music therapy and preliminary outcomes of a community-based research project that yielded increased communication in young children with ASD. Carpente elaborates on combining improvisational music therapy as used in Nordoff-Robbins music therapy with the DIR®/Floortime™ Model, and provides guidelines and considerations for music therapists, interdisciplinary team members, and parents. Humpal and Kern round out this part of the book by addressing instructional strategies (e.g., predictable routines, prompting, transitions, and peer-mediated interventions) that can be enhanced and strengthened by using common music therapy techniques adapted for young children with ASD.

Chapters 10 to 14 focus on collaborating and consulting with interdisciplinary team members, including parents. Kern introduces a case scenario of a four-year-old boy with ASD, illustrating a step-by-step music therapy intervention process embedded in an inclusive childcare program by early childhood educators. Lim discusses social communication and speech-language development in young children with ASD, and offers suggestions for collaborating with speech-language pathologists to support communication through music therapy interventions. Next, Wakeford explains sensory processing in young children with ASD by examining theoretical models, assessment, and intervention, and proposes applications for music therapy practice. Walworth addresses the need for family-centered practice, describing how parents can integrate music into family routines to improve the independent functioning of their child with ASD at home. By featuring four interviews, Humpal provides valuable insights from individuals who are professional music therapists and parents of children with ASD.

Finally, Kern presents selected high-quality online resources, including professional development websites, briefs, podcasts, blogs, and latest apps related to ASD, specifying how to stay informed in the rapidly evolving world of technology. Humpal concludes the resources section with an annotated bibliography of selected music therapy research and recommended practice literature found throughout the book.

Each chapter begins with an image and focus sentence by the authors that illustrate the content of the chapter. Reader-friendly terms are used to present current research, practical applications, and strategies useful for everyone who includes music for learning in the natural environment of young children with ASD. Case scenarios, examples, checklists, charts, tip sheets, and music scores further support the application of the knowledge-based content. Learning questions address key points of the chapters, making this book a valuable teaching tool for music therapy students, educators, and those in related professions.

We offer this practical book as a source of information and support for students, practitioners, educators, researchers, and parents. Our intent is for this publication to be contemplated and used for developing the potential of young children with ASD through music in everyday life.

PART 1

Introduction
and Research

Chapter 1

Autism Spectrum Disorders Primer

Characteristics, Causes, Prevalence, and Intervention

Petra Kern, Ph.D., MT-DMtG, MT-BC, MTA
MUSIC THERAPY CONSULTING
SANTA BARBARA, CA

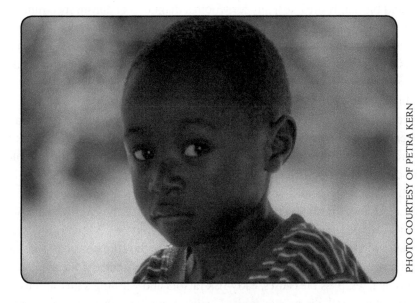

PHOTO COURTESY OF PETRA KERN

*The more we know about autism spectrum disorders, the better
we can provide efficient information and services to children
with autism spectrum disorders and their families.*
(Petra Kern)

Lucas is a 28-month-old boy who hardly ever looks into someone's eyes, cuddles with his parents, or imitates peers. He prefers playing alone, frequently spins objects, and rocks his body back and forth while vocalizing. Lucas shows little interest in others. He only communicates with adults to indicate his need for help, and he interacts with other children only when he is interested in the objects they have. However, Lucas pays close attention to sounds and likes to participate in movement activities. Lucas' parents are concerned about his overall development and well-being. They are seeking explanations for Lucas' behaviors and are worried that he might have an autism spectrum disorder.

Lucas and his family are like many for whom a diagnosis of autism spectrum disorder (ASD) is likely; they present a scenario that professionals working with young children and their families may face. Meeting families in this situation requires the professional to give precise and comprehensive information about ASD, and to lay out effective intervention options that are designed to have positive outcomes for the child. Professionals working in early childhood settings play a critical role in early identification of ASD, assessment, intervention planning, and providing early intervention services to children with ASD and their families. Therefore, it is crucial that professionals in early childhood education and early intervention are informed about the latest research outcomes and developments related to ASD.

This chapter provides key information about current diagnostic criteria and proposed changes in those criteria for the fifth edition of the *Diagnostic and Statistical Manual of Mental Disorders*, expected to be in effect by May, 2013 (American Psychiatric Association [APA], 2011), as well as an overview of the core characteristics of ASD. The chapter also summarizes the history of ASD and current information about prevalence rates, possible causes, early risk factors and warning signs, and frequently used screening and diagnostic tools. Finally, common categories of intervention, comprehensive treatment models, and current evidence-based focused interventions are briefly addressed. Web links are provided throughout the chapter to assist readers interested in finding more in-depth information.

Defining autism spectrum disorders
Current definition

The term "autism spectrum disorders" describes a group of lifelong developmental disabilities that share similar characteristics in various degrees of severity. Three core features define ASD:

1. impairments in social interaction
2. impairments in communication and language development
3. presence of repetitive, restricted, and/or stereotypic behaviors.

Because of this I found pleasure and comfort in doing the same thing over and over again" (Williams, 1992, p. 44). Persistent *preoccupations with parts of objects* and repetitive play behaviors (e.g., spinning the wheels of a tricycle or flicking a toy) are often evident as well. These behaviors can easily interfere with the child's learning and optimal development. Video examples representing repetitive behaviors and restricted interests of children with ASD (including restricted interests, insistence on sameness, repetitive mannerisms, and preoccupation with parts of objects) can be reviewed at the First Signs ASD Video Glossary (see www.firstsigns.org/asd_video_glossary/asdvg_about.htm).

OTHER SYMPTOMS AND DISORDERS

Children with ASD may have characteristics and disorders that are not currently listed among diagnostic criteria, but are often associated or co-morbid with a diagnosis of autism. For instance, many children with ASD demonstrate differences in sensory processing, including over-responsiveness and under-responsiveness to various forms of sensation, as well as sensory-seeking behaviors (Baranek, Boyd, and Poe, 2007; Baranek, David, and Poe, 2006). Temple Grandin describes her unusual responses to sound as follows: "Sometimes I heard and understood, and other times sounds or speech reached my brain like the unbearable noise of an onrushing freight train" (Grandin and Scariano, 1986, p. 145). In addition to sensory processing differences, the cognitive abilities of children with ASD may vary from mild to severe intellectual disabilities, and a few may present with exceptional musical or artistic talents, or with extraordinary calculation and memorization skills (i.e., Savant syndrome) (Treffert, 2012). A number of children with ASD also may have mental health issues, seizures, sleeping disorders, gastrointestinal disorders, and/or metabolic/nutritional deficiencies. These secondary, or associated, characteristics may create major challenges in the daily lives of children with ASD.

History, causes, and prevalence of ASD

History

In the late 1930s, child psychiatrist Leo Kanner received long, detailed letters from a number of parents whose children seemed "odd" to them in a way that they did not understand (Kanner, 1943). Among other things, these children did not behave as if they were attached or connected to their parents as reasonably might be expected, and did not communicate in a manner typical for children of their ages. In addition, these children seemed content to play alone, to avoid social interactions, to insist on sameness or routine, and to react with fear or extreme discomfort to various sensory stimuli, particularly sound and touch. Using both the parents' letters and statements, and his own observations and interactions with the children themselves, Kanner made note of the common characteristics described above. In 1943 Kanner published a review of 11 of these unusual cases, including both the common and individual aspects of their presentation that led to his naming and describing of "autism."

During almost the same time period, Austrian psychiatrist Hans Asperger also was called on to consult regarding children with characteristics very similar to those described by Kanner, and he, too, named it "autism." However, because Asperger's original work was in German and written during World War II, it remained unnoticed in the United States for years, and was recognized in the early 1990s once it was published in English (Murray, 2008). The descriptions of both Kanner and Asperger are notable for many similarities, including the facts that both related remarkable abilities and signs of intelligence in the children that they saw, in addition to the oddities, and that while the children certainly shared common general characteristics, there were significant individual variations related to the characteristics.

Autism initially posed a dilemma within the world of psychiatric medicine, however, over several decades it became increasingly a source of public fascination as well (Murray, 2008). This fascination was born of both intrigue and fear—its varied presentation within individuals, and the unique competencies and "oddities" that accompany it evoke interest and speculation, yet its unknown origins are also cause for fear. Those in medical science continue to study and theorize about autism, as do others, including parents, teachers, therapists, and researchers within a variety of fields. As a result, a number of theories about the causes of autism have emerged, some of which have been investigated and rejected, and some of which continue to be studied.

Among the more well-known theories is psychologist Bruno Bettelheim's assertion that cold, unaffectionate mothers ("refrigerator mothers") were responsible for childhood autism, particularly the seemingly "asocial" characteristics (Bettelheim, 1967). A series of studies disproved this theory (Capps, Sigman, and Mundy, 1994; Rogers, Ozonoff, and Maslin-Cole, 1993) and further asserted that ASD is not caused by a parent's life style, level of education, or by emotional factors in the child's environment. Another theory, more recently popularized in the United States by celebrity and mother Jenny McCarthy, is that childhood immunizations cause ASD, particularly in children with "fragile" immune systems (Wakefield *et al.*, 1998). Systematic studies have established that there is no epidemiological evidence for links between the measles, mumps, and rubella (MMR) vaccines and an increased risk for ASD (Fombonne *et al.*, 2006; Price *et al.*, 2010). In addition, it has recently been discovered that the initial research conducted by Wakefield was essentially fraudulent (Eggertson, 2010).

Causes

Autism is currently understood as a neurodevelopmental disorder with a strong genetic component (Geschwind, 2009; Lord and Bishop, 2010). Current twin and sibling studies suggest that ASD is highly heritable but genes are risk factors that appear to have environmental triggers (Hallmayer *et al.*, 2011). Furthermore, the presence of a broader autism phenotype (the presence of core characteristics at levels that do not meet diagnostic criteria) has been reported in some studies of parent characteristics (Losh and Piven, 2007; Piven *et al.*, 1997). However, no specific genetic link to ASD has yet been discovered within the majority of children diagnosed with ASD (Geschwind, 2009).

Researchers continue to pursue a better understanding of the cause(s) of ASD. For instance, current theories being tested include the exploration of the role of hormones (particularly androgens/testosterone) in ASD (Baron-Cohen, Knickmeyer, and Belmonte, 2005; Knickmeyer and Baron-Cohen, 2006), the mechanisms that may underlie differences in neural connectivity in various areas and pathways in the brain (Just *et al.*, 2007; Wan *et al.*, 2010), multiple genetic markers (Abrahams and Geschwind, 2008; Sanders *et al.,* 2012), autoimmunity (Goines and Van de Water, 2010), and attempts to identify environmental factors that may be interacting with biological or genetic mechanisms to cause autism (Bilder *et al.*, 2009; Edelson and Saudino, 2009; Hallmayer *et al.*, 2011; Mann *et al.*, 2010; Newschaffer *et al.*, 2007).

In addition to these theories, which tend toward a "medicalized" view of ASD, the relatively recent idea of a "spectrum" has led the way toward a view of autism as an aspect of human diversity, rather than as a disability. As a result there are those encouraging a move away from the idea of "cure" and toward an idea of "adaptation." These ideas have emerged based on the efforts to make the strengths of individuals with ASD better known, and their voices better heard (e.g., Bagatell, 2007, 2010; Broderick, 2009; Davidson, 2010).

Prevalence

The prevalence rate of ASD has increased over the past two decades. Once considered a rare disorder, ASD is now the second most frequently occurring developmental disability in the United States, after intellectual disability. Recent results from the CDC suggest that the overall prevalence rate for ASD is 1 in 88 in the United States (CDC, 2012a), and is about five times more common in boys (1 in 54) then in girls (1 in 252); ASD occur in all ethnic and socioeconomic groups. Study reports from Asia, Europe, and North America resulted in an average prevalence of about 1 percent (CDC, 2012b). Detailed information from other regions of the world is not readily available yet. To date, it remains unclear whether the rise in prevalence rates reflects an increased incidence of ASD in the population or is related to one or more of the following (Lord and Bishop, 2010; Odom, Schertz, and Wong, 2010; Weintraub, 2011):

- a broader definition of the diagnostic criteria in the *DSM-IV-TR*™
- a diagnostic shift where conditions are classified differently
- earlier identification as a result of improved screening approaches and diagnostic instruments
- an enhanced public awareness due to increased media attention.

The proposed changes in diagnostic criteria in the fifth edition of the *DSM* may also have an influence on future prevalence rates of ASD. For the most current information, one may access prevalence reports by the CDC (see www.cdc.gov/ncbddd/autism/data.html).

Early identification, screening, and diagnosis
Identifying early signs
Currently there is no valid biological marker or test to identify ASD (CDC, 2012a), and the diagnosis of ASD is based on observations or reports of the child's development and behavior using the *DSM-IV-TR*™ criteria (Lord and Bishop, 2010). However, early recognition of risk for ASD can be a key factor for access to early intervention services and potential achievement of better outcomes than are possible with later diagnosis.

Table 1.1 Early indicators signaling the need for screening for ASD
Possible signs of ASD
Children with ASD might: • not respond to their name by 12 months of age • not point at objects to show interest (point at an airplane flying over) by 14 months • not play "pretend" games (pretend to "feed" a doll) by 18 months • avoid eye contact and want to be alone • have trouble understanding other people's feelings or talking about their own feelings • have delayed speech and language skills • repeat words or phrases over and over (echolalia) • give unrelated answers to questions • get upset by minor changes • have obsessive interests • flap their hands, rock their body, or spin in circles • have unusual reactions to the way things sound, smell, taste, look, or feel.

Source: Centers for Disease Control and Prevention (2010). Signs and symptoms. Retrieved from www.cdc.gov/ncbddd/autism/signs.html.

Within a child's first year, early signs of ASD may be evident, making it imperative for parents of children with high risk (e.g., those with older siblings or other close relatives diagnosed with an ASD) and professionals working with infants and toddlers to recognize the early indicators of ASD risk. A campaign by CDC, "Learn the Signs, Act Early," established a user-friendly website which contains descriptions of typical developing children and early warning signs related to ASD (see www.cdc. gov/ncbddd/actearly). Table 1.1 summarizes common warning signs or "red flags" that suggest a need for screening or assessment for ASD.

Screening and diagnostic evaluation

A number of children can be reliably diagnosed with ASD as young as two years of age (Lord *et al.*, 2006), but without awareness of early warning signs and timely screening, many may not be diagnosed until 30–36 months or even later, delaying access to intervention. If "red flags" are evident, targeted screening (i.e., administration of an ASD standardized screening tool) should take place. Because routine pediatric care and general developmental screening usually do not identify subtle characteristics of ASD, the American Academy of Pediatrics (AAP) now recommends an ASD-specific screening routine for all children at 18 and 24 months during their well-child check-ups (Johnson, Myers, and the Council on Children with Disabilities, 2007).

Professionals in various medical, healthcare, or educational settings may conduct screening for ASD. Depending on the screening tool, this may involve a brief parental questionnaire, short interactions and observations of the child, or the evaluation of parent and teacher reports (Pretzel and Cox, 2008). When screening results indicate a high risk for ASD, a comprehensive diagnostic evaluation is necessary to confirm whether or not a child meets the full criteria for ASD. These evaluations should include a core battery of assessment measures to make sure that all aspects of the child's development are addressed (CDC, 2012a). Diagnostic evaluations for children at high risk of ASD are usually based on (a) family interviews, including the child's medical and developmental history as well as the child's current behaviors and activities, and (b) interacting with and observing the child in a series of play-based activities (Pretzel and Cox, 2008). Some of the most common ASD-specific screening tools and diagnostic instruments are listed in Table 1.2.

It is recommended practice that a multidisciplinary team (i.e., psychiatrist, neurologist, or developmental pediatrician, along with early interventionists, special educators, and therapists) participate in the diagnostic evaluation to guarantee a comprehensive perspective on the severity of ASD and levels of developmental functioning of the child. This holistic approach is important for subsequent individualized intervention planning with families (National Research Council [NRC], 2001), including access to early intervention services as well as to resources for parents (Lord and Reichler, 2006).

Unfortunately, reimbursement for this type of evaluation may not be covered, or may be restricted by the family's health insurance and other funding sources (Lord and Bishop, 2010). Access to timely and appropriate diagnostic evaluations continues to be a frequent subject of advocacy for the improvement of resources for children with ASD and their families.

Table 1.2 Sample of validated screening tools and diagnostic instruments for ASD	
Measurements	**Brief description and link**
Screening Tools	
Modified Checklist for Autism and Toddlers (M-CHAT™)	M-CHAT™ (Robins et al., 2001) is a short parent-completed questionnaire (23 items) that provides reliable information about risk of ASD in children between 16 and 30 months of age. The questionnaire takes about 5–10 minutes to administrate and is available in multiple languages. It can be downloaded for free at www2.gsu.edu/~psydlr/Diana_L._Robins,_Ph.D..html.
Screening Tool for Autism in Toddlers and Young Children (STAT™)	STAT™ (Stone et al., 2004) is an interactive measure (12 items) that assesses key social and communicative behaviors in children between 24 and 36 months of age who are at risk of ASD. The screening is conducted by trained community service providers and takes about 20 minutes. An online STAT™ Training Tutorial for professionals is available at http://kc.vanderbilt.edu/triad/training/page.aspx?id=821.
Infant–Toddler Checklist (ITC)	ITC (Wetherby and Prizant, 2002) is a parent-completed questionnaire (24 items) assessing developmental milestones of social communication in infants and toddlers between 6 and 24 months of age to screen for developmental risk and ASD. The checklist takes about 5–10 minutes to complete and should be scored by healthcare or childcare service providers. It is available in several languages and can be downloaded for free at http://firstwords.fsu.edu/index.php/early-identification-of-communication-delays/26-csbschecklist.
Diagnostic Instruments	
Autism Diagnostic Observation Schedule (ADOS)	ADOS (Lord et al., 2002) is a semi-structured, standardized assessment and coding of social interaction, communication, and behaviors relevant to ASD in individuals 24 months and older. The administration of ADOS takes about 30–45 minutes. ADOS is internationally recognized as a diagnostic instrument for ASD and widely used by trained professionals in clinical practice and research. Information on ADOS training workshops can be obtained at www.cornellpsychiatry.org/education/autism.html.

Autism Diagnostic Interview—Revised (ADI-R)	ADI-R (Rutter, Le Couteur, and Lord, 2003) is a semi-structured diagnostic interview with response coding based on the *DSM-IV-TR*™ and *ICS-10* criteria for autism and PDD. Professionals experienced in clinical interviewing and assessment administer the ADI-R to parents of children and adults (mental age above 24 months) who are at risk for ASD. The administration of ADI-R takes approximately 90 minutes to 3 hours. ADI-R is a reliable and validated diagnostic tool accepted by researchers and clinicians worldwide. ADI-R training information for researchers is available at www.cornellpsychiatry.org/education/autism.html.
Childhood Autism Rating Scale, Second Edition (CARS2™)	CARS2™ (Schopler *et al.*, 2009) is based on direct observation of behaviors in individuals 24 months and older who have been screened for high risk of ASD. CARS2™ generates symptom severity (i.e., mild, moderate, and severe) through quantifiable ratings and an unscored parental questionnaire. CARS2™ is administered by a trained clinician and takes about 5–10 minutes after information gathering. CARS2™ has been used widely and in various countries for many years. Additional information on training workshops and different versions of CARS2™ can be found at http://teacch.com/trainings.

Intervention

Approaches to intervention

Although there is no cure for ASD (as it is a disability and not a disease), research shows that early diagnosis followed by individualized intervention can significantly improve children's ability to function well and live meaningful lives (NRC, 2001). Because there are many types of interventions for ASD, it can be challenging for parents to find the right fit for their child. Experts recommend that intervention practices for individuals with ASD should (a) address the child's individual strengths and needs, (b) have scientific evidence supporting the value of the treatment, and (c) be structured and involve parents (NRC, 2001).

According to the CDC (2012a), treatment options for children with ASD can be placed into four general categories: Behavior and Communication Approaches, Dietary Approaches, Medication, and Complementary and Alternative Medicine. The CDC website provides brief descriptions of treatments falling under these categories plus resources for more in-depth readings (see www.cdc.gov/ncbddd/autism/treatment.html#2). Of the four categories listed above, Behavior and Communication Approaches currently has received the most support from research studies (NRC,

2001). However, there is no single approach or intervention that fits all children. In most cases, a combination of individualized interventions is the most beneficial for each child's learning and development (Lord and Bishop, 2010).

Early childhood intervention

In recent early childhood literature, interventions for young children with ASD and their families are divided into two categories that differ from those listed by the CDC. These two categories include focused intervention practices, and comprehensive treatment models (CTMs) (Boyd *et al.*, 2010; National Autism Center [NAC], 2009; Odom *et al.*, 2010). Focused intervention practices are designed to change a target behavior or improve developmental outcomes for a particular child with ASD in a relatively short period of time (Boyd *et al.*, 2010). Examples of evidence-based focused intervention practices include strategies such as prompting, reinforcement, Discrete Trial Training, Social Stories™, and peer-mediated interventions. In contrast, CTMs are a set of intensive, long-term practices designed to attain a broader impact on the three core features of ASD (Odom *et al.*, 2010). These also may be referred to as "programs." CTMs for children with ASD that have been appraised and supported by strong evidence include Early Childhood Denver Model, Pivotal Response Training (PRT), Treatment and Education of Autistic and Communication Handicapped Children (TEACCH), Learning Experiences and Alternative Programs for Preschoolers and Their Parents (LEAP), and Lovaas (Odom *et al.*, 2010). It should be noted that CTMs may include the use of one or more focused intervention practices (NAC, 2009; Odom *et al.*, 2003). Some of the focused intervention practices and comprehensive treatment models have been applied and studied in the field of music therapy and will be addressed in other chapters within this book.

Conclusion

The increased prevalence of ASD has triggered a call for action on the part of parents, professionals, organizations, and federal agencies. Strides have been made in research related to the causes of ASD, early identification, and the development of reliable diagnostic assessments. A number of early intervention practices based on behavioral and developmental approaches have been identified as effective, and programs using research-supported comprehensive treatment models are available for children with ASD and their families. However, children continue to be undiagnosed for a variety of reasons and their parents must struggle to find access to appropriate and effective interventions to support their engagement in everyday life. Therefore, ASD-related research must continue so that we may gain a better understanding of the causes of ASD, develop valid and reliable early screening tools, as well as provide approaches to intervention that create the best "fit" for young children with ASD, their families, and their daily life environments. As professionals working with children with ASD and their families, it is vital that we stay informed to ultimately make a difference in the lives of those children and families.

LEARNING QUESTIONS

1. What is meant by the term "autism spectrum disorders" and what are the core characteristics?

2. What is the current prevalence rate of ASD?

3. Describe a current theory about the causes of ASD.

4. Describe a proven misconception about the causes of ASD.

5. Name five common "red flags" of ASD.

6. What is the difference between screening and diagnostic evaluation?

7. Name two common screening or diagnostic instruments.

8. Name the four categories or approaches to intervention identified by the Centers for Disease Control and Prevention.

9. Name the two categories of early intervention available for children with ASD.

Author's note

The author wishes to thank Linn Wakeford for her contributions to the History and Causes sections and Dr. Gary Mesibov for his helpful review of this chapter.

References

Abrahams, B.S., and Geschwind, D.H. (2008). Advances in autism genetics: On the threshold of a new neurobiology. *Nature Reviews Genetics, 9*, 341–355.

American Psychiatric Association (APA) (2000). *Diagnostic and Statistical Manual of Mental Disorders (Fourth Edition). Text Revision.* Washington, DC: APA.

American Psychiatric Association (APA) (2011). DSM-5 Development: 299.0 autistic disorder. Retrieved from www.dsm5.org/proposedrevisions/pages/proposedrevision.aspx?rid=94#.

Bagatell, N. (2007). Orchestrating voices: Autism, identity and the power of discourse. *Disability and Society, 22*, 413–426.

Bagatell, N. (2010). From cure to community: Transforming notions of autism. *Ethos, 38*, 33–55.

Baranek, G.T., Boyd, B., and Poe, M.D. (2007). Hyperresponsive sensory patterns in young children with autism, developmental delay, and typical development. *American Journal on Mental Retardation, 112(4)*, 233–245.

Baranek, G.T., David, F.J., and Poe, M.D. (2006). Sensory Experiences Questionnaire: Discriminating sensory features in young children with autism, developmental delays, and typical development. *Journal of Child Psychology and Psychiatry, 47(6)*, 591–601.

Baron-Cohen, S., Knickmeyer, R.C., and Belmonte, M.K. (2005). Sex differences in the brain: Implications for explaining autism. *Science, 310*, 819–823.

Bettelheim, B. (1967). *The Empty Fortress: Infantile Autism and the Birth of the Self.* New York: The Free Press.

Bilder, D., Pinborough-Zimmerman, J., Miller, J., and McMahon, W. (2009). Prenatal, perinatal, and neonatal factors associated with autism spectrum disorders. *Pediatrics, 123*, 1293–1300.

Boyd, B.A., Odom, S.L., Humphreys, B.P., and Sam, A.M. (2010). Infants and toddlers with autism spectrum disorders: Early identification and early intervention. *Journal of Early Intervention, 32(2)*, 75–98.

Broderick, A.A. (2009). Autism, "recovery (to normalcy)" and the politics of hope. *Intellectual and Developmental Disabilities, 47*, 263–281.

Capps, L., Sigman, M., and Mundy, P. (1994). Attachment security in children with autism. *Development and Psychopathology, 6*, 249–261.

Centers for Disease Control and Prevention (2010). Signs and symptoms. Retrieved from www.cdc.gov/ncbddd/autism/signs.html.

Centers for Disease Control and Prevention (CDC) (2012a). Autism spectrum disorders (ASD). Retrieved from www.cdc.gov/ncbddd/autism/index.html.

Centers for Disease Control and Prevention (CDC) (2012b). Prevalence of autism spectrum disorders—Autism and developmental disabilities monitoring network. *MMWR Surveillance Summaries, 61(SS03)*, 1–19. Retrieved from www.cdc.gov/mmwr/preview/mmwrhtml/ss6103a1.htm?s_cid=ss6103a1_w.

Centers for Disease Control and Prevention (2012c). Summary of autism spectrum disorder (ASD) prevalence studies. Retrieved from www.cdc.gov/ncbddd/autism/documents/Autism_PrevalenceSummaryTable_2011.pdf.

Davidson, J. (2010). "It cuts both ways": A relational approach to access and accommodation for autism. *Social Science and Medicine, 70*, 305–312.

Edelson, L., and Saudino, K. (2009). Genetic and environmental influences on autistic-like behaviors in 2-year-old twins. *Behavior Genetics, 39(3)*, 255–264.

Eggertson, L. (2010). Lancet retracts 12-year-old article linking autism to MMR vaccines. *Canadian Medical Association Journal, 182*, E199–E200.

Fombonne, E., Zakarian, R., Bennett, A., Meng, L., and McLean-Heywood, D. (2006). Pervasive developmental disorders in Montreal, Quebec, Canada: Prevalence and links with immunizations. *Pediatrics, 118(1)*, 139–150.

Geschwind, D.H. (2009). Advances in autism. *Annual Review of Medicine, 60(1)*, 367–380.

Goines, P., and Van de Water, J. (2010). The immune system's role in the biology of autism. *Current Opinion in Neurology, 23*, 111–117.

Grandin, T. (1999). *Social Problems: Understanding Emotions and Developing Talents.* Retrieved from www.autism-help.org/story-emotions-talents-autism.htm.

Grandin, T., and Scariano, M.M. (1986). *Emergence: Labeled Autistic.* New York: Warner Books.

Hallmayer, J., Cleveland, S., Torres, A., Phillips, J., Cohen, B., Torigoe, T., Miller, J., Fedele, A., Collins, J., Smith, K., Lotspeich, L., Croen, L.A., Ozonoff, S., Lajonchere, C., Grether, J.K., and Risch, N. (2011). Genetic heritability and shared environmental factors among twin pairs with autism. *Archives of General Psychiatry, 68(11)*, 1095–1102.

Johnson, C.P., Myers, S.M., and the Council on Children with Disabilities (2007). Identification and evaluation of children with autism spectrum disorders. *Pediatrics, 120(5)*, 1183–1215.

Just, M.A., Cherkassky, V.L., Keller, T.A., Kana, R.K., and Minshew, N.J. (2007). Functional and anatomical cortical underconnectivity in autism: Evidence from an fMRI study of an executive function task and corpus callosum morphometry. *Cerebral Cortex, 17*, 951–961.

Kanner, L. (1943). Autistic disturbances of affective contact. *Nervous Child, 2*, 217–250.

Knickmeyer, R.C., and Baron-Cohen, S. (2006). Fetal testosterone and sex differences in typical social development and in autism. *Journal of Child Neurology, 21*, 825–846.

Lord, C., and Bishop, S.L. (2010). Autism spectrum disorders: Diagnosis, prevalence, and services for children and families. *Social Policy Report, 24(2)*, 1–27. Retrieved from www.srcd.org/index. php?option=com_contentandtask=viewandid=232andItemid=655.

Lord, C., and Reichler, J. (2006). Early diagnosis of children with autism spectrum disorders. In T. Charman and W. Stone (Eds.) *Social and Communication Development in Autism Spectrum Disorders.* New York: Guilford.

Lord, C., Risi, S., DiLavore, P.S., Shulman, C., Thurm, A., and Pickles, A. (2006). Autism from 2 to 9 years of age. *Archives of General Psychiatry, 63(6)*, 694–701.

Lord, C., Rutter, M., DiLavore, P.C., and Risi, S. (2002). *Autism Diagnostic Observation Schedule.* Los Angeles, CA: Western Psychological Services.

Losh, M., and Piven, J. (2007). Social-cognition and the broad autism phenotype: Identifying genetically meaningful phenotypes. *Journal of Child Psychology and Psychiatry, 48*, 105–112.

Mann, J.R., McDermott, S., Bao, H., Hardin, J., and Gregg, J. (2010). Pre-eclampsia, birth weight, and autism spectrum disorders. *Journal of Autism and Developmental Disorders, 40*, 548–554.

Murray, S. (2008). *Representing Autism: Culture, Narrative, Fascination.* Liverpool, UK: Liverpool University Press.

National Autism Center (NAC) (2009). *National Standards Report.* The National Standards Project— Addressing the need for evidence-based practice guidelines for autism spectrum disorders. Retrieved from www.nationalautismcenter.org/affiliates/reports.php.

National Research Council (NRC) (2001). *Educating Children with Autism.* Committee on Educational Interventions for Children with Autism. C. Lord and J.P. McGee (Eds.), Division of Behavioral and Social Science and Education. Washington, DC: National Academy Press.

Newschaffer, C.J., Croen, L.A., Daniels, J., Giarelli, E., *et al.* (2007). The epidemiology of autism spectrum disorder. *Annual Review of Public Health, 28*, 235–258.

Odom, S.L., Boyd, B.A., Hall, L., and Hume, K. (2010). Evaluation of comprehensive treatment models for individuals with autism spectrum disorders. *Journal of Autism and Developmental Disorders, 40*, 425–436.

Odom, S.L., Brown, W.H., Frey, T., Karasu, N., Smith-Carter, L., and Strain, P. (2003). Evidence-based practice for young children with autism: Evidence from single-subject research design. *Focus on Autism and Other Developmental Disabilities, 18*, 176–181.

Odom, S.L., Schertz, H.H., and Wong, C. (2010). Autism spectrum disorders in young children. In H.H. Schertz, C. Wong, and S.L. Odom (Eds.) Supporting young children with autism spectrum disorders and their families [Monograph]. *Young Exceptional Children, 12*, 1–11.

Piven, J., Palmer, P., Jacobi, D., and Childress, D. (1997). Broader autism phenotype: Evidence from a family history study of multiple-incidence autism families. *American Journal of Psychiatry, 154*, 185–190.

Pretzel, R.E., and Cox, A.W. (2008). Early identification, screening, and diagnosis of ASD, Parts A and B. In A.W. Cox, D. Hatton, G.A. Williams, and R.E. Pretzel (Eds.) *Foundations of Autism Spectrum Disorders: An Online Course* (Session 3). Chapel Hill, NC: National Professional Development Center on Autism Spectrum Disorders, FPG Child Development Institute, The University of North Carolina.

Price, C.S., Thompson, W.W., Goodson, B., Weintraub, E.S., Croen L., Hinrichsen V. L., Marcy, M., Robertson A., Eriksen E., Lewis E., Bernal, P., Shay, D., Davis, R.L., and DeStefano, F. (2010). Prenatal and infant exposure to thimerosal from vaccines and immunoglobulins and risk of autism. *Pediatrics, 126(4)*, 656–664.

Robins, D., Fein, D., Barton, M., and Green, J. (2001). The modified checklist for autism in toddlers: An initial study investigating the early detection of autism and pervasive developmental disorders. *Journal of Autism and Developmental Disorders, 31(2)*, 131–144.

Rogers, S.J., Ozonoff, S., and Maslin-Cole, C. (1993). Developmental aspects of attachment behavior in young children with pervasive developmental disorders. *Journal of the American Academy of Child and Adolescent Psychiatry, 36(6)*, 1274–1282.

Rutter, M., Le Couteur, A., and Lord, C. (2003). *ADI-R: The Autism Diagnostic Interview Revised*. Los Angeles, CA: Western Psychological Services.

Sanders, S. J., Murtha, M.T., Gupta, A.R., Murdoch, J.D., Raubeson, M.J., Willsey, A.J., Ercan-Sencicek, A.G., DiLullo, N.M., Parikshak, N.N., Stein, J.L., Walker, M.F., Ober, G.T., Teran, N.A., Song ,Y., El-Fishawy, P., Murtha, R.C., Choi, M., Overton, J.D., Bjornson, R.D., Carriero, N.J., Meyer, K.A., Bilguvar, K., Mane, S.M., Sestan, N., Lifton, R.P., Günel, M., Roeder, K., Geschwind, D.H., Devlin, B., and State, M.W. (2012). De novo mutations revealed by whole-exome sequencing are strongly associated with autism. *Nature, 485*, 237–41.

Schopler, E., Van Bourgondien, M.E., Wellman, G.J., and Love, S.R. (2009). *Childhood Autism Rating Scale (Second Edition)*. Los Angeles, CA: Western Psychological Services.

Stone, W.L., Coonrod, E.E., Turner, L.M., and Pozdol, S.L. (2004). Psychometric properties of the STAT for early autism screening. *Journal of Autism and Developmental Disorders, 34(6)*, 691–701.

Treffert, D.A. (2012). *Islands of Genius: The Bountiful Mind of the Autistic, Acquired, and Sudden Savant*. London and Philadelphia: Jessica Kingsley Publishers.

Wakefield, A.J., Murch, S.H., Anthony, A., Linnell, J., Casson, D.M., Malik, M., Berelowitz, M., Dhillon, A.P., Thomson, M.A., Harvey, P., Valentine, A., Davies, S.E., and Walker-Smith, J.A. (1998). Ileal-lymphoid-nodular hyperplasia, non-specific colitis, and pervasive developmental disorder in children. *Lancet, 351*, 637–641.

Wan, C.Y., Demaine, K., Zipse, L., Norton, A., and Schlaug, G. (2010). From music making to speaking: Engaging the mirror neuron system in autism. *Brain Research Bulletin, 82*, 161–168.

Weintraub, K. (2011). Autism counts. *Nature, 479*, 22–24.

Prizant, B.M. (2002). *Communication and Symbolic Behavior Scales Developmental Profile*. Baltimore, MD: Paul H. Brookes Publishing Co.

Wetherby, A.M., and Prizant, B.M. (2002). *CSBS DP Infant-Toddler Checklist™*. Baltimore, MD: Paul H. Brookes Publishing Co.

Williams, D. (1992). *Nobody Nowhere: The Extraordinary Autobiography of an Autistic*. New York: Times Books.

World Health Organization (WHO) (1993). *International Classification of Diseases and Related Health Problems (Tenth Edition)*. Geneva: WHO.

Chapter 2

Evidence-Based Practice for Young Children with Autism Spectrum Disorders

Implications for Music Therapy

Marcia Humpal, M.Ed., MT-BC
OLMSTED FALLS, OH

Petra Kern, Ph.D., MT-DMtG, MT-BC, MTA
MUSIC THERAPY CONSULTING
SANTA BARBARA, CA

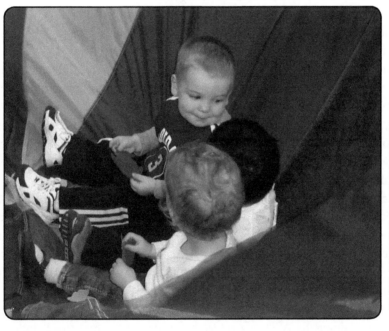

PHOTO COURTESY OF MARCIA HUMPAL

*Adhering to the principles of evidence-based practice will ensure
that we are offering the best possible services and supports to
children with autism spectrum disorders and their families as they
embark on a long journey of finding suitable treatment options.
(Marcia Humpal and Petra Kern)*

Early intervention offers hope for families faced with their young children's diagnoses of autism spectrum disorders (ASD) as it promises long-term success. There are many interventions, strategies, and supports available for children with ASD. However, parents and professionals often question if various services are effective or appropriate. This chapter provides a brief overview of evidence-based practice and its benefits, specific considerations from major players in ASD, and implications for music therapy practice.

What is evidence-based practice?
Overview of primary definitions

Evidence-based practice (EBP) is rooted in the medical profession. Evidence-based medicine (EBM) traces its philosophical framework to the mid-nineteenth century when medical decisions and treatment were usually dependent on the opinions and experiences of physicians. EBM emerged to fill the gap between research and practice, utilizing three different paths of acquiring information: best research evidence, clinical expertise, and the values of their patients (Else and Wheeler, 2010; Sackett *et al.*, 2000).

Other professions endorse EBP, though by slightly different terms. The American Psychiatric Association (APA) defines EBP as the "integration of the best available research and clinical experience with the context of patient characteristics, culture, values and preferences" (APA, 2006, p. 273). Early childhood professionals lean towards the following proposed definition: "…a decision-making process that integrates the best available research evidence with family and professional wisdom and values" (Buysse and Wesley, 2006, p. 12).

Recognizing the importance of this topic, the American Music Therapy Association (AMTA) states: "Evidence-based music therapy practice integrates the best available research, the music therapists' expertise, and the needs, values, and preferences of the individual(s) served" (AMTA, 2010). Additionally, individual music therapists continue to study how evidence informs music therapy practice (Abrams, 2010; Else and Wheeler, 2010; Kern, 2010).

The National Autism Center (NAC) identifies four factors of evidence-based practice pertaining to ASD: (1) research findings, (2) professional judgment, (3) values and preferences of parents, care providers, and the individual with ASD, and (4) capacity. The fourth factor directly impacts service providers and service delivery, noting the importance of adequate training and dedication to correctly implementing treatment to fidelity (NAC, 2009). This description of EBP aligns with the APA's 2006 version. Others invested in applying EBP with children with ASD concur, reiterating the need for EBP with ASD to incorporate flexibility of cultural variables as well as the client's unique circumstances (Mesibov and Shea, 2010).

Components of EBP

At the turn of the twenty-first century, EBP was often used synonymously with the term "best available research evidence." Weighted attention was given to "scientifically based research," described in the United States' No Child Left Behind Act of 2001 as "research that involves the application of rigorous, systematic, and objective procedures to obtain reliable and valid knowledge relevant to education activities and programs" (Title IX, SEC. 9101, 37 A).

In addition to research, other factors are now considered essential for the process of finding the best available services and supports for the individual with ASD. Thus, the melding of the three components (1) least biased research evidence, (2) clinical expertise, and (3) individual client factors along with their underpinnings creates today's evidence-based practice.

Being an EBP practitioner

Music therapists working with young children with ASD and their families can learn from established definitions and criteria that exist within their own profession as well as in early childhood education, psychology, and from ASD organizations. Although guided by specific standards and scope of practice, music therapists have a responsibility to look beyond their ranks, reflecting on the efficacy and effectiveness of intervention protocols that have evidence-based merit. Professionals must inform families about the most effective treatment options and strive to offer highly appropriate interventions when providing services. As outlined in Kern (2010, p. 116), subscribing to EBP is desirable because it:

- *maximizes beneficial outcomes for children and families* by offering the best available intervention options

- *responds to accountability demands* by providing data on one's own position and practice

- *expands one's own skills and competencies* by staying current on the latest developments and trends in the field

- *enhances political and financial support* from various stakeholders (i.e., administrators, policy makers, and funders) by providing evidence on the effectiveness of specific interventions

- *provides consumers with a rationale* for the service by making sound recommendations on effective practice.

Evidence-based practice and ASD

Major "players"

The publicity surrounding the increase in cases of ASD has resulted not only in a greater awareness of ASD, but also in many suggested treatment options, several still in experimental stages. Numerous organizations and programs have conducted research focusing on the many facets of ASD and surrounding issues. Some have been influential in identifying goal areas and evidence-based practices for young children with ASD and have created professional development resources for parents and professionals (see also Chapter 15).

NATIONAL RESEARCH COUNCIL

The U.S.-based National Research Council (NRC) is a non-profit institution that provides science, technology, and health policy. The NRC has been actively involved in studying ASD. Since 2001, its mission has been to integrate the scientific, theoretical, and policy literature surrounding ASD and create a framework for evaluating the scientific evidence concerning the effectiveness of educational programs for young children with ASD worldwide. The NRC advocates that goals for children with ASD should be the same as those for typically developing children. The goal areas should include personal independence and social responsibility. The NRC further implies that progress should be expected in social and cognitive abilities, verbal and non-verbal communication skills, and adaptive skills, as well as reduction of behavioral difficulties and generalization of abilities across multiple environments (NRC, 2001).

NATIONAL PROFESSIONAL DEVELOPMENT CENTER

ON AUTISM SPECTRUM DISORDERS

The National Professional Development Center on Autism Spectrum Disorders (see NPDC on ASD, n.d.) is funded by the Office of Special Education Programs in the United States Department of Education. Its major focus is to promote the use of EBP that produces optimal outcomes for learners with ASD. The NPDC on ASD's efforts towards identification of EBP mainly emphasize focused interventions rather than comprehensive treatment models (see Chapter 1 for further discussion of these terms) as well as the development of instructional modules.

NATIONAL AUTISM CENTER

The National Autism Center (NAC) is a non-profit organization in the United States that promotes EBP. The NAC launched the National Standards Project in 2005, guided by a renowned panel of scholars, researchers, and leaders representing various fields of study. In 2009, the NAC unveiled its *National Standards Report* that established a set of standards for effective, research-validated educational and behavioral interventions for children with ASD. The report includes 775 research studies that examine a wide range of applied treatments and identifies the level of scientific evidence for them. Guidelines for selecting treatment options are also provided (NAC, 2009).

Strength of evidence classification systems

Conclusions from research reviews based on quality indicators inform the level of EBP. Quality indicators usually describe core features of research designs and may evaluate the degree to which each core feature is met. Levels of EBP rank the strength of evidence that supports the effectiveness of a practice, strategy, or intervention (Snyder, 2006). However, different reviewers may have different criteria and therefore reach different conclusions (Else and Wheeler, 2010; Odom et al., 2005).

Reichow, Volkmar, and Cicchetti (2008) define two levels of EBP (*Established EBP* and *Promising Practice*) specifically pertaining to young children with ASD. The Council for Exceptional Children (CEC)'s 2006 ranking system recommends *Research-Based Practice* yet notes that *Promising Practice* may be applied while closely monitoring developing literature. *Emerging Practice* should be used with caution as there is not yet sufficient research to support generalization (CEC, 2006). The NAC's 2009 *National Standards Report* rankings reflect the level of quality, quantity, and consistency of research findings of specific ASD interventions and define four levels of effectiveness as follows:

- *Established*—Sufficient evidence is available to confidently determine that a treatment produces favorable outcomes; therefore, the treatment is established as effective.

- *Emerging*—Although some studies suggest that a treatment produces favorable outcomes, there is not enough evidence to meet the research criteria for being truly effective.

- *Unestablished*—There is little or no evidence to indicate a firm conclusion about the treatment's effectiveness.

- *Ineffective/Harmful*—Sufficient evidence is available to determine that a treatment is ineffective or harmful for individuals on the autism spectrum. No treatments reviewed in the *National Standards Report* fell into this category (NAC, 2009).

Under the CEC 2006 rating system, music therapy most likely falls under the *Promising Practice* category (Umbarger, 2007). The NAC 2009 report assigned music therapy under *Emerging Practice*. Although music therapy currently is not classified in the top tier of effective practices, one must keep in mind that guidelines for evaluating research and the rules and standards for systematic research review vary and change over time. Furthermore, inclusion in research reviews may depend on where reviewers search for studies and what kinds of research are included in the review (Else and Wheeler, 2010). It also remains unclear if evidence about the effectiveness of music therapy interventions can be measured on the discipline. A more appropriate evaluation might be to gauge how music can effectively impact focused interventions for children with ASD. Moreover, the increasing number of rigorous studies demonstrating the effectiveness of music therapy interventions for skill improvements of young children with ASD may change the classification of music therapy over time (see Chapter 3).

Considerations and implications for music therapy services
Considering research evidence in clinical practice

Making sound decisions on the best treatment modality for children with ASD and their families requires solid knowledge about latest research outcomes and their application in clinical practice. To contribute to enhancing the lives of children with ASD, music therapists must understand (a) early childhood development, (b) musical development, (c) early intervention and early childhood special education, and (d) the effectiveness of music therapy interventions for skill improvements in young children with ASD.

UNDERSTANDING EARLY CHILDHOOD DEVELOPMENT

Music therapists need to understand typical developmental milestones of young children as well as deviations from those norms. During the first five years, children do move through various stages of development, which provide windows of opportunity for skill improvements that lay the foundation for all later development (Bokova, 2010; National Scientific Council on the Developing Child, 2007). Developmental milestones do not depend only on chronological age but also on the child's developmental age. While children typically follow a certain pattern of development, some do not. To understand development that is delayed or splintered, one needs to have a frame of reference that guides the direction and intent of possible interventions. The Centers for Disease Control and Prevention (2010), in collaboration with other stakeholders in the United States, conducted a public awareness campaign regarding key developmental milestones in children aged three months to five years. The available resources (e.g., interactive milestones chart and checklist, a video, fact sheets, and resource kits) provide parents and professionals with a comprehensive overview on typical early childhood development and delayed development, including early signs of ASD.

KNOWING ABOUT MUSICAL DEVELOPMENT OF YOUNG CHILDREN

The development of music skills and responses to music also follows a typical sequence that is influenced by the stages of general development and learning (Briggs, 1991; Gordon, 2003). Music therapists need to know what and when musical skills and responses develop. Schwartz (2008) examined observable behaviors and physical changes from various developmental scales and checklists. Her blended compilation is organized into developmental milestones that note characteristics of children from birth to 60 months of age across physical, sensory, motor, cognitive, emotional/social, and language areas. Such information and knowledge about musical developmental milestones should be considered when selecting goals and designing appropriate music therapy interventions for children with ASD.

LEARNING ABOUT EARLY INTERVENTION FOR YOUNG CHILDREN WITH ASD

In the United States, early intervention (EI) refers to services for children who are at risk for or display developmental delays or disabilities in the first three years of life (National Dissemination Center for Children with Disabilities, 2010). At the age of three, children with ASD may become part of the Early Childhood Special Education (ECSE) system. Educational laws, definitions, and trends are not static, and eligibility for both EI and ECSE may vary across and sometimes within countries. Therefore, music therapists need to be aware and keep abreast of guidelines, regulations, and issues that may influence service delivery to young children with ASD within their professional context.

When planning for appropriate interventions for young children with ASD and their families, music therapists must consider both effective practices and how they should be implemented. Table 2.2 identifies evidence-based focused interventions and comprehensive treatment models (CTMs) that work. The following five principles recommended by the Division of Early Childhood (Schertz, 2010) describe how those interventions should be implemented:

- via a family-centered and strength-based approach
- in natural and inclusive environments
- with developmentally sound methodology
- by working towards goals that are functional and oriented toward active child engagement
- in a coordinated and systematic manner.

BEING AWARE OF THE EFFECTS OF MUSIC THERAPY INTERVENTIONS IN CHILDREN WITH ASD

Reschke-Hernández (2011) gives an historical overview of music therapy research and interventions for children with ASD from 1940 to 2009. The author notes that early pioneers in the field described the positive impact of using music for enhancing the lives of children with ASD, and numerous anecdotal case reports yielded valuable supportive information. Reschke-Hernández further explains that the impact of music therapy interventions in areas such as socialization, communication, and behavior were formally studied. Although the rigor of most of these studies is not optimal, recent review articles (e.g., Accordino, Comer, and Heller, 2007; Gold, Wigram, and Elefant, 2006; Simpson and Keen, 2011; Whipple, 2004) conclude that music therapy offers several positive benefits for improving the core features of ASD. Chapter 3 provides an in-depth examination of music therapy research that reflects its effectiveness in priority areas for young children with ASD. Music therapists and others using music as an intervention need to be aware of the outcomes of these studies to make informed practice decisions.

Clinical expertise of the practicing music therapist

In many countries, music therapists are certified, accredited, or licensed; they practice according to the professional competencies, clinical practice standards, and codes of ethics defined by professional organizations and government guidelines. Continued education requirements, plus professional experiences in the field, foster increased clinical expertise.

As of today, there are no practice guidelines established by professional music therapy organizations for working specifically with young children with ASD. Music therapy interventions, strategies, and supports are based on therapeutic frameworks and techniques that have been proven effective for specific populations. This means that music therapists working with young children with ASD and their families plan interventions on specific focused intervention practices and add music or its elements (i.e., rhythm, melody, harmony, timbre, dynamics, and form) to the intervention. Therefore, music therapy as an intervention can reinforce other therapies by adding the beneficial piece of music and its therapeutic aspects, but also can stand on its own. Because focused interventions are most effective when carefully adapted to the specific needs and children's unique abilities, music therapists provide ongoing assessment and adjust the intervention accordingly. Table 2.1 provides a sample of research-based music therapy interventions that support evidence-based focused intervention practices.

Table 2.1 Sample of focused intervention practices for young children with ASD supported by music therapy interventions

Sample of focused intervention practices for children with ASD identified by the NPDC on ASD (2010)	Supported by music therapy intervention research	References
Peer-Mediated Instruction	Peers modeled singing a unique song while playing instruments in the Music Hut (i.e., an outdoor music center) located at a childcare program. The songs targeted social skill improvements (i.e., turn-taking) of four children (ages 3–5) with ASD.	Kern, P., and Aldridge, D. (2006). Using embedded music therapy interventions to support outdoor play of young children with autism in an inclusive community-based child care program. *Journal of Music Therapy, 43(4)*, 270–294.
Picture Exchange Communication System (PECS)	Two children with ASD (age 3) exchanged a picture displaying a stick figure waving "hello" as a means to greet a teacher or peer while singing a song that guided them through the steps of a set morning greeting routine upon arrival at a childcare program.	Kern, P., Wolery, M., and Aldridge, D. (2007). Use of songs to promote independence in morning greeting routines for young children with autism. *Journal of Autism and Developmental Disorders, 37,* 1264–1271.
Social Narratives	Four children with ASD (ages 6–9) reduced the frequency of a target behavior by adding original music to a unique social story similar to the read version—in one case the sung version was more effective.	Brownell, M.D. (2002). Musically adapted social stories to modify behaviors in students with autism: Four case studies. *Journal of Music Therapy, 39(2),* 117–144.
Video Modeling	18 children with ASD (ages 3–5), especially those identified as low functioning, improved their verbal production after a music training using music videos with six songs and pictures of 36 target words.	Lim, H.A. (2010). Effects of "Developmental Speech and Language Training through Music" on speech production in children with autism spectrum disorders. *Journal of Music Therapy, 47(1),* 2–26.

Individual client factors: Early intervention for young children with ASD

Recognizing that each child with ASD is unique, educational and therapeutic services should be tailored to the individual needs and abilities of each child as well as the family's values and beliefs. However, children with ASD are first and foremost children and should be treated like their typically developing peers to the extent that is reasonable and feasible.

The NRC (2001) addressed this issue by identifying goals, areas of needs, and basic recommendations for professionals serving young children with ASD and their families. According to the NRC, goals for young children with ASD should mirror programming that is appropriate for children who are developing typically, specifically in the areas of personal independence and social responsibility. Targeted interventions should fall under the following priority areas of educational programming: (1) functional spontaneous communication, (2) social instruction, (3) play skills, (4) cognitive development, (5) proactive approaches to behavior, and (6) functional academic skills (Stansberry-Brusnahan and Collet-Klingenberg, 2010, p. 48).

In a multimedia article, Walworth (2010) addressed how priority areas and intervention recommendations of the NRC can be incorporated into music therapy practice, giving examples of a music therapy intervention for a young child with ASD in the home environment. An interview with the child's parents confirmed the positive response of the child and reflects the family's involvement.

Various other professions are recognizing that early intervention is essential for improving long-term outcomes, and are responding to the increasing number of young children diagnosed with ASD by offering diverse treatment options (Eikseth *et al.*, 2007; Smith-Miles *et al.*, 2009; Stansberry-Brusnahan and Collet-Klingenberg, 2010). However, many of these possibilities are not formally described as *effective practice* nor do they account for the wide range of needs or the developmental levels of the young child with ASD. The effectiveness of strategies is often questioned among professionals as well as parents. As an attempt to avoid confusion generated by debated issues and opinions, the National Professional Development Center on ASD and the National Autism Center (i.e., National Standards Project, 2009) conducted a literature review and identified current evidence-based practices for individuals with ASD. Both entities came to similar conclusions, which are reflected in Table 2.2.

The NRC (2001) also identified key features of early intervention programs that may be beneficial to an audience across borders concerned with designing, choosing, and evaluating programs for children with ASD. The educational programming recommendations delineate that interventions should:

1. begin as soon as a child is suspected of having ASD

2. include a child's active engagement in systematically planned, age and developmentally appropriate activities toward identified objectives (full day, five days a week (25 hours a week), year-round programming)

3. include teaching that is planned and organized around repeated short intervals individualized daily and in one-to-one as well as very small group instruction that focuses on meeting individualized goals

4. include the inclusion of a family component and parent training

5. include mechanisms for ongoing evaluation of the program and child's progress, with adjustments made accordingly

6. include inclusive opportunities to the extent that these lead to the acquisition of a child's educational goals.

Practicality and reality
Applying EBP in clinical work

Gathering research information is becoming less daunting due to rapid technological advances and avenues of information-sharing. However, practitioners might continue to struggle with the concept of EBP because terminology used by various sources may differ, appraisals are often quite complex, and the validity and reliability of the research itself may be questionable.

The issue becomes more manageable if practitioners consider how EBP can inform clinical work. Practitioners may be able to better address and support individual outcomes for children with ASD across multiple settings by centering on focused interventions rather than entire comprehensive treatment models (Odom *et al.*, 2010). Furthermore, a focused intervention approach may be more cost effective because comprehensive treatment models often require intensive staff training or the purchase of large amounts of materials specific to the model (Stansberry-Brusnahan and Collet-Klingenberg, 2010).

The question is: How can practitioners make informed practice decisions that directly benefit young children with ASD and their families? Buysse and Wesley (2006) recommend a five-step decision-making process that is based on the EBM model. Figure 2.1 summarizes the five steps of this decision-making process.

Kern (2010) further describes a comprehensive case scenario demonstrating how this process could be used in a music therapy practice setting serving a child with ASD. Detailed descriptions and resources for each step are included.

Table 2.2 Evidence-based practices identified by the NPDC on ASD and the NAC

Overlap between evidence-based practices by the NPDC on ASD and the National Standards Project (NSP)

Evidence-based practices identified by the NPDC on ASD	Established treatments identified by the NSP										
	Antecedent package	Behavioral package	Story-based intervention package	Modeling	Naturalistic teaching strategies	Peer training package	Pivotal response treatment	Schedules	Self-management	Comprehensive behavioral treatment for young children	Joint attention intervention
Prompting	x			x						The NPDC on ASD did not review comprehensive treatment models. Components of the comrehensive behavioral treatment of young children overlap with many NPDC-identified preactices.	The NPDC on ASD considers joint attention to be an outcome rather than an intervention. Components of joint attention interventions overlap with many NPDC-identifies practices.
Antecedent-based intervention	x										
Time delay	x										
Reinforcement		x									
Task analysis		x									
Discrete Trial Training		x									
Functional behavior analysis		x									
Functional communication training		x									
Response interruption/ redirection		x									
Differential reinforcement		x									

Intervention							
Social narratives	x						
Video modeling		x					
Naturalistic interventions			x				
Peer mediated intervention				x			
Pivotal response training					x		
Visual supports						x	
Structured work systems						x	x
Self-management							x
Parent-implemented intervention	The NSP did not consider parent-implemented intervention as a category of evidence-based practice. However, 24 of the studies reviewed by the NSP under other intervention categories involve parents implementing the intervention.						
Social skills training groups	Social skills training groups (social skills package) was identified as an emerging practice by the NSP.						
Speech-generating devices	Speech-generating devices (Augmentative and Alternative Communication Device) was identified as an emerging practice by the NSP.						
Computer-aided instruction	Computer-aided instruction (technology-based treatment) was identified as an emerging practice by the NSP.						
Picture exchange communication	Picture Exchange Communication System was identified as an emerging practice by the NSP.						
Extinction	Extinction (reductive package) was identified as an emerging practice by the NSP.						

Source: The National Professional Development Center (NPDC) on ASD. Available at http://autismpdc.fpg.unc.edu/content/national-standards-project. Reprinted with permission.

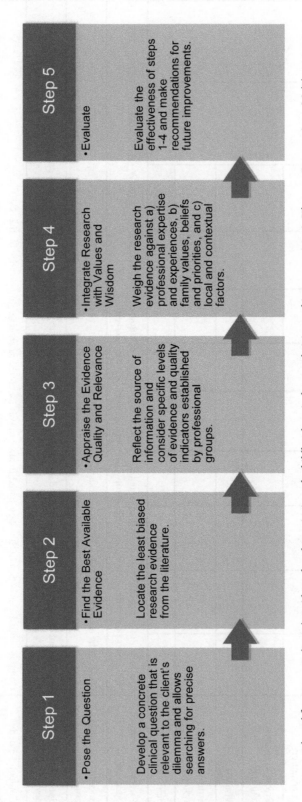

Step 1

- Pose the Question

Develop a concrete clinical question that is relevant to the client's dilemma and allows searching for precise answers.

Step 2

- Find the Best Available Evidence

Locate the least biased research evidence from the literature.

Step 3

- Appraise the Evidence Quality and Relevance

Reflect the source of information and consider specific levels of evidence and quality indicators established by professional groups.

Step 4

- Integrate Research with Values and Wisdom

Weigh the research evidence against a) professional expertise and experiences, b) family values, beliefs and priorities, and c) local and contextual factors.

Step 5

- Evaluate

Evaluate the effectiveness of steps 1-4 and make recommendations for future improvements.

Note: Adapted from Kern, P. (2010). Evidence-based practice in early childhood music therapy: desicion-making process. Music Therapy Perspectives, 28(2), 116–123.

Figure 2.1: Decision-making process of an EBP practitioner

From implementation to fidelity

Music therapy services in early childhood and early intervention settings are provided along a continuum ranging from direct to consultative services. Contemporary service delivery in early childhood education is often based on an integrated therapy model; therefore, many music therapists collaborate with parents and professionals from related fields (Kern, 2005). Hence, music therapists may act as consultants to a classroom teacher or be asked to provide musical components for interventions other team members have designed. This may include holding workshops for parents, suggesting instructional strategies and music therapy techniques that may help a child with ASD in the home environment, or offering guidance for accommodating children with ASD within the community. The role of the music therapy consultant may range from providing professional development to solely relaying information and presenting choices; it is necessary to understand that, in early childhood, parents still retain the final decision in their child's programming.

Even after effective interventions are determined, how they are implemented greatly affects child outcomes (Levy, Kim, and Olive, 2006). The research literature may not contain enough details for the intervention to be replicated (Stansberry-Brusnahan and Collet-Klingenberg, 2010). However, when designing music therapy interventions, the music therapist should be guided by available research outcomes and established recommendations. Providing consultative services to families and colleagues of the interdisciplinary team requires:

- careful planning of the music therapy intervention (i.e., materials, strategies, and techniques)

- precise training for parents and staff (i.e., step-by-step instruction and demonstration)

- close monitoring of the implementation and child's progress (i.e., implementation checklist and outcome data collection sheets)

- thorough evaluation of the intervention (i.e., child outcomes and suggestions for further improvements).

The checklist in Figure 2.2 offers considerations for providing evidence-based music therapy services to young children with ASD and their families.

Conclusion

Evidence-based practice presents an avenue for identifying the best available interventions, strategies, and supports for young children with ASD. Music therapists need to be aware of the latest research outcomes, apply evidence-based practice and recommended principles to clinical practice, and be available to various stakeholders. By focusing on the core components of EBP (i.e., sharing knowledge and clinical experiences with families and colleagues) while being ever vigilant advocates of the child's strengths and family's values, music therapists may bring children with ASD one step closer to the ultimate goal of living independent and fulfilled lives.

Checklist

1. Apply the five-step evidence-based decision-making ☐
   process to help identify the best available treatment option.

2. Provide accurate information about the research-based ☐
   benefits of music therapy interventions for young
   children with ASD.

3. Share your clinical experiences and assessment of the ☐
   strengths and abilities of the target child with ASD.

4. Respect the family's beliefs, values, and decisions. ☐

5. When providing music therapy services, plan the ☐
   intervention toward individualized goals, including age
   and developmentally appropriate music activities,
   engaging the child with ASD in a systemic manner.

6. Consider which service delivery model best ☐
   accommodates the need for daily repeated short
   intervals, one-to-one and small group involvement, and
   inclusive moments.

7. Present a family component and parental training. ☐

8. Include ongoing evaluation of the intervention ☐
   implementation (i.e., intervention fidelity) and
   child's progress.

Figure 2.2: Checklist for providing evidence-based music therapy services to young children with ASD

LEARNING QUESTIONS

1. What are the three components that define evidence-based practice?

2. Why is it desirable to be an evidence-based practitioner?

3. What is the difference between quality indicators and level of evidence-based practice?

4. Which level of evidence is recommended by the Council for Exceptional Children and under which level is music therapy currently listed?

5. Give an example of how music therapy interventions can support each of the priority areas for educational programming of children with ASD.

6. According to the NRC (2001), what should be considered when designing interventions for young children with ASD?

7. Using the five-step decision-making model by Buysse and Wesley (2006), describe the best intervention option for one of your clients and his or her family.

8. Summarize considerations for providing evidence-based music therapy services to young children with ASD and their families.

Authors' note

The authors wish to thank Dr. Gary Mesibov for providing valuable feedback during the development of this chapter.

References

Abrams, B. (2010). Evidence-based music therapy practice: An integral understanding. *Journal of Music Therapy, 4(4)*, 35–379.

Accordino, R., Comer, R., and Heller, W.B. (2007). Searching for music's potential: A critical examination of research on music therapy with individuals with autism. *Research in Autism Spectrum Disorders 1*, 101–115.

American Music Therapy Association (AMTA) (1999). *Music Therapy and the Young Child Fact Sheet*. Silver Spring, MD: AMTA.

American Music Therapy Association (AMTA) (2010). Definition: Evidence-Based Music Therapy Practice *(EBMTP)*. Retrieved from www.musictherapy.org/research/strategic_priority_on_research/ evidencebased_practice/.

American Psychiatric Association (APA) (2006). Evidence-based practice in psychology. *American Psychologist, 61*, 271–285.

Bokova, I. (2010). Opening address to the UNESCO World Conference on early childhood care and education. Retrieved from http://unesdoc.unesco.org/images/0018/001870/187000e.pdf.

Briggs, C.A. (1991). A model for understanding musical development. *Music Therapy, 10(1)*, 1–21.

Brownell, M.K. (2002). Musically adapted social stories to modify behaviors in students with autism: Four case studies. *Journal of Music Therapy, 39(2)*, 117–144.

Buysse, V., and Wesley, P.W. (2006). *Evidence-Based Practice in the Early Childhood Field*. Washington, DC: Zero to Three.

Centers for Disease Control and Prevention (CDC) (2010). *Learn the Signs: Act Early*. Retrieved from www.cdc.gov/ncbddd/actearly/about.html.

Council for Exceptional Children (CEC) (2006). *CEC Evidence-Based Professional Practice Proposal*. Arlington, VA: Professional Standards and Practice Committee.

Eikseth, S., Smith, T., Jahr, K., and Eldevik, S. (2007). Outcome for children with autism who began intensive behavioral treatment between ages 4 and 7: A comparison controlled study. *Behavior Modification, 31*, 264–278.

Else, B., and Wheeler, B. (2010). Music therapy practice: Relative perspectives in evidence-based reviews. *Nordic Journal of Music Therapy, 19(1)*, 29–50.

Gold, C., Wigram, T., and Elefant, C. (2006). Music therapy for autistic spectrum disorder. *Cochrane Database of Systematic Reviews, Issue 2*. Art. No.: CD004381. DOI:10.1002/14651858.CD004381. pub2.

Gordon, E.E. (2003). *A Music Learning Theory for Newborn and Young Children*. GIA Publications, Inc. (Originally published in 1990.)

Kern, P. (2005). Single case designs in an interactive play setting. In D. Aldridge (Ed.) *Case Study Designs in Music Therapy*. London and Philadelphia: Jessica Kingsley Publishers.

Kern, P. (2010). Evidence-based practice in early childhood music therapy: A decision-making process. *Music Therapy Perspectives, 28(2)*, 116–123.

Kern, P., and Aldridge, D. (2006). Using embedded music therapy interventions to support outdoor play of young children with autism in an inclusive community-based child care program. *Journal of Music Therapy, 43(4)*, 270–294.

Kern, P., Wolery, M., and Aldridge, D. (2007). Use of songs to promote independence in morning greeting routines for young children with autism. *Journal of Autism and Developmental Disorders, 37*, 1264–1271.

Levy, S., Kim, A., and Olive, M. (2006). Interventions for young children with autism: A synthesis of the literature. *Focus on Autism and Other Developmental Disabilities, 21(1)*, 55–62.

Lim, H.A. (2010). Effects of "Developmental Speech and Language Training through Music" on speech production in children with autism spectrum disorders. *Journal of Music Therapy, 47(1)*, 2–26.

Mesibov, G.B., and Shea, V. (2010). The TEACCH program in the era of evidence-based practice. *Journal of Autism and Developmental Disorders, 4(5)*, 570–579.

National Autism Center (NAC) (2009). *National Standards Report*. The National Standards Project— Addressing the need for evidence-based practice guidelines for autism spectrum disorders. Randolph, MA: NAC.

National Dissemination Center for Children with Disabilities (2010). Overview of early intervention. Retrieved from http://nichcy.org/babies/overview.

National Professional Development Center on Autism Spectrum Disorders (NPDC on ASD) (n.d.) Home. Retrieved from http://autismpdc.fpg.unc.edu.

National Research Council (NRC) (2001). *Educating Children with Autism*. Committee on Educational Interventions for Children with Autism. C. Lord and J. McGee (Eds.) Division of Behavioral and Social Sciences and Education. Washington, DC: National Academy Press.

National Scientific Council on the Developing Child (2007). The timing and quality of early experiences combine to shape brain architecture: working paper no. 5. Retrieved from www.developingchild. harvard.edu.

Odom, S.L., Brantliner, E., Gersten, R., Horner, R.H., Thompson, B., and Harris, K.R. (2005). Research in special education: Scientific methods and evidence-based practice. *Exceptional Children, 71(2)*, 137–148.

Odom, S.L., Collet-Klingenberg, L., Rogers, S.J., and Hatton, D.D. (2010). Evidence-based practices in interventions for children and youth with autism spectrum disorders. *Preventing School Failure: Alternative Education for Children and Youth, 54(4)*, 275–282.

Reichow, B., Volkmar, F.R., and Cicchetti, D.V. (2008). Development of the evaluation method for evaluative and determining evidence-based practice in autism. *Journal of Autism and Developmental Disorder, 38*, 1311–1319.

Reschke-Hernández, A.E. (2011). History of music therapy treatment interventions of children with autism. *Journal of Music Therapy, 48(2)*, 169–207.

Sackett, D.L., Straus, S.E., Richardson, W.S., Rosenberg, W., and Haynes, R.B. (2000). *Evidence Based Medicine: How to Practice and Teach EBM (Second Edition)*. London: Churchill Livingstone.

Schertz, H.H. (2010). Principles of interventions for young children: Implications for toddlers and preschoolers with autism spectrum disorders. In H.H. Schertz, C. Wong, and S.L. Odom (Eds.) Supporting young children with autism spectrum disorders and their families [Monograph]. *Young Exceptional Children, 12*, 12–24.

Schwartz, E. (2008). *Music, Therapy, and Early Childhood*. Gilsum, NH: Barcelona Publishers.

Simpson, K., and Keen, D. (2011). Music interventions for children with autism: Narrative review of the literature. *Journal of Autism and Developmental Disorders, 41*, 1507–1514.

Smith-Miles, B., Grossman, B., Aspy, R., and Henry, S. (2009). Planning a comprehensive program for young children with autism spectrum disorders. *International Journal of Early Childhood Special Education, 1(2)*, 164–180.

Snyder, P. (2006). Evidence-based research evidence: Impact on research in early childhood. In V. Buysse, and P.W. Wesley (Eds.) *Evidence-Based Practice in the Early Childhood Field*. Washington, DC: Zero to Three.

Stansberry-Brusnahan, L.L., and Collet-Klingenberg, L.L. (2010). Evidence-based practices for young children with autism spectrum disorders: Guidelines and recommendations for the National Resource Council and National Professional Development Center on Autism Spectrum Disorders. *International Journal of Early Childhood Special Education (INT-JECSE), 2(1)*, 45–56.

Umbarger, G.T. (2007). State of the evidence regarding complementary and alternative medical treatments for autism spectrum disorder. *Education and Training in Developmental Disabilities, 42(2)*, 437–447.

Walworth, D. (2010). Incorporating music into daily routines: Family education and integration. *imagine, 1(1)*, 28–31. Retrieved from http://imagine.musictherapy.biz/Imagine/imagine__online_magazine. html.

Whipple, J. (2004). Music in intervention for children and adolescents with autism: Meta-analysis. *Journal of Music Therapy, 41(2)*, 90–106.

Chapter 3

Music Therapy as an Effective Treatment for Young Children with Autism Spectrum Disorders

A Meta-Analysis

Jennifer Whipple, Ph.D., MT-BC
CHARLESTON SOUTHERN UNIVERSITY
CHARLESTON, SC

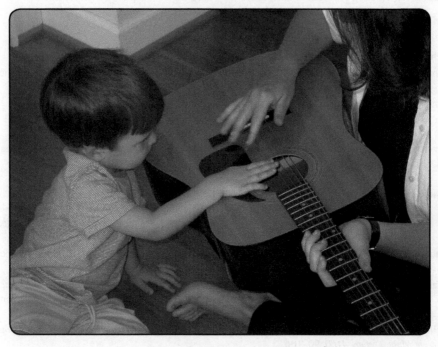

PHOTO COURTESY OF PETRA KERN

Music therapists must continue documenting to validate what we intuitively know to be true—that music therapy is extremely beneficial for young children with autism spectrum disorders.
(Jennifer Whipple)

The existing literature base regarding music therapy in treatment for individuals with autism spectrum disorders (ASD) already boasts numerous independent studies as well as two systematic reviews related to music in treatment for individuals with ASD (Gold, Wigram, and Elefant, 2006; Whipple, 2004). The purpose of this meta-analysis chapter is to address the limitation of the previous two, focus specifically on music therapy treatment for ASD in early childhood, and incorporate more recently published research studies. Results of this study provide support for offering music therapy services as an effective treatment option to young children and their families.

Introduction: Evaluating the research
Do children with ASD have exceptional music skills?

Since the first documented descriptions of ASD by Kanner in 1943, discussions of advanced musical memory and other music behaviors within this population have been addressed in various research studies. Heaton (2009) points out in a review of related studies that much of the focus on advanced music and auditory discrimination skills of individuals with ASD has been on those considered to be musical savants.

The term "autistic savant," first introduced in 1978, refers to individuals with ASD who have seemingly organic abilities more advanced than those typically exhibited by the general population. Savant abilities most commonly appear in the areas of math, memory, art, and music. The estimated prevalence of these abilities in individuals with ASD is 10 percent, compared to less than 1 percent in the remainder of the population. The reasons are not known (Treffert, 2012).

More recent studies investigating music perception, cognition, and learning in musically untrained children with ASD who do not meet savant criteria have revealed a pattern of enhanced abilities. Increased sensitivity to musical pitch and timbre has been observed frequently in children with ASD, and perhaps surprisingly, children with ASD perform as well as their typically developing peers in perception of musical structure and emotions. Most of the available studies specifically assessing musical abilities of children (and not simply the broader population of individuals of all ages with ASD) include an age range beginning with seven years and a mean age of 10 to 12 years. None of these studies includes the early childhood population; nevertheless, the following examples may yield information that may have ramifications for music therapy service delivery with young children.

Heaton (2003) documented that high-functioning children with ASD have significantly better pitch memory for individual tones and for identifying tones missing from chord structures than their typically developing peers. In a subsequent study, Heaton (2005) exposed high-functioning children with ASD to 48 melodic pitch intervals ranging from a minor second to an octave apart. The children with ASD detected pitch direction over small pitch distances significantly better than their age- and intelligence-matched controls.

These studies also conversely indicated that children with ASD are unskilled at determining whether a particular tone is part of a chord they had just heard, indicating that like their typically developing peers, children with ASD tend to focus on the Gestalt (i.e., perception of the whole without perceiving or processing all the details) qualities of chords (Heaton, 2003). High-functioning children with ASD who demonstrated advanced skills in detecting pitch direction were no better than their matched peers at determining musical contours, being unable to indicate if pairs of six-note melodies were the same or different from one another (Heaton, 2005). Heaton *et al.* (2007) played hymn-like seven-chord sequences for both children with ASD and age- and intelligence-matched children without ASD to examine processing of higher-level, structural aspects of music. The children were then asked to judge whether the eighth and final target chord sounded correct (i.e., if it seemed to relate to the preceding harmonic context) or incorrect. Results indicated no significant difference in performance between the two groups.

Regardless, it is the opinion of these researchers that many children with ASD possess musical potential that should be developed (Heaton, 2003, 2005, 2009; Heaton *et al.*, 2007). Enhanced sensitivity to and memory for musical pitch and timbre as documented above are neither the only aspects of music nor the only indicators of an individual's musical success, and advanced natural musical ability is not necessary for music therapy treatment to be beneficial for a client. This previous research supports the need for further investigation into how children with ASD of all functioning levels process music, and how music therapists subsequently may help them achieve the greatest outcome benefits through music.

Why a meta-analysis?

Numerous studies pertaining to the use of music therapy for individuals with ASD have been conducted (Gold, Wigram and Elefant, 2006; Simpson and Keen, 2011; Whipple, 2004). Studies are not always easily compared due to such factors as their varied methodologies, sample sizes, and data analyses. A systematic review of research related to the topic of interest can aid the reader in assessment of the efficacy of certain treatments. One type of systematic review is the meta-analysis, which uses a set of statistical procedures to compile quantitative research data, resulting in an effect size. This resulting figure allows comparison and summary of research findings across studies, thereby making large bodies of literature more manageable, differentiating clinically relevant research findings from others that may be less meaningful, and providing greater confidence in conclusions about the efficacy of treatment (Gold, 2004; Whipple, 2004).

The use of effect size originated in psychotherapy research (Gold, 2004). Over the past 25 years, meta-analyses have been published within the field of music therapy to evaluate its benefits in the following areas:

- in general medical and dental settings (Standley, 1986, 1992, 1996, 2000)

- in pediatric medical settings (Standley and Whipple, 2003)

- in child and adolescent mental health settings (Gold, Voracek, and Wigram, 2004)

- for premature infants (Standley, 2002)

- for adults with symptoms of psychosis (Silverman, 2003)

- for individuals with dementia (Koger, Chapin, and Brotons, 1999)

- to decrease arousal during periods of stress (Pelletier, 2004).

All music therapy meta-analyses cited medium to large effect sizes, indicating that based on the existing published research at the time of publication, music therapy can be an effective treatment for each studied population. In addition to a strictly narrative review of literature related to music interventions for children with ASD (Simpson and Keen, 2011), two systematic reviews have been published related to music therapy in the treatment of ASD (Gold, Wigram, and Elefant, 2006; Whipple, 2004). Both resulted in small to medium effect sizes.

Purpose: What do we already know?

The existing research literature boasts two systematic reviews related to music in treatment for individuals with ASD, yet both reveal limitations within existing publications. Whipple (2004) compared music to no-music conditions in treatment of children and adolescents with ASD by analyzing 12 dependent variables (divided into the three categories of cognitive skill, communication, and social behavior) from nine quantitative studies, which tallied 76 total subjects. Studies were not limited to those in which treatment was implemented by music therapists, but instead included intervention provided by educators, psychologists, and occupational therapists as well. The number of subjects per study ranged from 1 to 20, and ages of subjects varied widely among studies (2.1 to 21 years) and also within individual studies. While research relies on a sharpened focus for drawing conclusions about efficacy of intervention, meta-analysis procedures take these variations into account. Therefore, all were included in the overall evaluation in order to encompass as many studies as possible to best represent the literature base. Results indicated that all music interventions, regardless of client outcomes addressed or specific treatment implemented, were effective for children and adolescents diagnosed with ASD. The meta-analysis cited the need for future research to include larger sample sizes, greater clarity in research and treatment designs, and increased focus on assessment of specific music therapy applications.

Similarly, in their Cochrane review of music therapy intervention for children with ASD, Gold, Wigram, and Elefant (2006) identified only three small randomized controlled trials and controlled clinical trials comparing music therapy to "placebo" therapy, no treatment, or standard care which met their inclusion criteria, with all included subjects totaling 24 (ranging per study from 4 to 10 subjects). Results indicated that music therapy was significantly more effective than "placebo" therapy, no treatment, or standard care for addressing verbal and gestural communicative skills, but not for behavioral problems. The authors noted that the three included studies examined only the short-term effect of brief music therapy interventions (i.e., daily sessions over a period of one week) for children with ASD; despite the revealed treatment benefits, the studies seem to be of limited applicability to clinical practice.

Several years have passed since both the meta-analysis (Whipple, 2004) and Cochrane review (Gold, Wigram, and Elefant 2006) were conducted. Both were limited by the availability of published literature meeting the studies' criteria, and neither specifically examined music therapy treatment for ASD in early childhood. Simpson and Keen (2011) addressed this specific focus to a certain extent in their narrative review of 20 experimental music intervention studies targeting communication, socialization, and behavioral skills of children with ASD. To keep pace with the developing literature base, the purpose of this meta-analysis is to review all, including recently published, literature related to music therapy in treatment for young children diagnosed with ASD.

Method: What were the steps?
Study inclusion: What studies were included?
Only studies that met the following criteria were included in this meta-analysis:

1. Used group or individual subject experimental treatment designs.

2. Design, procedures, and results allowed replicated data analysis.

3. Used subjects who were children five years or younger diagnosed with ASD, but did not include studies that incorporated diverse special education populations regardless of inclusion of students with ASD.

4. Utilized music as a separate, independent variable contrasted with a no music control condition (e.g., no contact control condition; standard care; or other treatment condition, such as play therapy or spoken instructions only).

5. Music treatment procedures were conducted by a music therapist.

6. Quantitative results were reported with sufficient information to extract an effect size.

7. Were in the form of articles published worldwide in peer-reviewed journals (i.e., dissertations, theses, and research poster session presentations were not included).

Studies related to assessment of music skills or appropriateness of music therapy for children with ASD also were not included in the effect size analysis, nor were articles that described treatment techniques for children with ASD, but did not include quantitative data. In addition, studies were excluded in which data analysis focused on parents or caregivers of children with ASD, or in which the data for young children could not be divided from data for older children and adolescents or adults with ASD.

Based on accepted meta-analysis procedures (Johnson and Wood, 2006), an exhaustive literature search was conducted to find all studies meeting the defined criteria. Characteristics of the collected studies were identified and described. Each study's results were statistically analyzed and converted to computed effect sizes using meta-analysis software (Johnson and Wood, 2006).

The identification of applicable literature included searches of the *Journal of Music Therapy* (1964–2011), *Music Therapy Perspectives* (1982–1984, 1986–2011), *Music Therapy* (1981–1996), and Academic Search Premier, a database for the social sciences, using "music," "autism," and "children" as keywords. Reference lists of all collected articles were searched, as were the music therapy focus issue of *Early Childhood Connections* (Humpal, 2001), an analysis of music research with disabled children and youth from 1975 to 1999 (Jellison, 2000), and the *National Standards Report* by the National Autism Center (2009).

Study descriptions: What do the studies say?

Of the treatment studies located, eight met criteria for inclusion in the meta-analysis. They are described in Table 3.1, Parts A and B, in terms of type of dependent variables measured; study design; number of subjects in treatment sessions; participation in and use, selection, and presentation of music; and subject age and gender. Each study's scientific merit was rated based on two rating systems (National Autism Center, 2009; Reichow, Volkmar, and Cicchetti, 2008). Included studies are summarized by variable addressed below.

- Communication: Kern, Wolery, and Aldridge (2007) incorporated the concept of caregiver training by teaching classroom teachers a routine and original morning greeting song to ease individual children's morning transitions into the classroom and facilitate peer interaction. Lim (2010) compared the effect of a video with six original songs and pictures of 36 vocabulary words viewed by children twice a day for three days to (a) a video with six stories and pictures of the same words and to (b) no intervention on the verbal production of the target words. Lim and Draper (2011) compared the effect of developmental speech-language training using an Applied Behavior Analysis Verbal Behavior approach and the same approach paired with music in which instruction was sung *a cappella* rather than spoken. They assessed the impact of both interventions on speech production of target words, including immediate echolalia of target phrases.

- Interpersonal: Finnigan and Starr (2010) examined the use of individual music play sessions involving various instruments and toys as well as original "piggyback" songs and guitar to increase social responsive behaviors of eye contact, imitation, and turn-taking. Decreasing avoidant behaviors of gaze aversion, pushing away toys and people, and moving away also were investigated. Responses to these sessions were compared to individual play therapy sessions that also incorporated instruments and toys but no singing, melodic, or rhythmic play. Kern and Aldridge (2006) constructed a "Music Hut" on a preschool playground to encourage active music play and peer interaction. Incorporating caregiver training, the researchers taught teachers original compositions and a procedure to use to help initiate music play and peer interaction. Kim, Wigram, and Gold (2008) compared the effect of individual improvisational music play sessions versus individual play therapy sessions, both partially child led and partially therapist directed. The researchers focused on joint attention behaviors and duration of both eye contact and turn-taking. Wimpory, Chadwick, and Nash (1995) addressed social acknowledgement and eye contact by providing several music therapy sessions incorporating games, movement, singing, and musical accompaniment of activities.

- Personal responsibility: Kern, Wakeford, and Aldridge (2007) explored the use of an original song outlining the steps of three self-care tasks (i.e., hand-washing, toileting, and cleaning up) taught to the classroom teacher to guide a preschool child with ASD through the daily tasks. This study incorporated caregiver training as in the Kern and Aldridge (2006) communication study already described.

- Play: Kern and Aldridge (2006) also addressed this category in their previously described "Music Hut" study.

Wimpory, Chadwick, and Nash (1995) is the only study included in the Whipple (2004) meta-analysis of music in treatment for children and adolescents with ASD that also met the additional criterion of early childhood included for this meta-analysis. It was actually an outlier (a value that deviates markedly from the remainder of the sample) in the 2004 meta-analysis and was therefore not included in the final effect size analysis at that time. One of its variables is again an outlier here.

Table 3.1 Study descriptors—Part A

Study authors and year	Variable analyzed	Type of variable	Subject age	Subject gender	Study design	Scientific merit rating	Evidence-based practice rating
Finnigan and Starr (2010)	Eye contact Imitation and turn-taking	Interpersonal	3y, 8m	Female	Single case experimental (music vs non-music interventions)	1	Strong
Kern and Aldridge (2006)	Play and engagement Peer interaction	Play Interpersonal	3y, 4m–4y, 9m; M = 3y; 11.5m	Male	Multiple baseline (community-based inclusive playground)	4	Strong
Kern, Wakeford, and Aldridge (2007)	Hand-washing, toileting, and cleaning up	Personal responsibility	3y	Male	Alternating treatment (musical vs verbal presentations)	1	Adequate
Kern, Wolery, and Aldridge (2007)	Independent responses Greetings by peers	Communication	3y, 5m and 3y, 2m; M = 3y; 2.5m	Male	ABAB withdrawal (morning greeting routine, music vs non-music)	3	Adequate
Kim, Wigram, and Gold (2008)[1]	Joint attention Eye contact and turn-taking	Interpersonal	3–5y; M = 4y, 4m	Male	Randomized controlled trial single subject (improvisational music therapy vs play)	1	Strong
Lim (2010)	Verbal production	Communication	3–5y; M = 4y, 8m	Unknown	Experimental (music vs speech vs no-training conditions)	1	Adequate
Lim and Draper (2011)	Verbal production	Communication	3–5y; M = 4y, 3m	Male (n = 17), Female (n = 5)	Within subjects experimental (Applied Behavior Analysis Verbal Behavior approach, music vs developmental speech-language vs no training)	1	Adequate
Wimpory, Chadwick, and Nash (1995)	Social acknowledgment Eye contact	Interpersonal	3y, 3m	Female	ABC, single case experimental (music vs non-music)	1	Strong

1 This study's data was also reported in a later publication (Kim, Wigram, and Gold, 2009) in terms of emotional synchronicity between child and therapist and initiation of engagement, among other variables. The later publication is not included within this meta-analysis in order to be consistent with the procedures outlined within this chapter and avoid weighting one group of subjects over others.

Note: Type of variable is consistent with treatment sub-classification categories described in the National Autism Center's *National Standards Report* (2009). The Scientific Merit Rating (scale: 1 to 5; 5 is best) was determined by the rubric provided in the same report for the purpose of determining if methods used in each study were strong enough to determine whether a treatment was effective for participants. The evidence-based practice rating (i.e. weak, adequate, strong) was determined based on standards described within Reichow, Volkmar, and Cicchetti (2008) related to determining evidence-based practices in ASD.

Table 3.1 Study descriptors—Part B

Study author and year	Session type	Music use	Music selection	Music presentation	Music involvement
Finnigan and Starr (2010)	Individual	Music-making/play; cue	Original lyrics to familiar children's melodies	Live	Active
Kern and Aldridge (2006)	Group	Music-making/play; cue	Original compositions	Live	Active
Kern, Wakeford, and Aldridge (2007)	Individual	Cue; carrier of information	Original lyrics to familiar children's melodies; original compositions	Live	Active
Kern, Wolery, and Aldridge (2007)	Group	Cue; carrier of information	Original lyrics to familiar children's melodies; original compositions; precomposed songs	Live	Active
Kim, Wigram, and Gold (2008)	Individual	Music-making/play	Not specified	Live	Active
Lim (2010)	Individual	Carrier of information	Original compositions	Recorded	Passive
Lim and Draper (2011)	Individual	Carrier of information	Original compositions	Live	Passive
Wimpory, Chadwick, and Nash (1995)	Individual	Music-making/play	Spontaneously composed simple songs; background	Live	Active

Examination of included studies indicates that music therapists, at least within published empirical research, are not addressing outcomes within the majority of the treatment sub-classification areas described within the *National Autism Centre* (NAC) report (those italicized below are not addressed within the studies included in the meta-analysis):

- Skills increased
  - *Academic*
  - Communication
  - *Higher cognitive functions*
  - Interpersonal
  - *Learning readiness*
  - *Motor skills*
  - Personal responsibility
  - *Placement*
  - Play
  - *Self-regulation*
- *Behaviors decreased*
  - *General symptoms*
  - *Problem behaviors*
  - *Restricted, repetitive, nonfunctional patterns of behavior, interests, or activity*
  - *Sensory or emotional regulation.*

Skill categories like *Academic* are probably more appropriate for older children. However, no studies were found that addressed *Self-regulation* or *Motor skills*, both appropriate for early childhood. Most identified articles focused on increasing skills rather than decreasing challenging behaviors; perhaps more challenging behaviors may tend to emerge later in childhood and adolescence and those seen in early childhood are often tied to typical development. Further, music therapy treatment naturally focuses and builds on client strengths, and therapists write goals and objectives using positive (e.g., increase or improve a skill), rather than negative (e.g., decrease an undesirable behavior), language. Finnigan and Starr (2010) did observe two types of avoidant behaviors (pushing a toy away and moving away). These were not included in the actual effect size analysis as both occurred infrequently within the study observations, so adequate data was not available.

Additional study design and implementation factors beyond those used as meta-analysis study inclusion criteria may be important to consider when supporting the benefits of music therapy for young children with ASD. These currently are best measured by the NAC (2009) scientific merit rating and the Reichow, Volkmar, and

Cicchetti (2008) evidence-based practice rating systems. Ratings for each study are found in Table 3.1, Part A. Due to adherence to the strict NAC (2009) rubric criteria, all but two of the eight studies received the lowest rating of 1, with one study receiving a rating of 3, one receiving 4, and none receiving the highest possible rating of 5. The Reichow, Volkmar, and Cicchetti (2008) evaluation system allowed more individualization of evaluation based on specific study aspects, resulting in the highest possible ratings (strong) for half of the studies and the mid-rating (adequate) for the other half.

A variety of outcomes were addressed through diverse methodologies across the included studies, yet there were quite a few similarities. All but one study incorporated live music and active involvement of participants and most used music play/music-making and/or original songs composed specifically for the children in the studies. While child-appropriate, these were not child-preferred songs and only three incorporated "piggyback" (i.e., altered lyrics) versions of familiar melodies.

Data extraction: How were the effect size data obtained?

When selecting variables for analysis, the following decision-making procedure was employed:

- The single variable with quantitative data was recorded.

- The primary variable based on the title of the study or otherwise identified by the authors as the focus of the intervention was selected if more than one variable was available.

- The data were combined into one variable if several variables met that criterion, meaning that all were of the same type of data (e.g., frequency of behavioral observations) and in the same category of variable measured (i.e., communication, interpersonal, play, or personal responsibility), and adequate raw data could be extracted.

- The two most important variables based on the already identified focus of the study were selected when it was not possible to select or create one single or combined variable, limiting total variables per study to two to avoid disproportional weighting of studies.

This process resulted in selection of 13 variables from eight studies. Variables were then converted to an estimated effect size, Cohen's *d*, using meta-analytic statistical software (Johnson and Wood, 2006). The allowance for varied comparisons (see Study Inclusion Criteria Item 4 described previously) is not a clean research design and therefore not ideal for analysis. Within the meta-analysis, music therapy treatment was compared to no contact control or standard care conditions for some studies; for others, music therapy treatment was compared to play or speech therapy or spoken instructions only. However, anticipating that only a relatively small sample of empirical studies would meet the other inclusion criteria for the meta-analysis, all such comparison options were included. When possible, music therapy treatment comparisons were made to other types of treatment (e.g., play therapy), rather than to no contact or baseline. This type of data was most frequently recorded, thereby allowing for the most consistency from one study to the next. Finally, a Pearson Product Moment Correlation was used to assess the correlation among Cohen's d, the NAC (2009) scientific merit rating, and the Reichow, Volkmar, and Cicchetti (2008) evidence-based practice rating systems for each of the determined variables. Two evaluators provided reliability, concurring with both ratings assigned by the author for each study, as well as data extraction for each study variable and meta-analysis procedures.

Results and discussion: What did we learn?

Table 3.2 includes sample size, Cohen's d, 95 percent confidence interval, Pearson r, and probability for each selected study variable. Effect sizes ranged from .00 to 5.98, with an overall effect size of $d = .79$ ($p < .0001$). Since the confidence interval did not include 0, results were considered to be significant. However, the largest outlier was the social acknowledgment variable studied by Wimpory, Chadwick, and Nash (1995), with an effect size ($d = 5.98$) more than one standard deviation larger than the next effect size for peer interaction studied by Kern, Wolery, and Aldridge (2007) ($d = 4.63$). Since the Wimpory, Chadwick, and Nash (1995) social acknowledgment variable was the largest outlier, it was marked for exclusion from data analysis. Reanalysis without this outlier resulted in an overall effect size of $d = .76$ ($p < .0001$), with effect sizes for included study variables now ranging from $d = .00$ to $d = 4.63$. Since the overall effect size confidence interval once again did not include 0, results were considered to be significant.

It is important to note the importance of study design (see Table 3.1, Part A), not only to the two scientific integrity ratings, but also to meta-analysis. Several studies within this meta-analysis have a sample size of only one or a small sample and incorporate a single case experimental design. Appropriately, these often report data using graphic rather than statistical analysis. However, these aspects do not translate well to data extraction and meta-analysis calculations and comparisons.

Table 3.2 Meta-analysis results

Study (Variable)	N	d	95% CI	r	p
Finnigan and Starr (2010) (eye contact)	1	1.79	.63 ± 2.95	.71	.001
Finnigan and Starr (2010) (imitation and turn-taking)	1	1.53	.62 ± 2.44	.64	.0005
Kern and Aldridge (2006) (play and engagement)	4	1.59	-.0003 ± 3.18	.74	.02
Kern and Aldridge (2006) (peer interaction)	4	4.63	1.91 ± 7.28	.95	.0003
Kern, Wakeford, and Aldridge (2007) (hand-washing, toileting, and cleaning up)	1	.22	-.41 ± 86	.11	.48
Kern, Wolery, and Aldridge (2007) (independent responses)	2	.00	−1.96 ± 1.96	.65	.007
Kern, Wolery, and Aldridge (2007) (greetings by peers)	2	.89	.02 ± 1.77	.44	.03
Kim, Wigram, and Gold (2008) (joint attention)	10	.97	0.04 ± 1.90	.47	.03
Kim, Wigram, and Gold (2008) (eye contact and turn-taking)	10	2.06	.97 ± 3.14	.75	<.0001
Lim (2010) (verbal production)	50	.24	-.42 + .89	.12	.47
Lim and Draper (2011) (verbal production)	22	.09	-.49 ± .69	.05	.74
Wimpory, Chadwick, and Nash (1995) (social acknowledgment)[1]	1	5.98	2.74 ± 9.22	.97	.0002
Wimpory, Chadwick, and Nash (1995) (eye contact)	1	3.64	1.38 ± 5.89	.93	.0005
Overall:		.76	.53 ± 1.06	Z = 5.84	<.0001

1 This study was the largest outlier and is not included in the overall analysis results.

$N = 8$ studies, 12 variables.

$Q(11) = 37.63$, $p < .0001$.

Total $N = 91$ subjects in studies, 108 subjects by variables.

Mean N/study = 11.38. Mean N/variable = 9.

While multiple meta-analysis methodologies and variables exist (particularly within the behavioral sciences), effect size is often expressed as Cohen's d (Gold, 2004; Johnson and Wood, 2006; Whipple, 2004). The further away from 0 an effect size is, the larger the effect. Within the behavioral sciences, an effect size of .20 is considered to be a small effect, while .50 meets the benchmark for a medium effect, and an effect size of .80 or larger constitutes a large effect. To determine actual efficacy, the cost of treatment to achieve a given effect as well as the importance of the particular outcome for the individual must be considered (Gold, 2004). Based on these criteria, the overall effect size revealed within this meta-analysis can be considered to be medium–large, indicating that music therapy is an effective treatment for improving communication, interpersonal, play, and personal responsibility skills of young children with ASD. The homogeneity Q value was significant ($p < .0001$), meaning the studies are not considered to be entirely homogeneous and therefore may not be explained by the overall effect size. Varied sample sizes, types of data analysis, and broad standard deviations within each study's reported data also must be considered. The original homogeneity Q prior to reanalysis without the outlier displayed even greater significance ($Q = 47.52$, $df = 12$, $p < .0001$), supporting the exclusion of the Wimpory, Chadwick, and Nash (1995) social acknowledgment outlier. Furthermore, four study variables from Kern, Wakeford, and Aldridge (2007), Kern, Wolery, and Aldridge (2007), Lim (2010) and Lim and Draper (2011), had only small effect sizes, while all other included variables had resulting effect sizes in the large effect range. For most, that was true even when considering their 95 percent confidence intervals.

Regarding scientific integrity of the studies, correlation analysis indicated a significant positive correlation ($r = .72$, $p = .008$) between the Cohen's d values ($M = 1.47$, $SD = 1.44$) and the Reichow, Volkmar, and Cicchetti (2008) evidence-based practice ratings ($M = 2.58$, $SD = .51$) for the final 12 variables analyzed; as evidence-based practice rating increased, d values also increased. However, there was no significant correlation between the scientific merit ($M = 1.83$, $SD = 1.27$) and evidence-based practice ratings ($r = .02$, $p = .94$), nor between the scientific merit ratings and d values ($r = .29$, $p = .37$).

The NAC (2009) scientific merit rating uses a detailed rubric to assess research design (i.e., number of groups, random assignment or pre-treatment significant differences, sample size, and data loss), measurement of dependent variable (i.e., type of measurement, standardization of protocol, type of measurement, and inter-rater reliability), measurement of independent variable (procedural integrity and treatment fidelity), participant ascertainment (diagnostic criteria and confirmation), and generalization of treatment effect (objectiveness of data, maintenance data, and incorporation of generalization). The lack of correlation with these ratings is probably explained by the little variation among the ratings assigned to the studies (i.e., only 2 of the 8 studies and 4 of the 12 final variables received a rating other than 1), limiting opportunities for correlation. Often one factor within one of the five rubric categories prevented the study from receiving a higher rating. For example, both Finnigan and Starr (2010) and Wimpory, Chadwick, and Nash (1995) would have received a mid-scale rating of 3, but because each only had a sample size of one, they warranted only the lowest rating of 1. Kim, Wigram, and Gold (2008), Lim (2010), and Lim and Draper (2011) had larger samples ($N = 10$, $N = 22$, and $N = 10$, respectively), but none included any generalization or maintenance data, thus reducing the ratings for those studies from the highest possible (5) to the lowest possible (1).

Deficits in these two areas of sample size and generalization/maintenance within published studies historically have plagued music therapy studies (Whipple, 2004). This is especially true for studies that focus on the unique aspects of music therapy used with populations as diverse as ASD. Difficulty in initially gaining access to enough clients, then maintaining access or funding long enough, become ongoing challenges. Because of these issues regarding sample sizes and generalization/ maintenance, the Reichow, Volkmar, and Cicchetti (2008) evidence-based practice rating system is a more accurate measure of scientific rigor within the field of music therapy, at least for the current time. Further, scientific rigor criteria and rating systems change over time; research initially considered strong at the time of publication may be viewed differently in the future.

Recommendations: What's next?

Based on results of the current meta-analysis, music therapy may be considered an extremely effective treatment for young children with ASD for developing communication, interpersonal, personal responsibility, and play skills. While this review focused on a more specific population than the two before (Gold, Wigram, and Elefant, 2006; Whipple, 2004), the resulting homogeneity Q from this study was surprisingly significant; this was not the case in the two previous reviews. To remedy this variation, music therapists must focus on increasing sample sizes while continuing to incorporate single case and group experimental designs, and also assess the efficacy of even more specific applications of music therapy. Compared to Whipple (2004) and Gold, Wigram, and Elefant (2006), the current review includes far more studies with a sample of only one (3 of 8, or 37.5%). Reichow, Volkmar, and Cicchetti (2008) recognize that a treatment can be representative of an *Established Evidence-Based Practice* with a minimum of five single case experimental studies of strong scientific integrity (or ten of adequate quality) related to the same topic with demonstrable benefits. A *Promising Evidence-Based Practice* rating would require only three studies of adequate quality. However, small samples are not ideal for meta-analysis and may have contributed to the lack of homogeneity. In addition, sophisticated studies might consider limiting the ages of subjects so that those addressing early childhood do not veer outside of that accepted range. In addition, researchers might wish to include only children with ASD, rather than mix in those with other developmental delays and diagnoses. Music therapists should further investigate music skills and preferences of young children and evaluate specific interventions. By designing better studies and clinical practice, music therapists can spotlight and capitalize on the children's music strengths.

Similarly, music therapists should familiarize themselves with the NAC (2009) scientific merit rating and/or the Reichow, Volkmar, and Cicchetti (2008) evidence-based practice rating systems and then focus specifically on adequate samples and the incorporation of generalization/maintenance into treatment. This will not only ensure the scientific integrity of their research designs, but also may lead to the inclusion of even more studies in future reviews and naturally enhance homogeneity ratings.

One hundred percent of the studies within this current analysis are from published sources. Refereed, yet unpublished, theses, dissertations, and research poster presentations were included previously, with only 22.2 percent published (Whipple, 2004). More music therapists are publishing about the use of music therapy in treatment for this growing population. To further enhance this improving publication record, music therapists should document the use of music therapy treatment for the remainder of the NAC (2009) outcome categories; only 4 of the 14 (28.6%) were able to be evaluated within this meta-analysis. It is likely that many more are being addressed daily in clinical practice.

LEARNING QUESTIONS

1. What are three musical skills that may be more advanced among high-functioning children with ASD than their typical developing peers?

2. What are four sub-classification areas (defined by the NAC) that empirical research documents as being addressed by music therapists working with young children with ASD?

3. Summarize the interventions used and research findings from one study within each of those four sub-classification areas.

4. What is the purpose of a meta-analysis?

5. Summarize the findings of the previously conducted meta-analysis (Whipple, 2004) and Cochrane review (Gold, Wigram, and Elefant 2006).

6. What is now known about music therapy treatment for young children with ASD that was not recognized prior to the completion of this meta-analysis?

7. What is one recommendation for future music therapy research with this population (based on limitations discovered during the meta-analysis process)?

Author's note

The author wishes to thank Dr. Jayne Standley and Dr. Petra Kern for providing valuable insights during the development of this chapter.

References

Finnigan, E., and Starr, E. (2010). Increasing social responsiveness in a child with autism: A comparison of music and non-music interventions. *Autism, 14(4),* 321–348.

Gold, C. (2004). The use of effect sizes in music therapy research. *Music Therapy Perspectives, 22(2),* 91–95.

Gold, C., Voracek, M., and Wigram, T. (2004). Effects of music therapy for children and adolescents with psychopathology: A meta-analysis. *Journal of Child Psychology and Psychiatry and Allied Disciplines, 45,* 1054–1063.

Gold, C., Wigram, T., and Elefant, C. (2006). Music therapy for autistic spectrum disorder. *Cochrane Database of Systematic Reviews, Issue 2.* Art. No.: CD004381. doi:10.1002/14651858.CD004381. pub2.

Heaton, P. (2003). Pitch memory, labeling and disembedding in autism. *Journal of Child Psychology and Psychiatry and Allied Disciplines, 44(4),* 543–551.

Heaton, P. (2005). Interval and contour processing in autism. *Journal of Autism and Developmental Disorders, 25(6)*, 787–793.

Heaton, P. (2009). Assessing musical skills in autistic children who are not savants. *Philosophical Transactions of the Royal Society B: Biological Sciences, 364(1522)*, 1443–1447.

Heaton, P., Williams, K., Cummins, O., and Happe, F.G.E. (2007). Beyond perception: Musical representation and on-line processing in autism. *Journal of Autism and Developmental Disorders, 27(7)*, 1355–1360.

Humpal, M. (2001). Music therapy and the young child. *Early Childhood Connections, 7(2)*, 9–15.

Jellison, J. (2000). A content analysis of music research with disabled children and youth (1975–1999): Application in special education. In D.S. Smith (Ed.) *Effectiveness of Music Therapy Procedures: Documentation of Research and Clinical Practice.* Silver Spring, MD: American Music Therapy Association.

Johnson, B.T., and Wood, T. (2006). *DSTAT 2.00: Software for Meta-Analysis.* Storrs, Connecticut.

Kern, P., and Aldridge, D. (2006). Using embedded music therapy interventions to support outdoor play of young children with autism in an inclusive community-based child care program. *Journal of Music Therapy, 43(4)*, 270–294.

Kern, P., Wakeford, L., and Aldridge, D. (2007). Improving the performance of a young child with autism during self-care tasks using embedded song interventions: A case study. *Music Therapy Perspectives, 25(1)*, 43–51.

Kern, P., Wolery, M., and Aldridge, D. (2007). Use of songs to promote independence in morning greeting routines for young children with autism. *Journal of Autism and Developmental Disorders, 37*, 1264–1271.

Kim, J., Wigram, T., and Gold, C. (2008). The effects of improvisational music therapy on joint attention behaviors in autism children: A randomized controlled study. *Journal of Autism and Developmental Disorders, 38*, 1758–1766.

Kim, J., Wigram, T., and Gold, C. (2009). Emotional, motivational and interpersonal responsiveness of children with autism in improvisational music therapy. *Autism, 13(4)*, 389–409.

Koger, S.M., Chapin, K., and Brotons, M. (1999). Is music therapy an effective intervention for dementia? A meta-analytic review of literature. *Journal of Music Therapy, 36*, 2–15.

Lim, H.A. (2010). Effect of "Developmental Speech and Language Training Through Music" on speech production in children with autism spectrum disorders. *Journal of Music Therapy, 48(1)*, 2–26.

Lim, H.A., and Draper, E. (2011). The effects of music therapy incorporated with Applied Behavior Analysis Verbal Behavior approach for children with autism spectrum disorders. *Journal of Music Therapy, 48(4)*, 532–550.

National Autism Center (NAC) (2009). *National Standards Report. The National Standards Project—Addressing the Need for Evidence-Based Practice Guidelines for Autism Spectrum Disorders.* Randolph, MA: NAC.

Pelletier, C.L. (2004). The effect of music on decreasing arousal due to stress: A meta-analysis. *Journal of Music Therapy, 41(3)*, 192–214.

Reichow, B., Volkmar, F.R., and Cicchetti, D.V. (2008). Development of the evaluative method for evaluating and determining evidence-based practices in autism. *Journal of Autism and Developmental Disorders, 38*, 1311–1319.

Silverman, M.J. (2003). The influence of music on the symptoms of psychosis: A meta-analysis. *Journal of Music Therapy, 40(3)*, 27–40.

Simpson, K., and Keen, D. (2011). Music interventions for children with autism: Narrative review of the literature. *Journal of Autism and Developmental Disorders, 41*, 1507–1514.

Standley, J.M. (1986). Music research in medical/dental treatment: Meta-analysis and clinical applications. *Journal of Music Therapy, 23*, 56–122.

Standley, J.M. (1992). Meta-analysis of research in music and medical treatment: Effect size as a basis for comparison across multiple dependent and independent variables. In R. Spintge and R. Droh (Eds.) *Music Medicine.* St. Louis: MMB, Inc.

Standley, J.M. (1996). Music research in medical/dental treatment: An update of a prior meta-analysis. In C. Furman (Ed.) *Effectiveness of Music Therapy Procedures: Documentation of Research and Clinical Practice (Second Edition)*. Silver Spring, MD: National Association for Music Therapy.

Standley, J.M. (2000). Music research in medical treatment. In C. Furman (Ed.) *Effectiveness of Music Therapy Procedures: Documentation of Research and Clinical Practice (Third Edition)*. Silver Spring, MD: National Association for Music Therapy.

Standley, J.M. (2002). A meta-analysis of the efficacy of music therapy for premature infants. *Journal of Pediatric Nursing, 17(2)*, 107–113.

Standley, J.M., and Whipple, J. (2003). Music therapy with pediatric patients: A meta-analysis. In S. Robb (Ed.) *Music Therapy in Pediatric Healthcare: Research and Best Practice*. Silver Spring, MD: American Music Therapy Association, Inc.

Treffert, D.A. (2012). *Islands of Genius: The Bountiful Mind of the Autistic, Acquired, and Sudden Savant*. London and Philadelphia: Jessica Kingsley Publishers.

Whipple, J. (2004). Music in intervention for children and adolescents with autism: A meta-analysis. *Journal of Music Therapy, 41(2)*, 90–106.

Wimpory, D., Chadwick, P., and Nash, S. (1995). Brief report. Musical interaction therapy for children with autism: An evaluative case study with two-year follow-up. *Journal of Autism and Developmental Disorders, 25(5)*, 541–552.

PART 2

Assessment and Goals

Chapter 4

Assessment and Goals

Determining Eligibility, Gathering Information, and Generating Treatment Goals for Music Therapy Services

Linda K. Martin, MME, MT-BC
COAST MUSIC THERAPY
SAN DIEGO, CA

Angela M. Snell, MS, MT-BC
MONROE COUNTY INTERMEDIATE SCHOOL DISTRICT
MONROE, MI

Darcy Walworth, Ph.D., MT-BC
UNIVERSITY OF LOUISVILLE
LOUISVILLE, KY

Marcia Humpal, M.Ed., MT-BC
OLMSTED FALLS, OH

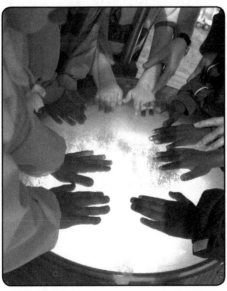

PHOTO COURTESY OF DON TRULL

Strong assessment tools reach beyond simply determining qualification for services; they extend to serving as a means for establishing appropriate goals to facilitating successful treatment outcomes.
(Linda K. Martin, Angela M. Snell, Darcy Walworth, and Marcia Humpal)

Assessment of children with an autism spectrum disorders (ASD) provides a comprehensive perspective of all aspects of the children's development and substantiation for determining appropriate services and treatment goals to best meet their unique needs. Although a music therapy assessment for young children with ASD can take many forms, it may yield unique information that other members of the child's interdisciplinary team have not yet discovered. This chapter examines the rationale for conducting assessments, the role of the music therapist in the assessment process, considerations for assessing young children with ASD, and an overview of various approaches to music therapy assessment. Representative music therapy assessments currently in use with young children with ASD are featured.

Introduction
Rationale for conducting assessments
Assessments provide important information to assist professionals in making informed decisions related to several specific purposes. Young children may be assessed (McLean and Snyder, 2011; NPDC on ASD, 2011) to:

- determine developmental risks (i.e., screening) or developmental delays/ disabilities (i.e., diagnostic evaluation) (see Chapter 1)

- identify eligibility for specialized services

- identify the child's present level of functioning for intervention planning

- determine the type and intensity of service delivery (i.e., within a response-to-intervention framework)

- monitor the child's progress in learning functional skills.

A contemporary approach to assessment with young children further emphasizes gathering of information about the family (e.g., family routines, cultural influences, and language used in the home). Conducting assessments in environments that include activities, adults, and peers that are familiar to the child is highly encouraged. Recent trends advocate utilizing various means to ensure authentic and ongoing information gathering (e.g., video technology) that can be stored and reviewed throughout time by families as well as service providers (McLean and Snyder, 2011).

Assessors
Uneven and inconsistent skills in communication, social interaction, and sensory processing in children with ASD may mask abilities as well as deficits (NPDC on ASD, 2011). Therefore, a comprehensive team, including members from different disciplines who understand the complexity and unique aspects of ASD, should conduct the assessment. Family involvement in the assessment process is essential for gathering a true picture of the child in the environment in which he or she spends the majority of time. The evaluation should include a variety of assessment measures,

both standardized and informal (Nagel, 2007), to ensure that all areas of the child's development are addressed (Centers for Disease Control and Prevention, 2012). Assessors must be culturally responsive while striving to identify and be guided by the needs of the family (McLean and Snyder, 2011).

Information gained from assessment should lead to the development of functional goals that support the delivery of early intervention services. It is paramount to identify and provide supports and services that can be embedded in natural environments and daily family and classroom activities and routines (DEC/NAEYC, 2009; McLean and Snyder, 2011). Supporting socialization, communication, and independence is especially critical for children with ASD. Both goal-planning and services for young children with ASD should consider information from all interdisciplinary team members and ensure that family resources, priorities, values, and beliefs are met (Buysse and Wesley, 2006; Wolery, 2004).

Role of the music therapist in the assessment process

SCOPES OF PRACTICE AND CREDENTIALING

Music therapists can bring unique perspectives to the assessment process and can be a vital part of a comprehensive approach to assisting children with ASD to meet early intervention and treatment goals. Music therapists are held to high standards by scopes of practice as well as credentialing regulations of the country, province, or state in which they work. For example, the *Scope of Practice* (Certification Board for Music Therapists [CBMT], 2010) of the CBMT defines the skills held by board-certified music therapists, providing "legally defensible" support for board-certified music therapists' ability to assess and treat conditions through the music medium. Specifically listed skills include identifying and interpreting human responses to the elements of music (e.g., tempo, melody, rhythm) to reveal functioning levels and strengths and weaknesses in the following domains: perceptual, sensory, physical, affective, cognitive, communicative, social, and spiritual. The *Scope of Practice* also delineates the music therapist's ability to integrate theoretical orientations (e.g., behavioral, cognitive, psychodynamic) into music therapy practice. Governments may require music therapists to obtain specific licenses for working with various populations or within certain facilities. These credentials might be supported by additional standards and scopes of practice. Additionally, professional organizations often have established standards of practices that speak to the unique skills and attributes that outline appropriate service delivery.

RAMIFICATIONS OF GOVERNMENT REGULATIONS AND LEGAL ISSUES

The representative examples in this chapter are practiced in the United States and therefore legally are bound to federal, state, and local laws and regulations. In the United States, music therapists need to know about and understand the Individuals with Disabilities Education Act (IDEA) (U.S. Department of Education, 2006).

IDEA assures access to a free and appropriate public education for any child age three and older with a disability. Legally, this means children with a qualifying disability receive access to the general education curriculum in the least restrictive environment alongside same-age peers without disabilities to the greatest extent possible. Qualifying students must receive an Individualized Education Program (IEP) developed collaboratively by an IEP team. Evaluation and re-evaluation are mandated, and the process is the basis for IEP team decisions. The IEP not only acts as a legal contract between the families and school districts to ensure an appropriate education based on information gained through a multi-factored assessment, but it also provides extensive information for the educational team working with that child. The United States Department of Education has published a Question and Answers document, which clarifies that music therapy can be considered a related service under IDEA (U.S. Department of Education, 2011a).

Regulations for early intervention programs for children from birth to age three are provided in IDEA Part C (U.S. Department of Education, 2011b). Implications of IDEA for this age group are similar to those for older children; however, family involvement is essential and directly specified. Assessment is required to develop both the Individual Family Service Plan (IFSP) and the IEP. Goals reflect information gained from this process and guide the selection of services.

While the aforementioned legal mandates are specific to the United States, other countries may have similar laws and regulations that pertain to young children. Music therapists practicing in other countries should become familiar with laws specific to where they reside and work, and recognize the ramifications for music therapy service delivery.

Music therapy assessment tools for ASD

A survey conducted by Walworth (2007) revealed that music therapists serving individuals with ASD used no consistent assessment tool to determine eligibility, goals, and services. Some music therapists reported no use of any assessment tools. Others reported using Coleman and Brunk's (2000) Special Education Music Therapy Assessment Process (SEMTAP) to determine eligibility of services; the SEMTAP allows music therapists to compare a child's performance on his or her IEP objectives both with and without music therapy intervention, justifying the recommendation for or against music therapy services. Other music therapists reported assessing client goals on agency-specific forms. No one assessment method was reported with any higher frequency. As of this writing there is no one validated music therapy assessment tool for ASD.

Wigram (1999a) noted that many assessments used by music therapists with individuals with ASD rely on subjective opinion. He adapted the Autonomy Profile Scale and the Variability Profile Scale from Bruscia's Improvisation Assessment Profiles (1987) to investigate and analyze musical materials within the assessment process, uncovering not only the child's interests and preferences, but also the child's response to change (Wigram, 1999b).

A team at the Nordoff-Robbins Center for Music Therapy in New York developed the Music Therapy Communication and Social Interaction (MTCSI) scale (Hummel-Rossi *et al.*, 2008) to rate social and communication behaviors in young children with ASD observed during Nordoff-Robbins music therapy sessions. Coded behaviors include an individual's simultaneous or sequential participation in musical activity with the music therapists or peers; joint attention and turn-taking; reciprocal verbal exchange and reciprocal musical exchange, either instrumental or vocal; communication of affect via facial expression, gesture, movement, or touch; and other indicators of the client's response to or initiation of communication and interaction. The assessment is administered by reviewing selected videotaped sessions in one-minute time intervals. More details of the clinical process of Nordoff-Robbins music therapy with young children with ASD can be found in Chapter 7.

The Individualized Music-Centered Assessment Profile for Neurodevelopmental Disorders (IMCAP-ND®) (Carpente, 2011) is a music-centered assessment tool consistent with outlined domain areas of the DIR®/Floortime™ Model. The seven targeted music domain areas are pertinent to the child's ability to musically engage, relate, and communicate in musical play. The assessment is administered within the context of interactive improvisational music therapy while observing the child through various modes of musical expression (i.e., instruments, voice, movement, and gestures). Each music domain area is evaluated based on the duration and quality of the client's musical responses in musical play, taking into consideration the type of support (i.e., visual cues, verbal, gestural cues, high-affect) used to assist the client in a particular music domain area. Additional information pertinent to improvisational music therapy and the DIR®/Floortime™ Model is available in Chapter 8.

The following sections of this chapter will spotlight three representative examples of music therapy assessment tools for children with ASD served in special education settings: (1) the Four-Step Assessment Model (Lazar, 2007), (2) the Music Therapy–Music Related Behavior (MT-MRB) assessment tool (Snell, 2002), and (3) the SCERTS® Model as applied in music therapy (Walworth, 2007).

Determining eligibility: A Four-Step Assessment Model

Overview

This section reviews the Four-Step Assessment Model developed by Lazar (2007) for determining a child's eligibility for music therapy services within the Individual Education Plan (IEP) and integrating legal requirements. Based on field-testing in several school districts in Southern California (of over 80 students with special needs per year), this non-standardized assessment model has proven to be successful in providing a consistent and comprehensive rationale for making music therapy service recommendations.

The purpose of the Four-Step Assessment Model is to illustrate whether a child with special needs (including ASD) enrolled in a special education program:

a.   requires music-based support (designed or implemented by a certified music therapist) to make progress on his or her IEP goals

b.   does not need music therapy services in order to benefit from his or her educational programming.

Utilizing a consistent assessment process (whether for young children with ASD whose programming falls under the auspices of public school districts, or within private agencies) demonstrates validity of the eligibility assessment results. Therefore, parents, educators, and other stakeholders may have greater confidence in the recommendations. However, any non-standardized assessment tool may be unable to produce a steadfast conclusion within the constraints of the assessment period. In such a case, a trial period of music therapy services should be recommended.

Applying the Four-Step Assessment Model

Obtaining several critical pieces of information prior to working directly with a child with ASD will ensure more reliable results from the assessment. The setting, communication tools, present levels, behavioral intervention strategies, reinforcement systems, and sensory needs are necessary considerations when planning activities and gathering materials relevant to the assessment. Much of this information may be gathered directly from members of the interdisciplinary team or found within the child's IEP.

STEP 1

Careful review of a child's IEP is the first step necessary for determining whether a music therapy eligibility assessment is appropriate for the child. The IEP documents essential information regarding diagnosis, medical history, relevant educational history, current goals, objectives, baselines, plus the services provided to the child. If the child's interdisciplinary team has identified music as an area of strength or preference, it may be documented as such in the IEP. Information on continued areas of need as indicated in the IEP will provide helpful insights as to whether goal areas could be appropriately and functionally supported through the use of evidence-based music therapy interventions.

This first step in this assessment procedure examines whether the child's IEP goal areas can be functionally supported through music therapy and music-assisted learning strategies (Lazar, 2007). Most school districts require the implementation of evidence-based strategies to support achievement of educational goals (U.S. Department of Education, 2010). For music therapy to be considered a necessary service documented within the IEP, the music therapist should utilize research-supported music strategies to address the child's goals. Common goal areas for young children with ASD in which music therapy interventions have shown to be effective include communication, interpersonal, personal responsibility, and play skills (refer to Chapter 3 for more details and supporting information). Music also may be used to work on speech articulation, in areas requiring increased on-task attention (e.g., matching or sorting), and as a mnemonic tool (e.g., for memorizing rote information).

STEP 2

The second step of this assessment process examines whether additional support is required to address relevant goals based on factors such as slow or insufficient progress, interfering behaviors, or a limited number of instructional approaches to which the child has been responsive (Lazar, 2007). For example, behavioral issues or lack of motivation may be lessened when the child is engaged in music-based strategies developed by a certified music therapist. Unchecked, these behaviors may impede progress on goals. Therefore, music therapy services may provide a necessary support. Music therapists must be aware that music serves as an additional prompt. To achieve independence and eventually demonstrate generalization of the skill, the prompt eventually must be faded (Grow et al., 2009; MacDuff, Krantz, and McClannahan, 2001). Therefore, prompts provided through music should only be added when necessary for the child to achieve the goal.

STEP 3

Many young children enjoy music. Yet, for the purposes of a music therapy eligibility assessment, the child must demonstrate more than mere enjoyment of music. Therefore, the third step examines whether music is a documented learning strength for the child (i.e., the child is able to respond to directions presented within the music, or attend to tasks embedded in a song). He or she should remain engaged in music-based activities for extended periods of time and show a willingness to comply with instructions given through music cuing. Enjoyment of music may provide motivation to engage in music-based activities, thereby increasing the amount of time spent participating in learning opportunities. However, if the child does not display active learning during music activities, music therapy services would not be justified as an IEP-based service. In these cases, suggestions may be made to the IEP team to perhaps utilize preferred music as a reinforcer or earned reward.

STEP 4

The fourth step identifies whether modifications or additional supports are necessary to access a child's learning strength through music. Music therapists may need to consult with the interdisciplinary team about how to best include a child with ASD in musical experiences. Music resources already may be available within the child's current program (Lazar, 2007). For example, facilities may have access to a variety of precomposed children's music. If so, the music therapist should make sure that the music is applied intentionally to (a) address the child's current goals, and (b) to adhere to the child's individual learning needs (e.g., extended response time, simplified language). Figure 4.1 illustrates the fundamental steps of the Four-Step Assessment Model.

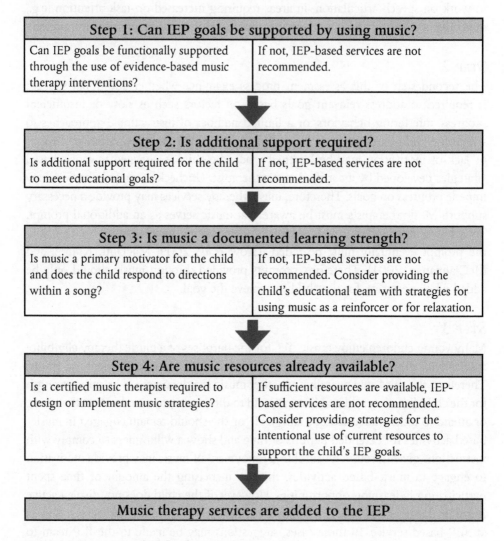

Step 1: Can IEP goals be supported by using music?	
Can IEP goals be functionally supported through the use of evidence-based music therapy interventions?	If not, IEP-based services are not recommended.

Step 2: Is additional support required?	
Is additional support required for the child to meet educational goals?	If not, IEP-based services are not recommended.

Step 3: Is music a documented learning strength?	
Is music a primary motivator for the child and does the child respond to directions within a song?	If not, IEP-based services are not recommended. Consider providing the child's educational team with strategies for using music as a reinforcer or for relaxation.

Step 4: Are music resources already available?	
Is a certified music therapist required to design or implement music strategies?	If sufficient resources are available, IEP-based services are not recommended. Consider providing strategies for the intentional use of current resources to support the child's IEP goals.

Music therapy services are added to the IEP

Figure 4.1: Determining eligibility for music therapy services

Recommendations

Following examination of the four steps, recommendations regarding music therapy service provision are made to the child's interdisciplinary team. A music therapy recommendation should be considered only if all four criteria are deemed necessary and appropriate. If music therapy services are recommended and the interdisciplinary team is in agreement, the type of service (i.e., from direct to consultative), frequency, and duration of sessions should be discussed. These determinations are based on the child's individual needs as well as the requirements of applicable laws (e.g., IDEA's policy calling for educating in the least restrictive environment). Music-based strategies developed by the music therapist can be implemented throughout the child's educational programming as well as across settings and disciplines to maximize the child's learning through music and to provide multiple opportunities for generalization of skills. Given appropriate service recommendations, children receiving music therapy may have the opportunity to improve their skills; families and other service providers thereby may gain an increased appreciation for the benefits of music therapy services for young children with ASD.

Gaining information: The MT-MRB assessment
Overview
This section describes the Music Therapy–Music Related Behavior (MT-MRB) assessment tool (Snell, 2002). This tool utilizes unique assessment information obtained through a child's musical behavior, and the music therapist's professional interpretation of that behavior as it relates to non-musical functioning; it shows how musical behavior exposes strengths and weaknesses, and stands up to legal scrutiny in determining the need for music therapy services. The assessment has been successfully applied within a special education agency that provides services to nine public school districts, and also within many individual cases across the United States.

The purpose of the MT-MRB assessment is to:

a. evaluate music-related behaviors (MRBs)

b. interpret the music-related behaviors' relevance to non-musical functioning

c. determine if music therapy is a needed service

d. give information and recommendations to the interdisciplinary team.

The way music therapy assessments are conducted, documented, and reported can make a difference in how school districts and agencies utilize the resulting information for service provision.

Applying the MT-MRB assessment
The MT-MRB assessment process has the same general outline as found in many assessment reports of other service providers. It follows four major steps:

1. gathering of background information

2. documenting current functioning levels

3. assessing, evaluating, and interpreting

4. forming conclusions and recommendations.

Gathering of background information

Prior to administering the MT-MRB assessment, music therapists should collect background information by:

- reviewing medical and educational documents (e.g., the child's IFSP or IEP)

- conducting initial interviews with early childhood educators, parents, and the child (if appropriate).

Music therapists should then summarize the preliminary information, briefly documenting family, medical, and educational history, as well as existing test scores and evaluations. Background information that further details the child's current skills and areas of need is set forth in the "Present Level of Academic and Functional Performance" section of the MT-MRB.

Documenting current functioning levels

In addition to collecting evidence found in documents and interviews, the music therapist should gather first-hand information on the child's level of functioning by:

- observing the child in natural learning environments (e.g., the preschool classroom, playground, or home)

- observing how the child responds to supports and adaptations currently provided.

This information is crucial for understanding the child's current level of functioning and eventually preparing an assessment session that is appropriate to the child's age, diagnosis, functioning level, and socio-cultural background. This information may also yield clues about the child's reactions to various musical or sensory stimuli.

Assessing, evaluating, and interpreting

Various service providers typically assess the child using tools and expertise specific to their disciplines (e.g., speech and language tests, occupational therapists' sensory or fine motor evaluations, psychology evaluations). In the MT-MRB, music therapists gather information through the child's MRBs, using assessment skills outlined in the professional standards of practice and scope of practice (AMTA, 2010; CBMT, 2010).

Utilizing the background information and current functioning levels, music therapists should create musical opportunities that will allow the child to demonstrate potential strengths and weaknesses in all developmental areas. By focusing on responses and non-responses to musical elements (e.g., tempo, rhythm, melody, harmony, timbre), the MT-MRB assessment allows the therapist to (a) musically build rapport, (b) elicit MRBs, and (c) be flexible in supporting the child through in-the-moment prescriptive use of musical elements while gathering assessment data. The child may reveal personality traits, interests, abilities, and weaknesses through musical expressions and responses to music that otherwise might go unnoticed.

A MT-MRB assessment session for young children with ASD typically takes 20–30 minutes to administer. Conducting group sessions within the child's daily routines (e.g., during circle time) is preferable as social skills may be better assessed when peers are present. If a one-to-one session is needed, the assessment can be done in a dedicated area or within a more individually specific and appropriate part of the child's routine (e.g., during playground time). With young children a comprehensive assessment usually can be completed in one to three sessions.

The evaluation and interpretation of the assessment data is the most important part of the MT-MRB assessment process. The child's responses and non-responses to the in-the-moment prescriptive music experiences are interpreted related to their relevance to non-musical functioning in all skill areas. Music therapists should base their interpretation on research and knowledge about typical child development, musical development, and core characteristic of ASD, always adhering to the principles of evidence-based practice.

The following sample questions may guide the interpretation process:

- Did the child demonstrate developmentally appropriate musical responses?

- Was the child able to sing or hum along? Was there melodic or rhythmic relevance?

- How did the child musically interact or respond to peers?

- Were there differences in responses to familiar versus unfamiliar music?

- How did the child respond to rhythms, tempi, phrasing, and cadences? Were actions synchronized, delayed (how many beats?), or inconsistent?

- Was the child able to play similar rhythms on different instruments?

- Were there differences in the child's functioning during the MT-MRB assessment session compared to baseline functioning?

Figure 4.2 gives examples of MRBs that might be observed in the assessment process as well as implications that might be revealed through these observations.

Assessment response	Response quality
☑ Tempo changes	☐ Increases physical actions ☐ Decreases physical actions ☑ Synchronizes physical actions
☑ Volume changes	☑ Covers ears ☐ Looks to sound source ☐ Listens attentively when volume decreases
☑ Melody lines/pitches	☐ Hums in monotone manner ☑ Hums in key of presented song ☐ Matches isolated pitches
☑ Harmonic progression	☐ Is disconnected to harmonic events ☑ Anticipates musical resolutions
☑ Musical surprises	☐ Engages in joint attention when music changes unexpectedly ☑ Responds with emotional expression
☑ Interactive musical play	☐ Playing/responding is inconsistent ☑ Responsive playing is delayed (for 4 seconds) ☐ Takes and waits turns, synchronized with music activity

Implications

Child's responses indicate an underlying understanding of the structure of music. He is sensitive to tempo, dynamics, melody, harmonic progressions, and cadences. Covering of ears to loud volume may indicate auditory hyper-sensitivity. Humming along in key and his anticipation to the ending of musical resolutions refers to being attuned to the activity and therapists. Child giggles when presented with a musical surprise; could mean that his mood can be impacted by use of musical elements. Child's two to four beat delayed physical response possibly indicates need for extended time for processing information.

Overall, child demonstrates potential to develop adaptive social-emotional skills, increased attention span, and self-organization skills given tailored music therapy supports.

Figure 4.2: Examples of MRBs in the assessment process

FORMING CONCLUSIONS AND RECOMMENDATIONS

Music therapists should summarize the interpretation of the MRBs and highlight support and non-support for other team members' findings, including any new information that may provide insight about the child's functioning. Recommendations may include suggestions for intervention strategies or additional tests, and whether music therapy services are indicated. A child's musical ability or lack thereof does not necessarily signify or negate the need for music therapy services.

Service recommendations are justified under the following conditions: (1) if the child is not progressing as expected through his or her current educational program or (2) therapeutic services and the MT-MRB assessment demonstrates that music therapy interventions improve baseline performance or show the potential to support needed skills. Music therapists should then suggest appropriate goals and objectives based on information gleaned from the child's musical behavior, and propose a level of music therapy service for consideration by the child's interdisciplinary team.

Generating treatment goals: The SCERTS® Model
Overview

This section, describes how the SCERTS® Model (designed to generate developmentally grounded goals and objectives for children with ASD and related disabilities) may be effectively applied within the music therapy intervention arena. This validated systematic assessment process has been developed by Prizant, *et al.* (2005) and is consistent with current evidence-based practice guidelines (Prizant, *et al.* 2010).

The purpose of the SCERTS® Model is to:

a. evaluate social and emotional development of children with ASD

b. promote social and emotional development of children with ASD

c. generate measureable and achievable goals that link transactional support with social communication and emotional regulation for children with ASD.

For the remainder of this chapter, the SCERTS® Model will be briefly overviewed to highlight the unique benefits of using the SCERTS assessment process in music therapy practice. Training options for practitioners interested in applying this comprehensive, multidisciplinary, educational approach within their settings are provided through:

• self-study of the two SCERTS® Model clinical manuals,

• attendance at SCERTS® Model training sessions, seminars, and presentations offered by the creators throughout the United States.

Applying the SCERTS® Model

After determining eligibility for music therapy services, the music therapist may further evaluate the child to create treatment goals. This process can take many forms ranging from an unstructured and informal assessment of client ability level and needs to the use of a standardized assessment tool. Some music therapists may argue that using standardized assessment tools does not allow enough individuality for children's needs. However, a comprehensive assessment tool may yield highly benficial information for determining the child's present level and thereby developing appropriate goals. Music therapists may further examine the child's unique responses to music and utilize this information to better facilitate specifically identified progressive components and hierarchical steps of areas of need.

The SCERTS® Model acronym represents three domain areas for development:

1. social communication

2. emotional regulation

3. transactional support.

Within each domain area, there are objectives and sub-objectives listed which contribute to the enhancement of each developmental domain. The objectives and sub-objectives are assigned to two domain areas within each overall domain.

For example, within the *social communication* overall domain, objectives and sub-objectives are listed either under joint attention or under symbol use. Within the *emotional regulation* overall domain, objectives and sub-objectives are listed within either the self-regulation or the mutual regulation domains. For the *transactional support* overall domain, objectives and sub-objectives are assigned to either interpersonal support or learning support.

The sub-objectives are the specific steps needed to achieve an objective. Having each step listed for successfully demonstrating a skill gives the added benefit of having a ready-made list of children's specific achievements over time.

Ideally, the SCERTS® Model is utilized by a multidisciplinary team. When used as designed, the treatment goals generated by the tool are a culmination of multiple observations from multiple people in a variety of settings. Having a multidimensional view of the child provides a comprehensive picture of the child's strengths and challenges that need to be addressed by the music therapists, early childhood educators, other specialists, and caregivers to best support the child's development. The administration of the SCERTS® Model assessment process takes about four hours of observations in at least two different settings. It may be challenging to find team members to contribute due to lack of knowledge of this assessment tool, time constraints, or lack of reimbursement.

Nevertheless, in the assessment process, music therapists may overlook pertinent goals or those used as underpinnings to future goal attainment. Being able to more accurately specify the objectives of each session and steps leading up to goal attainment might be highly beneficial for providing music therapy services to young children with ASD and their families. The following two studies substantiate this assumption.

RELATED STUDIES

When surveyed about the specific goals addressed in music therapy sessions, 21 music therapists working with 135 clients at risk or diagnosed with ASD reported a total of 27 different goals targeted over the course of the children's treatment (Walworth, 2007). The discrepancy between 27 reported goals and the over 300 possible goals delineated within the SCERTS® Model highlights the greater specificity of treatment goals that may be possible when music therapists use this model.

In a different study, music therapists submitted videos of music therapy intervention sessions with 33 children (Walworth, Register, and Engel, 2009). The sessions were evaluated by researchers trained on the SCERTS® Model to identify specific goals addressed within the sessions. When the actual music therapy goals submitted by the music therapists were compared with the researchers' video evaluation, researchers saw that the highest number of goals actually addressed fell within the transactional support domain within the SCERTS® Model. Interestingly, none of the music therapists had listed interventions that fell within this domain.

TRANSLATING RESEARCH INTO PRACTICE

The playground research conducted by Kern and Aldridge (2006) may be used as an example of how research findings can be translated into clinically achievable objectives and sub-objectives within the SCERTS® Model. In this study, an outdoor music center (i.e., Music Hut) was built on the playground at an inclusive university-affiliated childcare program for the purpose of providing meaningful interactions for young children with ASD. The researchers first observed the children with ASD on the playground before the Music Hut was installed. These children typically spent the majority of playground time in solitary play or in a dysregulated state when attempting to have peer interactions. The music therapy researcher composed unique songs for each child with ASD, and also taught these songs to the early childhood educators and classroom peers. The music therapist then trained the early childhood educators and peers on how to support and interact with the child with ASD in the Music Hut.

This protocol can be evaluated with the SCERTS® Model. While it is beyond the scope of this chapter to demonstrate a full assessment, brief examples of SCERTS® Model objectives and sub-objectives can be applied in all three domain areas as outlined in Table 4.1.

This extraction of possible SCERTS® Model objectives and sub-objectives observed within specific music therapy intervention protocols could be discussed relative to many other studies. Utilizing the SCERTS® Model assessment tool may provide greater specificity and achievable goals within a targeted timeframe for music therapists working with young children with ASD and their families.

Conclusion

A music therapy assessment for young children with ASD can provide much valuable information that may lead to unique learning opportunities. Assessment for eligibility may give rationale for inclusion of music therapy as an effective treatment modality. Assessment may uncover information gained exclusively through musical responses and music-related behaviors. A validated systematic assessment also may offer specific information that can lead to the development of appropriate goals that may be musically tailored to the precise needs of each individual. While currently no validated music therapy assessment tool for young children with ASD exists, music therapists have at their disposal examples from within and outside their profession that may be applicable for use in their particular settings. Music therapists have a responsibility to the young child with ASD, the family, the child's team, and to their profession to use assessment tools and processes that yield consistent and appropriate information that may lead to the facilitation of successful treatment outcomes through the distinctive use of music.

Table 4.1 Brief examples of the SCERTS® Model sub-categories identified in Kern and Aldridge (2006) (applications by Darcy Walworth)	
Domain areas	**Applicable music therapy objectives**

Social Communication: Shared Attention (SCERTS® Model Objective)	Sub-objectives addressed increasing shared attention skills of the child with ASD via monitoring the:
	
	 • **attentional focusing of a social partner**
	    ◦ focuses on the partner to play instruments in turn
	    ◦ joins in singing the song with peers
	
	 • **securing attention to himself prior to expressing his intention**
	    ◦ conveys desire to play a specific instrument in the Music Hut
	    ◦ early childhood educator facilitates skill in Music Hut intervention
	
	 • **understanding non-verbal cues of shifts in attentional focus developed by early childhood educator in Music Hut by**
	    ◦ stopping and starting songs
	    ◦ changing instruments being played in different areas of the Music Hut.

Emotional Regulation	Sub-objectives addressed in the Music Hut included: • **mutual regulation** • **responding to assistance offered by partners and responding to feedback and guidance regarding their behavior.** Note: Structure of the intervention gave many opportunities for the child with ASD to regulate his emotional state due to increased positive interactions between peers and teachers while in the Music Hut.

Transactional Support	The entire Music Hut project was aimed at increasing meaningful social interactions, structured with optimal supports to aid the child's regulation and successful communication with others.
	Interpersonal support objective was addressed through the playground intervention by:
	• **being responsive to the child** as the instruments were chosen and songs were requested
	• **fostering initiation with the child** by taking the child into the Music Hut to begin music play
	• **respecting the child's independence** when a choice was made to play a instrument that did not require sharing.
	Fostering initiation sub-objectives were structured by:
	• early childhood educators and peers **non-verbally and verbally offering choices**
	◦ indicating where in the Music Hut the play would begin
	◦ handing the child with ASD an instrument without a verbal request
	• the early childhood educator's **waiting and encouraging initiation** between the peers via not stepping in and interrupting
	• the early childhood educator's **providing a balance of initiated and respondent turns** within songs and instrument play.
	Learning support was accomplished by:
	• **structuring the activity for active participation**—teacher and peer (trained to facilitate interaction in the Music Hut) employed specific strategies for increasing child's interaction and activity level by following the same sequence used in the introduction to the Music Hut stage
	• **defining clear beginning and ending to activities** (the song's structure naturally cued its beginning and ending)
	• **providing predictable sequences to activities** (addressed in the protocol for intervention techniques in the Music Hut)—e.g. singing the same song when entering the Music Hut to initiate and cue that the Music Hut time had started
	• a partner's **using augmentative systems to foster development**—design of the Music Hut allowed for augmentative communication to be built into the choice areas for each instrument and song.

LEARNING QUESTIONS

1. What are the main reasons to assess a child with ASD?

2. What is the role of the music therapist in the assessment process?

3. Why is it important to involve the family in the assessment process?

4. Why should assessment for young children take place in natural settings?

5. Are there any validated music therapy assessments for use with young children with ASD?

6. What determines a child's eligibility for music therapy services?

7. What is the main function of the Four-Step Assessment Model?

8. What are the major steps of the Four-Step Assessment Model?

9. What is the purpose of the MT-MRB assessment?

10. What does the MT-MRB assessment use as its main source for gathering information about the child with ASD?

11. What are the three domain areas addressed by the SCERTS® Model?

12. How can using the SCERTS® Model help music therapists develop specific treatment goals and objectives for young children with ASD?

References

American Music Therapy Association (AMTA) (2010). *AMTA Standards of Clinical of Practice*. Silver Spring, MD: American Music Therapy Association.

Bruscia, K. (1987). *Improvisational Models of Music Therapy*. Springfield, IL: Charles C. Thomas Publishers.

Buysse, V., and Wesley, P.W. (2006). *Evidence-Based Practice in the Early Childhood Field*. Washington, DC: Zero to Three.

Carpente, J. (2011). *The Individual Music-Centered Assessment Profile for Neurodevelopmental Disorders (IMCAP-NDR) for Children, Adolescents, and Adults: A Clinical Manual*. Unpublished manual.

Centers for Disease Control and Prevention (CDC) (2012). *Learn the Signs: Act Early*. Retrieved from www.cdc.gov/ncbddd/actearly/index.html.

Certification Board for Music Therapists (CBMT) (2010). *CBMT Scope of Practice*. Downington, PA: Certification Board for Music Therapists.

Coleman, K., and Brunk, B. (2000). Development of a special education music therapy assessment process. *Music Therapy Perspectives, 18(1)*, 59–68.

DEC/NAEYC (2009). *Early Childhood Inclusion: A Joint Position Statement of the Division for Early Childhood (DEC) and the National Association for the Education of Young Children (NAEYC)*. Chapel Hill, NC: The University of North Carolina.

Grow, L.L., Carr, J.E., Gunby, K.V., Charania, S.M., *et al.* (2009). Deviations from prescribed prompting procedures: Implications for treatment integrity. *Journal of Behavioral Education, 18*, 142–156.

Hummel-Rossi, B., Guerrero, N., Selim, N., Turry, A. *et al.* (2008). *Music Therapy Communication and Social Interaction Scale—Group*. Unpublished instrument, Nordoff-Robbins Center for Music Therapy, New York University.

Kern, P., and Aldridge, D. (2006). Using embedded music therapy interventions to support outdoor play of young children with autism in an inclusive community-based child care program. *Journal of Music Therapy, 43(4)*, 270–294.

Lazar, M. (2007). When is music therapy necessary? Determining eligibility through the IEP. Presented at *The Autism Agenda: An Evidence-Based Approach to Music Therapy*, The Ninth AMTA Conference, 14 November. Louisville, KY.

MacDuff, G.S., Krantz, P.J., and McClannahan, L.E. (2001). Prompts and prompt-fading strategies for people with autism. In C. Maurice, G. Green, and R.M. Foxx (Eds.) *Making a Difference: Behavioral Intervention for Autism*. Austin, TX: Pro-Ed.

McLean, M.E., and Snyder, P.A. (Eds.) (2011). Gathering information to make informed decisions: Contemporary perspectives about assessment in early childhood special education. *Young Exceptional Children Monograph Series 13*. Missoula, MT: DEC.

Nagel, R. (2007). Issues in preschool assessment. In B.A. Bracken and R.J. Nagle (Eds.) *Psychoeducational Assessment of Preschool Children (Fourth Edition)*. Mahwah, NJ: Lawrence Earlbaum Associates, Inc.

National Professional Development Center on Autism Spectrum Disorders (NPDC on ASD) (2011). Session 3: Assessment for ASD. In *Foundations of Autism Spectrum Disorders: An Online Course*. Chapel Hill: FPG Child Development Institute, The University of North Carolina.

Prizant, B.M., Wetherby, A.M., Rubin, E., Laurent, A.C., and Rydell, P.J. (2005). *The SCERTS® Model: A Comprehensive Educational Approach for Children with Autism Spectrum Disorders* (Vols. 1–2). Baltimore, MD: Brookes.

Prizant, B.M., Wetherby, A.M., Rubin, E., and Laurent, A.C. (2010). The SCERTS model and evidence-based practice. Retrieved from www.scerts.com/docs/SCERTS_EBP%20090810%20v1.pdf.

Snell, A.M. (2002). Music therapy for learners with autism in a public school setting. In B.L. Wilson (Ed.) *Models of Music Therapy Interventions in School Settings (Second Edition)*. Silver Spring, MD: The American Music Therapy Association, Inc.

U.S. Department of Education (2006). (14 August) Rules and regulations. *Federal Register, 71(156)*. Retrieved from http://idea.ed.gov/download/finalregulations.pdf.

U.S. Department of Education (2010). (August) *Building the Legacy: IDEA 2004*. Retrieved from http://idea.ed.gov.

U.S. Department of Education (2011a). Questions and answers on Individualized Education Programs (IEPs), evaluations, and revaluations. Retrieved from http://idea.ed.gov/explore/view/p/,root,dynamic,QaCorner,3.

U.S. Department of Education (2011b). (28 September) *Federal Register*. Early intervention programs for infants and toddlers with disabilities. Retrieved from https://www.federalregister.gov/articles/2011/09/28/2011-22783/early-intervention-program-for-infants-and-toddlers-with-disabilities.

Walworth, D.D. (2007). The use of music therapy within the SCERTS® Model for children with autism spectrum disorder. *Journal of Music Therapy, 44(1)*, 2–22.

Walworth, D., Register, D., and Engel, J.N. (2009). Using the SCERTS® Model assessment tool to identify music therapy goals for clients with autism spectrum disorder. *Journal of Music Therapy, 46(3)*, 204–216.

Wigram, T. (1999a). Analysis and interpretation of musical material. Presented at *Music Therapy and the Autistic Spectrum: An International Perspective,* Ninth World Congress of Music Therapy, Washington, DC, November 1999.

Wigram, T. (1999b). Contact in music: The analysis of musical behavior in children with communication disorder and pervasive developmental disability for differential diagnosis. In T. Wigram and J. DeBacker (Eds.) *Music Therapy Applications in Developmental Disability, Pediatrics and Neurology.* London and Philadelphia: Jessica Kingsley Publishers.

Wolery, M. (2004). Monitoring children's progress and intervention implementation. In M. McLean, M. Wolery, and D. Bailey, Jr. (Eds.) *Assessing Infants and Preschoolers with Special Needs (Third Edition).* Upper Saddle River, NJ: Pearson Education, Inc.

PART 3

Treatment Approaches

Chapter 5

Applied Behavior Analysis

Introduction and Practical Application in Music Therapy for Young Children with Autism Spectrum Disorders

Linda K. Martin, MME, MT-BC
Coast Music Therapy
San Diego, CA

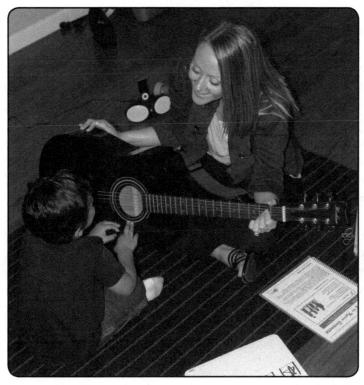

PHOTO COURTESY OF ZAP MARTIN

For most music therapists, designing sessions within an ABA framework will not require a shift in philosophy, but rather a proper understanding of the various principles and practical application sof ABA.
(Linda K. Martin)

Applied Behavior Analysis (ABA) is a widely recognized treatment modality for young children with autism spectrum disorders (ASD). Numerous studies support its effectiveness in modifying behaviors in children with ASD. However, practitioners and parents may be distracted by the great variety of treatment approaches based on ABA, and thus may not grasp the major principles central to the modality. This chapter will provide a brief overview of ABA, examining four major principles, highlighting three common treatment approaches, and offering illustrations for applications in music therapy practice.

Introduction

ABA and several ABA-based approaches are recognized by the National Autism Center (NAC) as *Established Treatments* for children with ASD; this means "they have been thoroughly researched and have *sufficient* evidence for us to confidently state that they are effective" (NAC, 2009b, p. 38). The US Surgeon General's report states, "Thirty years of research demonstrated the efficacy of applied behavioral methods in reducing inappropriate behavior and in increasing communication, learning, and appropriate social behavior" (U.S. Department of Health and Human Services, 2011). Many educational institutions and autism agencies internationally now are providing ABA education and services (Association for Behavior Analysis International, n.d.).

Because ABA treatment approaches are evidence-based and used extensively by professionals working with children with ASD, music therapists should familiarize themselves with the major principles of ABA. Consistency is crucial to the educational program of a child with ASD; if ABA approaches are being implemented within the child's natural environments, music therapists should be able to infuse common ABA approaches into their music therapy interventions. Upon gaining a better understanding of ABA and the techniques that comprise an ABA program, music therapists may find that they already are naturally implementing components of ABA within their sessions. For most music therapists, designing a music therapy session within an ABA framework will not require a shift in philosophy, but rather a desire to apply its principles to music therapy service delivery.

What is Applied Behavior Analysis?

Behavior analysis studies behavior and learning and examines how biological and environmental factors affect changes in behavior. ABA is the applied science of studying and modifying behavior to promote desired change (Baer, Wolf, and Risley, 1968). For young children with ASD, ABA is often used to promote improved quality of life or socially relevant behaviors (Leach, 2010).

The science of behavior analysis was first recognized following pivotal research by Igor Pavlov (1927) who searched to understand why dogs salivated upon seeing the person who delivered their food, even before any food was present. In this well-known study, Pavlov paired a neutral stimulus (i.e., a bell) with an unconditioned stimulus (i.e., a dog's natural salivation when presented with food). Each time food was given to the dog, the bell was rung. Over time, simply hearing the bell caused the dog to salivate. Through what is now called classical conditioning, the dog was taught to salivate even without the presence of food.

B.F. Skinner (1957) continued the study of behavior through his research on the use of rewards and punishments to promote learning or change. Known as operant conditioning, Skinner's studies revealed that a voluntary behavior could be changed by adding or removing positive or negative stimuli (Skinner, 1957). ABA typically utilizes techniques based on the fundamentals of operant conditioning and focuses on behaviors that are both observable and measurable (Baer, Wolf, and Risley, 1968; Bailey and Burch, 2002). Reliable measurement requires that each goal, skill, or behavior be clearly broken down and defined so that each element can be individually observed and measured. For example, a goal to increase a child's self-confidence would be neither observable nor measurable. However, when clearly broken down and defined, a similar goal could read: "Child will demonstrate improved self-confidence by raising his hand in response to a teacher's question during circle time activities on at least one occasion per day for three consecutive days." Creating goals that can be reliably measured also ensures that multiple people tracking data on the same goal would obtain identical results.

Music therapists need to understand the definitions of common terms used within the context of this theoretical framework. For instance, the term "behavior" refers to a breadth of actions, skills, and responses. While often presupposed to be only inappropriate or maladaptive actions, a behavior also may indicate a positive action or response such as waving hello to a neighbor or playing on a drum. Likewise, the term "environment" may refer to a social situation or event that influences behavior as well as to a setting or particular surroundings.

Four major principles of Applied Behavior Analysis

This section will examine reinforcement, prompting, task analysis, and generalization, four major principles of ABA; three common evidence-based ABA approaches using the four principles are also highlighted (see Figure 5.1 for how these principles relate to the treatment approaches). Corresponding Autism Internet Modules addressing the selected principles and approaches can be found at www.autisminternetmodules. org/mod_list.php.

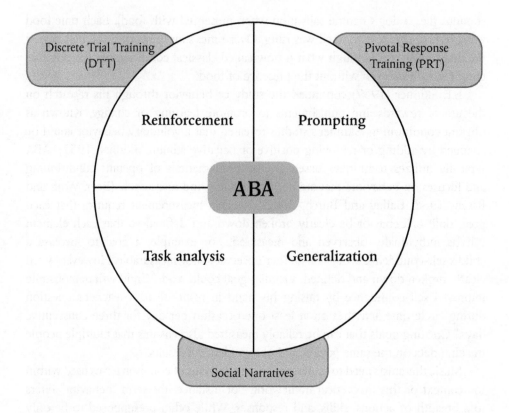

Figure 5.1: Major principles of ABA and related treatment approaches

Reinforcement

Reinforcement techniques are identified as one of the evidence-based practices for children with ASD (NAC, 2009; NPDC on ASD, n.d.). Research indicates that their purposeful and timely use can greatly influence changes in children's behavior (Neitzel, 2009). Just as effective reinforcement is likely to increase desired behavior, inadvertent reinforcement of undesired behavior may lead to an increase in negative behavior (Fisher *et al.*, 1996). Therefore, it is important to carefully consider how and when reinforcement techniques are implemented.

Likewise, music therapists need to understand the similarities and differences between positive and negative reinforcement and punishment. Reinforcement seeks to increase desired behavior through the addition of an item or activity that is pleasurable or through the removal of an undesired or unpleasant stimulus. Conversely, the goal of punishment is to decrease undesired behavior through the addition of a negative stimulus or by the removal of a positive stimulus (Neitzel, 2009).

Reinforcement techniques are often preferred over punishment within educational settings because their effective use can largely accomplish the same desired outcomes as systems of punishment. Implementation of reinforcement strategies focuses on positive change and provides the child with input on desirable behavior.

A preference assessment may effectively determine specific items or activities that have the most reinforcement potential. The overarching purpose of a preference assessment is the systematic comparison of highly preferred items to determine which one the child most consistently chooses (e.g., favorite toys, food items, objects, or even musical instruments) (Carr, Nicolson, and Higbee, 2000; DeLeon and Iwata, 1996). Repeating the assessment over a period of a few days determines consistency in responding. Preference assessments should be re-administered on a regular basis because each child's preferences may change over time.

The token economy system is one effective positive reinforcement strategy. The child earns a token following appropriate targeted behavior. Once the child has earned a specified number of tokens, they are exchanged for access to a highly reinforcing object or activity (Matson and Boisjoli, 2009; Neitzel, 2009). Table 5.1 provides brief definitions, applications, and examples of these most prominent reinforcement techniques applied in music therapy.

MUSIC AS A REINFORCER

Music may be utilized as a reinforcer for children with ASD who enjoy listening to music, playing instruments, singing, or dancing to favorite tunes (Finnigan and Starr, 2010; Standley, 1996). By conducting a music-specific preference assessment, the music therapist may discover the child's preferred recorded music, musical instruments, and dance or movement songs and thereby determine the most effective music strategy to use as a reinforcer. The following guidelines may be applied to this assessment process:

1. Consider the environment where the reinforcement strategy will be used.

2. Determine if the reinforcer will be functional.

3. Observe how the child responds to the music (avoid overstimulation).

4. Have musical equipment and materials readily available.

5. Determine whether the reinforcement will be used immediately following the desired behavior or intermittently.

Furthermore, the music therapist should differentiate between music that is being used as reinforcement and music that is being utilized to teach a skill. Music as a reinforcer is only effective if it remains highly preferred and motivating for the child. Task demands should not be requested of the child during music activities being used as reinforcement. However, when music is being utilized to teach a skill, the child should clearly understand the expectations associated within the music-based learning task. If directions are being given within the song or responses are required, the child should become accustomed to consistently responding within the song. The child may become confused if a song is used as a learning task and also as a reinforcement tool, and may even resist responding to prompts within the song when used as a learning support.

Table 5.1 Reinforcement and punishment techniques

Strategies	Definition	Implementation	Examples
Positive Reinforcement	The addition of a consequence in response to learner behavior that will increase the likelihood of that behavior recurring or at least maintaining (Neitzel, 2009).	• Generally offered immediately following the desired behavior. • Must be an item or activity that is highly preferred by the child. • Note: Offering a reward that is aversive for the child may ultimately set back progress toward achieving desired behavior.	• Giving a sticker or other reinforcing item. • Giving verbal praise. • Giving the opportunity to listen to a favorite song.
Negative Reinforcement	The removal of an undesired object or activity to increase target behavior (Neitzel, 2009).	• Removal of undesired object or activity directly following desired behavior. • Consequence must be an object or activity that is unpleasant and aversive to the child. • Note: If a child is particularly sensitive to negative feedback or consequences, it may be anxiety-provoking to have the constant presence of negativity.	• Not having to remain seated. • Removal of a work task or chore. • Being able to skip a counting song to play a preferred instrument.
Token Economy	The provision of tokens following desired behavior. When a specified number of tokens are collected, they are exchanged for a highly reinforcing object or activity (Neitzel, 2009).	• Can be used in combination with other forms of reinforcement including verbal praise or social reinforcement. • Is most effective when tokens can be exchanged without delay (Tarbox, Ghezzi, and Wilson, 2006). • Note: Token economy systems are especially beneficial for children requiring a dense schedule of reinforcement (Tarbox, Ghezzi, and Wilson, 2006).	• Child earns a star after each correct response. After earning five stars, he gains access to a favorite book. • Child earns a smiley face each time he raises his hand appropriately. Ten smiley faces earns time on the computer. • Child earns a penny for sharing an instrument. After earning three pennies, he can play his favorite drum.

Prompting

Prompting and prompt fading are integral components of any ABA approach and have been identified as established evidence-based practice for children with ASD (NPDC on ASD, n.d.). Prompting is the purposeful provision of help or cues to facilitate acquisition of the desired task or skill (MacDuff, Krantz, and McClannahan, 2001). Helping the child attain independent functioning is the main goal when selecting the prompting method to be used. The level and type of prompt should be based on the task being taught, the needs of the child, and the plan for prompt fading (MacDuff, Krantz, and McClannahan, 2001). Three basic prompting methods that may be considered by music therapists, parents, and other practitioners are: (1) graduated guidance, (2) simultaneous prompting, and (3) least-to-most prompts (Neitzel and Wolery, 2009).

The *graduated guidance* strategy ensures errorless learning by starting with a controlling prompt that guarantees the correct response or action. Once the child has shown success, the prompt is faded by altering its intensity or changing the type of prompt. Facilitators must continually evaluate the level of prompt used and scale back the level of assistance provided to ensure the child remains successful. This continues until the child can complete the task independently.

In *simultaneous prompting*, the teacher or practitioner provides a cue for the child to complete a target skill or task while simultaneously providing a controlling prompt to ensure successful completion of the task (e.g., stating "Get the red bell" while helping the child pick up the red bell). Then, when the cue is provided a second time, the teacher or practitioner waits for the child to respond independently.

The strategy of *least-to-most prompts* uses a minimum level of prompt to ensure the child's successful response or completion of the given task; a more intense level of prompting is provided until the child is able to accurately respond. Prompts are then faded until eventual independence is achieved.

Within these prompting strategies, the intensity of prompts is varied through more or less intrusive prompting strategies. According to Neitzel and Wolery (2009), five main types of prompts may be given: physical, verbal, visual, model, and gestural prompts.

Physical prompts require direct contact with the child to complete the desired skill or task. Examples of physical prompts are using hand-over-hand assistance to beat the drum with a mallet or touching a child's chin to cue opening the mouth and imitating a sound.

Verbal prompts facilitate correct responses through auditory sounds or statements that provide clues or direction (e.g., producing the initial consonant sound of a desired response or saying "sit down"). Verbal prompts often are over-utilized because people initially tend to rely on giving verbal direction; substituting visual or gestural prompts may reduce the likelihood of dependence on verbal directions or cues to complete tasks.

Visual prompts are cues received via sight. Visual prompts include schedule boards, a visual timer, or picture icons placed in strategic locations.

When a skill or task is first demonstrated by the practitioner, it is referred to as a *model prompt*. It may be verbal or physical in nature (e.g., verbally providing the correct answer to a question or raising a hand to demonstrate desired behavior).

Gestural prompts are the least intrusive prompting strategies, only requiring a simple gesture to facilitate successful achievement of the desired task or skill. Gestural prompts include pointing in a certain direction, toward an object, or nodding the head to cue the child.

Practitioners must be very intentional when using prompts and prompt fading techniques. Fading should begin as soon as the child has successfully completed each component part of a task or skill. Until the child has mastered the task or skill independently, practitioners and parents of children with ASD might consider utilizing the least intrusive prompt (e.g., a visual or gestural prompt), reducing the number of prompts simultaneously offered, and continue fading prompts.

MUSIC AS A PROMPT

Graduated guidance techniques are effective for using music as a mnemonic device to teach a skill. The music therapist may first present information within the rhythmic and melodic framework of a song. After the child has memorized the information within the context of the song, lyric cues may be faded, leaving only the melodic and rhythmic cues intact. When the child can supply relevant information without the provision of lyric cues, melodic song cues also may be faded. Utilizing the same rhythmic cues taught within the song can then trigger the child's recall of information learned. Ultimately, the child will provide the information learned within the song independent of any musical cues.

Music acts as an additional prompt when used to teach certain developmental skills because it can function as a tool to facilitate learning of information (Kern, Wolery, and Aldridge, 2007). As prompts are faded, the music therapy strategies also must be faded for the child with ASD to independently master the skill; incorporating *prompt fading* may greatly increase the likelihood for the child to retain information and generalize across environments. Figure 5.2 provides an example of how the *graduated guidance* technique and *prompt fading* procedure can be implemented in music therapy interventions.

Step 1
Embed a child's address and phone number within a catchy, repetitive song and include visual supports for the child to follow.

Step 2
Once the child is able to fully recite the information within the context of the song, remove the lyric prompts from the song, leaving only the same melodic and rhythmic cues, along with the visual supports.

Step 3
Once the child is able to provide his or her personal information when given only melodic, rhythmic, and visual cues, remove all melodic components of the song. The child will now be chanting the address and phone number within the rhythmic context of the song. Provide visual cues only if needed.

Step 4
Remove all rhythmic and visual cues once the child has reached independent mastery of the personal information.

Figure 5.2: Example of applying the graduated guidance technique and prompt fading technique in music therapy

Task analysis

Task analysis, the thorough breaking down of a task or activity into individual component parts that together comprise the whole (NAC, 2009a), meets the evidence-based practice criteria and therefore is a valuable ABA principle to consider when providing services for young children with ASD (Franzone, 2009). Each step should be a single, manageable task or direction. The steps should be placed in sequential order, noting all steps that are required for completion of the task (Matson *et al.*, 1990). For instance, the task of tooth-brushing may be presented in a basic task analysis as such: (1) Get toothbrush, (2) Put water on toothbrush, (3) Put toothpaste on toothbrush, (4) Brush teeth, (5) Spit out toothpaste, (6) Rinse out mouth, (7) Rinse toothbrush, and (8) Dry mouth and hands.

MUSIC AND TASK ANALYSIS

Task analysis principles can be implemented in song-writing along with other music therapy techniques (Kern, Wakeford, and Aldridge, 2007). For example, each verse of a song could be organized to teach a component part of the task while the chorus section reiterates the task and its function; or each line of a verse could describe an individual component, with the entire verse describing the task in its entirety. Each verse would then repeat the same instruction to provide opportunities for practicing and repeating the task.

Generalization

Generalization allows children to apply skills learned in a structured teaching situation across settings, people, subject, behaviors, materials, or time (Stokes & Baer, 1977). Evidence suggests that many children with ASD have physiological processing difficulties that hinder the generalization of skills (Plaisted, 2001); they may have difficulty adjusting their skills to meld in with new or different frameworks or circumstances (NAC, 2009). Hence, generalization is difficult for them, and is a process that must be planned for and facilitated through specific advanced programming (Mesibov, Shea, and Schopler, 2005).

Stokes and Baer (1977) summarize seven key strategies that may be implemented to promote generalization of learned skills or behaviors:

1. Embed teaching within natural environments.

2. Diversify the setting, context, and facilitator when teaching a skill.

3. Institute loose training principles, include less rigid responses, and train multiple examples concurrently.

4. Incorporate intermittent reinforcement schedules or delayed reinforcement to set less rigid boundaries on when the skill is to be targeted.

5. Implement stimuli (e.g., peers, materials, environmental noise) into training sessions that will be found in generalization settings.

6. Encourage self-reporting and self-reinforcement when applicable.

7. Reinforce desired behaviors across settings, situations, and people.

Considering these suggestions at the onset of teaching a new skill may ensure that the implementation of the chosen strategy is timely and purposeful. Note that when targeted skills or learning is carried over in the home environment, the child's ability to generalize and maintain the information may improve (Lovaas *et al.*, 1973).

Music and generalization

Music therapists can apply the above principles to music therapy settings. Whenever possible, specific skills should be taught in the natural environment in which they will occur (Kern, 2008). For example, implement a song designed to teach a young child with ASD to appropriately request a snack during the child's actual snack time. The skill is then presented in context and takes on meaning within the environment. If teaching the skill during snack time is not feasible, the song should be brought into that environment after being learned in a separate setting.

Music therapists can use common props, visuals, and other supports to provide opportunities for generalizing skills to other settings and environments (Walworth, 2010). If specific picture cards are being used in the classroom and at home to teach the concept of opposites, facilitate generalization of the skill by using those same cards within the music therapy setting. Likewise, when teaching a behavioral script through music, implement the same visual sequence within the classroom and at home to ensure carry-over and generalization.

Practicing a learned skill in a variety of environments can also promote generalization (Kaplan and Steele, 2005). A young boy with ASD may learn a song about washing and drying his hands in the classroom setting. He then should practice the steps learned from the script within the song in a variety of situations and settings, using the song cues as needed to assist in generalizing learned information to other environments.

Related treatment approaches using principles of ABA
Discrete Trial Training

Discrete Trial Training (DTT) and ABA are not synonymous. DTT is an approach utilizing the principles of ABA (e.g., implementing consequences to effect desired change and systematic observation and measurement of desired outcomes) (Smith, 2001). The principles of DTT are based on studies first published by Igor Lovaas (1987) showing educational progress made by individuals with ASD who received direct one-to-one treatment and systematic presentation of information. DTT is a teaching procedure that breaks down skills into discrete, individual components. Each discrete trial is comprised of the following five steps and is provided in an environment with limited distractions and one-on-one support by a teacher or facilitator with specialized training (Smith, 2001):

1. *Cue:* The child is presented with a brief, clear instruction.

2. *Prompt:* A model or assist is given to ensure the child's successful response to the cue.

3. *Response:* The child responds to the cue, either correctly or incorrectly.

4. *Consequence:* Correct responses are immediately reinforced while incorrect responses are presented with a consequence of *no, try again,* or other indication that the response was incorrect.

5. *Intertrial interval:* Following the consequence, a brief pause is given before presenting the next trial.

Discrete trials are repeated consecutively allowing the child multiple opportunities to practice the skill (i.e., "mass trialing"). In DTT, mastery of the skill must be obtained before moving on to the next sequential skill (Smith, 2001).

MUSIC AND DISCRETE TRIAL TRAINING

Due to the inherent repetitive nature of music, the principles of DTT may be easily implemented within song interventions. Furthermore, incorporating music strategies into DTT may be an effective means of engaging children who are motivated by music in DTT tasks. For instance, instead of singing a song that incorporates multiple colors, the song may be adapted to simply mass trial a single color. Once the child has mastered the ability to label that individual color, the song lyrics can be changed to mass trial a different color. Colors can be "randomly rotated" into the same song for generalization and maintenance purposes.

Pivotal Response Training

Continued research in the field of ABA has led to the development of different approaches for meeting the various learning needs of children with ASD. Over the past two decades, Pivotal Response Training (PRT) has become a widely recognized approach in teaching young children with ASD (Koegel and Koegel, 2006). Vismara and Bogin (2009) examined the effectiveness of PRT in teaching social interaction and social play skills, demonstrating its relevance for inclusion in educational settings. Stahmer (1995) showed significant increases in the children's ability to perform complex and creative symbolic play actions and also in their ability to generalize play skills across settings, people, and toys when taught through PRT.

While DTT is a systematic approach to teaching new skills within a controlled environment, PRT is also a structured method of teaching. However, PRT focuses on using the natural environment and naturally occurring consequences to improve skills in young children with ASD (Koegel and Koegel, 2006). PRT is based on the premise that four pivotal areas affect other non-targeted areas: (1) responsivity to multiple cues, (2) motivation, (3) self-management, and (4) self-initiations (Koegel *et al.*, 1999). By arranging the environment, setting up opportunities for social interaction or turn-taking, and following the child's lead, adults embed teaching opportunities into activities initiated by the child. Reinforcement of behavior is instituted in a way that is natural to the environment as opposed to giving verbal praise or an unrelated reinforcer (e.g., if a child says "bubbles," bubbles are provided).

MUSIC AND PIVOTAL RESPONSE TRAINING

In many ways music therapy is very similar to PRT. Within the music environment and via musical improvisation, a child's natural reinforcement is the music with which he or she is surrounded, fulfilling a pivotal area of PRT, and also providing opportunities for self-management, self-initiation, and responding to multiple cues within the music therapy setting. Target behaviors or skills can be addressed naturally by giving the child freedom to explore sounds and textures through various musical instruments.

Social narratives

Social narratives, often referred to as social scripts or Social Stories™, are short stories about social situations, activities, or tasks that have been broken down into a format designed to teach specific social skills or desired behaviors (Gray and Garand, 1993). Often scripts are implemented when the child with ASD becomes anxious over certain situations or tasks that may lead to socially inappropriate responses or reactions (Bledsoe, Smith Myles, and Simpson, 2003). Systematically breaking difficult tasks or situations into concrete, manageable steps with clear behavioral expectations leads to improved social functioning in children with ASD (Crozier and Tincani, 2011; Test et al., 2011).

MUSIC AND SOCIAL NARRATIVES

Using music as a mnemonic device is an effective way to facilitate memorization and retention of information presented within scripts (Brownell, 2002; Pasiali, 2004). Lyrics to many traditional children's songs are, in essence, scripts about life situations and handling difficult circumstances. While a script is a much abbreviated and simplified version, it is easily transformed into song lyrics. A script put into song format may motivate the child to practice, memorize and internalize concepts. See Chapter 6 for a more detailed description of social narratives and their application in music therapy.

Conclusion

ABA is an evidence-based approach that is utilized extensively with children with ASD. Therefore, music therapists, educators, and parents should become familiar with the major principles of this approach and its relevance for implementation in music therapy sessions, the classroom, and other environments. This chapter has provided a brief overview of ABA; however, readers are encouraged to further explore the enormous amount of literature and research that is available on this topic. By keeping informed about current research and evidence-based practice, music therapists may be better equipped to deliver treatment that reflects a common goal of all who work with young children with ASD and their families: To provide the best and most efficacious treatment for children with ASD.

LEARNING QUESTIONS

1. In one sentence, how would you describe Applied Behavior Analysis to someone who is unfamiliar with this approach?

2. Applied Behavior Analysis focuses on behaviors that are _____ and _____.

3. What is the difference between positive and negative reinforcement?

4. Give an example of how to conduct a preference assessment within the music therapy setting.

5. Why is it important to set up specific prompt fading strategies at the onset of teaching a skill?

6. Name five types of prompts and provide an example of each.

7. Describe strategies for ensuring that a child who learns to identify numbers within the context of music will be able to generalize the skill across environments and settings.

8. Give an example of how the principles of Discrete Trial Training could be implemented within a music therapy session.

9. In what ways is Pivotal Response Training similar to music therapy?

References

Association for Behavior Analysis International (n.d.). *Affiliated Chapters.* Retrieved from www. abainternational.org.

Baer, D.M., Wolf, M.M., and Risley, T.R. (1968). Some current dimensions of Applied Behavior Analysis. *Journal of Applied Behavior Analysis, 1,* 91–97.

Bailey, J.S., and Burch, M.R. (2002). *Research Methods in Applied Behavior Analysis.* Thousand Oaks, CA: Sage Publications, Inc.

Bledsoe, R., Myles, B.S., and Simpson, R.L. (2003). Use of a social story intervention to improve mealtime skills of an adolescent with Asperger syndrome. *Autism, 7(3),* 289–295.

Brownell, M.D. (2002). Musically adapted social stories to modify behaviors in students with autism: Four case studies. *Journal of Music Therapy, 39,* 117–144.

Carr, J.E., Nicolson, A.C., and Higbee, T.S. (2000). Evaluation of a brief multi-stimulus preference assessment in a naturalistic context. *Journal of Applied Behavioral Analysis, 33,* 353–357.

Crozier, S., and Tincani, M. (2007). Effects of social stories on prosocial behavior of preschool children with autism spectrum disorders. *Journal of Autism and Developmental Disorders, 37(9),* 1803–1814.

DeLeon, I.G., and Iwata, B.A. (1996). Evaluation of a multiple-stimulus presentation format for assessing reinforcer preferences. *Journal of Applied Behavior Analysis, 29(4)*, 519–533.

Finnigan, E., and Starr, E. (2010). Increasing social responsiveness in a child with autism: A comparison of music and non-music interventions. *Autism, 14(4)*, 321–348.

Fisher, W.W., Ninness, H.A., Piazza, C.C., and Owen-DeSchryver, J.S. (1996). On the reinforcing effects of the content of verbal attention. *Journal of Applied Behavior Analysis, 29*, 235–238.

Franzone, E. (2009). *Overview of Task Analysis.* Madison, WI: National Professional Development Center on Autism Spectrum Disorders, Waisman Center, University of Wisconsin. Retrieved from http://autismpdc.fpg.unc.edu/sites/autismpdc.fpg.unc.edu/files/TaskAnalysis_Overview_0.pdf.

Gray, C.A., and Garand, J.D. (1993). Social Stories™: Improving responses of students with autism with accurate social information. *Focus on Autistic Behavior, 8(1)*, 1–10.

Kaplan, R.S., and Steele, A.L. (2005). An analysis of music therapy program goals and outcomes for clients with diagnoses on the autism spectrum. *Journal of Music Therapy, 42(1)*, 2–19.

Kern, P. (2008). Singing our way through the day: Using music with young children during daily routines. *Children and Families, 22(2)*, 50–56.

Kern, P., Wakeford, L., and Aldridge, D. (2007). Improving the performance of a young child with autism during self-care tasks using embedded song interventions: A case study. *Music Therapy Perspectives, 25(1)*, 43–51.

Kern, P., Wolery, M., and Aldridge, D. (2007). Use of songs to promote independence in morning greeting routines for young children with autism. *Journal of Autism and Developmental Disorders, 37*, 1264–1271.

Koegel, L.K., Koegel, R.L., Harrower, J.K., and Carter, C.M. (1999). Pivotal Response Intervention, I: Overview of approach. *Journal of Applied Behavior Analysis, 25*, 341–354.

Koegel, R.L., and Koegel, L.K. (2006). *Pivotal Response Treatments for Autism: Communication, Social and Academic Development.* Baltimore, MD: Paul H. Brookes Publishing Co.

Leach, D. (2010). *Bringing ABA into Your Inclusive Classroom: A Guide to Improving Outcomes for Students with Autism Spectrum Disorders.* Baltimore, MD: Paul H. Brookes Publishing Co.

Lovaas, O.I. (1987). Behavioral treatment and normal educational and intellectual functioning in young autistic children. *Journal of Counseling and Clinical Psychology, 55*, 3–9.

Lovaas, O.I., Koegel, R., Simmons, J.Q., and Stevens Long, J. (1973). Some generalization and follow-up measures on autistic children in behavior therapy. *Journal of Applied Behavior Analysis, 6(1)*, 161–165.

MacDuff, G.S., Krantz, P.J., and McClannahan, L.E. (2001). Prompts and prompt-fading strategies for people with autism. In C. Maurice, G. Green, and R.M. Foxx (Eds.) *Making a Difference: Behavioral Intervention for Autism.* Austin, TX: Pro-Ed.

Matson, J., and Boisjoli, J.A. (2009). The token economy for children with intellectual disability and/or autism: A review. *Research in Developmental Disabilities, 30(2)*, 240–248.

Matson, J., Taras, M., Seven, J., Love, S., and Fridley, D. (1990). Teaching self-help skills to autistic and mentally retarded children. *Research in Developmental Disabilities, 11*, 361–378.

Mesibov, G. B., Shea, V., and Schopler, E. (2005). *The TEACCH Approach to Autism Spectrum Disorders.* New York: Plenum Press.

National Autism Center (NAC) (2009a). *National Standards Report.* The National Standards Project— Addressing the need for evidence-based practice guidelines for autism spectrum disorders. Randolph, MA: NAC.

National Autism Centre (NAC) (2009b). *Evidence-Based Practice and Autism in the Schools: A Guide to Providing Appropriate Interventions to Students with Autism Spectrum Disorders.* Randolph, MA: NAC.

National Professional Development Center on Autism Spectrum Disorders (NPDC on ASD) (n.d.) *The NPDC on ASD and the National Standards Project.* Retrieved from http://autismpdc.fpg.unc.edu.

Neitzel, J. (2009). Overview of reinforcement. Chapel Hill, NC: The National Professional Development Center on Autism Spectrum Disorders, Frank Porter Graham Child Development Institute, the University of North Carolina. Retrieved from http://autismpdc.fpg.unc.edu/sites/autismpdc.fpg.unc.edu/files/Reinforcement_Overview.pdf.

Neitzel, J., and Wolery, M. (2009). Overview of prompting. Chapel Hill, NC: The National Professional Development Center on Autism Spectrum Disorders, Frank Porter Graham Child Development Institute, the University of North Carolina. Retrieved from http://autismpdc.fpg.unc.edu/sites/autismpdc.fpg.unc.edu/files/Prompting_Overview.pdf.

Pasiali, V. (2004). The use of prescriptive therapeutic songs in a home-based environment to promote social skills acquisition by children with autism: Three case studies. *Music Therapy Perspectives, 22,* 11–20.

Pavlov, I.P. (1927). *Conditioned Reflexes: An Investigation of the Physiological Activity of the Cerebral Cortex.* (G.V. Anrep (ed. and trans.)). London: Oxford University Press.

Plaisted, K.C. (2001). Reduced generalization in autism: An alternative to weak centeral coherence. In J.A. Burack, T. Charman, N. Yirmiya, and P.R. Zelazo (Eds.) *The Development of Autism: Perspectives from Theory and Research.* Mahwah, NJ: Lawrence Erlbaum Associates Publishers.

Skinner, B.F. (1957). *Verbal Behavior.* Englewood Cliffs, NJ: Prentice Hall.

Smith, T. (2001). Discrete Trial Training in the treatment of autism. *Focus on Autism and Other Developmental Disabilities, 16(2),* 86–92.

Stahmer, A.C. (1995). Teaching symbolic play skills to children with autism using Pivotal Response Training. *Journal of Autism and Developmental Disorders, 25(2),* 123–141.

Standley, J. (1996). A meta-analysis on the effects of music as reinforcement for education/therapy objectives. *Journal of Research in Music Education, 44,* 105–133.

Stokes, T.F., and Baer, D.M. (1977). An implicit technology of generalization. *Journal of Applied Behavior Analysis, 10(2),* 349–367.

Tarbox, R.S.F., Ghezzi, P.M., and Wilson, G. (2006). The effects of token reinforcement on attending in a young child with autism. *Behavioral Intervention, 21(3),* 155–164.

Test, D.W., Richter, S., Knight, V., and Spooner, F. (2011). A comprehensive review and meta-analysis of the Social Stories literature. *Focus on Autism and Other Developmental Disabilities, 26(1),* 49–62.

U.S. Department of Health and Human Services (2011). Office of the Surgeon General. Retrieved from www.surgeongeneral.gov.

Vismara, L.A., and Bogin, J. (2009). Overview of Pivotal Response Training (PRT). Sacramento, CA: The National Professional Development Center on Autism Spectrum Disorders, The M.I.N.D. Institute, the University of California at Davis School of Medicine. Retrieved from http://autismpdc.fpg.unc.edu/sites/autismpdc.fpg.unc.edu/files/PRT_Overview.pdf.

Walworth, D. (2010). Incorporating music into daily routines: Family education and integration. *imagine, 1,* 28–31.

Chapter 6

Social Stories™

Pairing the Story with Music

Mike D. Brownell, MME, MT-BC
MUSIC THERAPY SERVICES OF ANN ARBOR
ANN ARBOR, MI

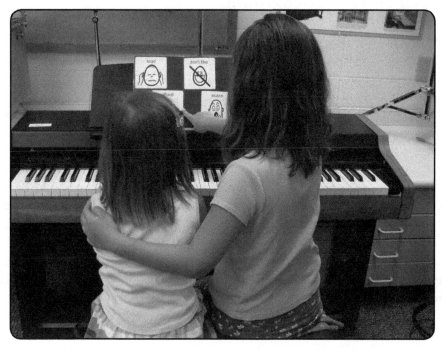

*Setting Social Stories™ to music provides an engaging additional
way to impart relevant social information and context.
(Mike D. Brownell)*

Anyone who learned to recite the alphabet using the melody to "Twinkle, Twinkle, Little Star" is familiar with music's capacity as an information conduit and mnemonic device. This chapter describes the creation of a musical adaptation of Social Stories™—a frequently used tool designed to impart pertinent social information to students with autism spectrum disorders (ASD)—to take advantage of music's ability to provide a memorable, engaging backdrop. Basic constructions of Social Stories™ and considerations when setting them to music are discussed; musical examples are provided.

Social Story™ background

Social Stories™ were first described by Carol Gray in 1993 (Gray and Garrand, 1993). Typically they are individualized stories written and presented according to specified guidelines with the aim of providing a student with ASD with specific information about how to react in a particular social scenario. The stories often include answers to many of the wh- questions (e.g., who, when) as well as how others are likely to respond and react in a given environment. Since their original description, Social Stories™ or social narratives have been used in countless situations and now are among the identified evidence-based practices (see Chapter 2). Numerous research studies have found them to be an efficacious tool in a variety of conditions (Ali and Frederickson, 2006) including teaching appropriate play skills (Barry and Burlew, 2004), decreasing disruptive behaviors (Crozier and Tincani, 2005; Scattone *et al.*, 2002), improving levels of physical activity (Zimbelman *et al.*, 2007), reducing precursors to tantrum behavior (Kuttler, Myles, and Carlson, 1998; Lorimer *et al.*, 2002), changing problematic lunchtime behavior (Toplis and Hadwin, 2006), improving mealtime skills (Bledsoe, Myles, and Simpson, 2003), and increasing prosocial behavior (Ivey, Heflin, and Alberto, 2004; Norris and Dattilo, 1999).

While Gray's original intention was for Social Stories™ to be used for students with ASD, their clinical and research usage has extended beyond this population. Soenksen and Alper (2006) used a Social Story™ to teach a child diagnosed with hyperlexia to appropriately gain peers' attention. In their extensive survey of teachers who use Social Stories™, Reynhout and Carter (2009) found that educators implement Social Stories™ for students across the full range of ASD, cognitive, and expressive language abilities, and for students with low-level receptive language abilities. These teachers found Social Stories™ to be an intervention that was both effective and easy to create and to personalize.

While the bulk of research has focused on a typical presentation of Social Stories™, other investigators have devised variants in implementation. Sansosti and Powell-Smith (2008) combined a computer-presented Social Story™ along with video models to improve social communication skills. Hagiwara and Myles (1999) employed a multi-media Social Story™ intervention while Thiemann and Goldstein (2001) paired Social Stories™ with video feedback. A further adaptation, setting Social Stories™ to music, is the focus of this chapter.

Music therapy interventions to modify behavior

The use of music therapy interventions to modify behaviors in individuals with ASD is well documented in the research literature. Children within this population are often regarded as having a strength for visual learning (Grandin, 1995), but an auditory preference can be observed when the stimulus is music (Kolko, Anderson, and Campbell, 1980). As early as 1943, Leo Kanner mentioned high musical abilities and capacity to memorize and sing songs; Sherwin (1953) documented a memory for melody and preference for singing over speech in children with ASD. Blackstock (1978) noted a partiality for sung over spoken versions of song lyrics while Thaut (1987) observed that children with ASD favored listening to music over looking at visual slides for significantly longer periods of time than did typically developing peers. Thaut (1988) also found that children in this population perform well in musical tasks and respond more frequently and appropriately to music as opposed to other auditory stimuli. More recent studies (Heaton, 2003, 2005; Heaton *et al.*, 2007) report that high-functioning children with ASD have significantly better skills than their age- and intelligence-matched controls in some areas of musical aptitude but not in others. Building on these musical interests and abilities to memorize both melodies and song lyrics, researchers have incorporated pertinent information into song lyrics, using them to help sequence, categorize, and generalize tasks (Gfeller, 1983; Jellison and Miller, 1982; Wolfe and Horn, 1993). To increase the independence and memorization of multiple-step self-care tasks, Kern, Wakeford, and Aldridge (2007) added songs into a classroom routine designed to prompt the necessary steps toward task completion. Individually composed songs were implemented by Kern, Wolery, and Aldridge (2007) to prompt morning greeting behavior. Music has also been used to help children with ASD better understand emotional states (Hinze, Larkin, and Stanton, 2008; Katagiri, 2009; Ziv and Goshen, 2006), providing an auditory context for the emotional content of stories.

Salient to the rationale for incorporating music with Social Stories™ is research suggesting that singing along with song texts can help students remember rules of social and emotional interaction with others (Brownell, 2002; Buday, 1995; Pasiali, 2004; Wimpory, Chadwick, and Nash, 1995). Pasiali (2004) used "piggyback" songs (whereby the lyrics of familiar, well-known songs are altered) to convey pertinent social information and appropriate responses. Results suggested that children with ASD tend to follow directions embedded in song lyrics. Brownell (2002) utilized Gray's recommendation for Social Story™ construction, setting the stories to original music. The sung versions of these stories were found to be at least as effective in modifying problem behaviors as their traditionally read counterparts; in one instance, the sung version was found to be more effective than the read version.

Building a basic Social Story™

Four basic sentence types form the backbone of a Social Story™ (Gray, 1998; Gray and Garrand, 1993). *Descriptive Sentences* are one of the most important types. They objectively describe the context in which the target behavior is occurring. These sentences typically answer *who, where, when,* and *why* questions. They should be written with room for variability, for example, "We usually go to music class on Tuesday" as opposed to "We go to music class on Tuesday." *Directive Sentences* define the expectations of the student. These sentences are used sparingly because Social Stories™ should not be a long list of directions and orders. The wording of *Directive Sentences* should be positive and flexible. Wording such as "I will try…" is preferred over the more rigid "I will…" *Perspective Sentences* describe how other people might feel, act, or respond in a given situation, for example, "When I yell, Mom might feel angry." The final sentence type, *Control Sentences,* may not be used in every story. These are sometimes written by older students and function as a mnemonic to recall the content of the story. All sentences should be written with the student's reading and cognitive levels in mind.

Table 6.1 Social Story™ Example 1: "Personal Space in Playground Line"	
Original sentence	**Sentence type**
At playground time, my teacher will tell all the kids to go line up by the door.	Descriptive
No one can go outside until everyone is in line.	Descriptive
All of my friends are very excited to go out and play.	Perspective
Some of them might be jumping around while waiting in line.	Descriptive
If I stand too close to my friends while they're jumping, they might bump into me.	Descriptive
Sometimes this makes me feel like they're being mean to me.	Perspective
They're not trying to hurt me or be mean.	Perspective
They're just feeling very excited to go out to play with each other and me.	Perspective
If I don't want them to bump into me, I can go stand at the end of the line.	Directive
I can also take a few steps away from my friends.	Directive
When I'm standing further away, I won't get bumped into.	Descriptive
Then we can all go out and play on the playground.	Descriptive
Social Story™ ratio maintained: Descriptive (6) + Perspective (4) = 10; Directive = 2	

To ensure that Social Stories™ are used primarily for describing a social situation as opposed to providing a list of rules, Gray (1997) created the basic Social Story™ ratio of 0–1 *Directive* or *Control Sentences* for every 2–5 *Descriptive* and/or *Perspective Sentences*. As an example, two basic Social Stories™ are used throughout this chapter. Notice the importance of adhering to the Social Story™ ratio, resulting in stories that spend most of their time describing the environment and the actions of others. The first story example, "Personal Space in Playground Line" (see Table 6.1), deals with maintaining distance from peers in a crowded, excitable situation. "Quiet Times at School" (see Table 6.2) discusses when it is appropriate to talk at school.

Table 6.2 Social Story™ Example 2: "Quiet Times at School"	
Original sentence	**Sentence type**
There are lots of people I know at school.	Descriptive
I might see friends, teachers, and parents.	Descriptive
Sometimes it's okay for me to talk, like during play group or circle time.	Descriptive
Nap time and story time are quiet times at school.	Descriptive
I should just listen during nap and story times.	Directive
Other kids are trying to rest during nap time.	Perspective
The kids are trying to hear the teacher during story time.	Perspective
If I talk during quiet times, I might be bothering my friends.	Perspective
We can talk when quiet time is over.	Descriptive
I should just listen during quiet times at school.	Directive
Social Story™ ratio maintained: Descriptive (5) + Perspective (3) = 8; Directive = 2	

Swaggart *et al.* (1995, pp. 14–15) developed a ten-step procedure for producing a Social Story™, implementing the story into children's daily routines and evaluating its efficacy:

1. Identify a target behavior or problem situation for Social Story™ intervention.

2. Define target behaviors for data collection.

3. Collect baseline data on the target social behavior.

4. Write a short story using descriptive, directive, perspective, and control sentences.

5. Place one to three sentences per page.

6. Use photographs, hand-drawn pictures, or pictorial icons.

7. Read the Social Story™ to the student and model the desired behavior.

8. Collect intervention data.

9. Review intervention data.

10. Review the findings and related Social Story™ procedures.

When creating the pages of the story themselves, base the level of detail upon the individual needs of the child. Photographs may be too detailed for some children who would be unable to generalize if the depicted environment changed in some way (Gray, 1994). Icons are easily added and allow for a more general representation of the story. The content of the story, not the sophistication of the book or pages, is most important to students and should be the focus of their attention.

Setting the story to music

Just as the visual appeal of a traditional Social Story™ is secondary to the actual descriptive content of the story, a musical adaptation of a Social Story™ is not about creating the most sophisticated, complicated rhythms, melodies, or harmonies. Melodies should be simple and memorable. Harmonies should be straightforward and reflect the mood of the story.

Katagiri (2009) found that appropriately matched background music succeeded in improving emotional understanding of song texts. The musical component functions to supplement the content of the story by:

1. encouraging student engagement

2. promoting active participation

3. serving as an additional tool to aid in memory and recall

4. providing a natural and appropriate environment for repetition.

The same visuals used in a traditional Social Story™ can be incorporated into the musical presentation, making for a truly multisensory intervention. A musically adapted Social Story™ can be created by anyone: music therapists and/or educators, special education team members, or parents, to name a few. They also can be created as part of an interdisciplinary team approach, with the story being written by a team member trained in their writing and the musical adaptation being composed by another with musical inclinations.

Original or "piggyback"

In creating a Social Story™ set to music, the question of whether to use original music or a "piggyback" song is significant. Brownell (2002) and Kern, Wolery, and Aldridge (2007) used original music and Pasiali (2004) used "piggyback" songs; both were found to be effective conduits of information. Kern, Wakeford, and Aldridge (2007) utilized both original and "piggyback" songs, but suggested that familiar music promoted greater learning than unfamiliar. The final decision should be based on a number of factors:

1. *The musical skill and comfort level of the clinician:* While music therapists may have more flexibility in this regard, teachers, other professionals, and parents should feel confident in creating songs of their own. If creating original melodies seems daunting, utilizing a familiar melody from a song already known to the child is a convenient, effective alternative.

2. *Adaptability of lyrics:* Maintaining the basic Social Story™ ratio and appropriately utilizing the four basic sentence types is paramount. However, after the story is complete it may be necessary to slightly alter the wording of sentences to make them fit comfortably into the contours of a melody. This is especially true if using a "piggyback" song, where significant alteration of the story text may be necessary. The length and complexity of the story, as well as the degree to which the wording can be realistically and successfully altered, will have a bearing on whether or not to use an original melody. If the story's wording cannot fit into a known melody without distorting its meaning or compromising the Social Story™ ratio, a different melody or song may have to be used.

3. *Preference of the student:* Some children may be naturally drawn to familiar, recognizable melodies while others may display an ability to pick up and retain original tunes. Age appropriateness of songs used for piggybacking should be considered.

4. *Length of time the story/song will be used:* If the Social Story™ and its musical adaptation are to be used for a short-term behavioral intervention, a song that is more recognizable and immediately memorable may be preferred. Long-term usage may warrant the composition of an original melody.

Both an original and "piggyback" version of the two basic Social Stories™ presented earlier are included here (see Figures 6.1–6.4). Notice how the lyrics are slightly different in each version; nevertheless, the Social Story™ ratio is maintained.

Personal Space in Playground Line

to the tune of "Take Me Out to the Ball Game"

Adapted Lyrics: Mike D. Brownell, MME, MT-BC   Original Melody: Albert von Tilzer

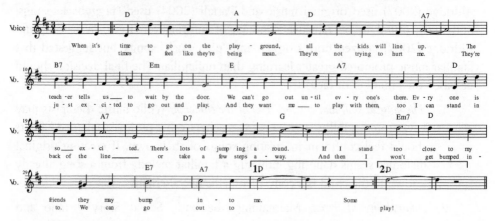

Figure 6.1: Song example for "Personal Space in Playground Line"—"Piggyback"

Personal Space in Playground Line

Words and Music by: Mike D. Brownell, MME, MT-BC

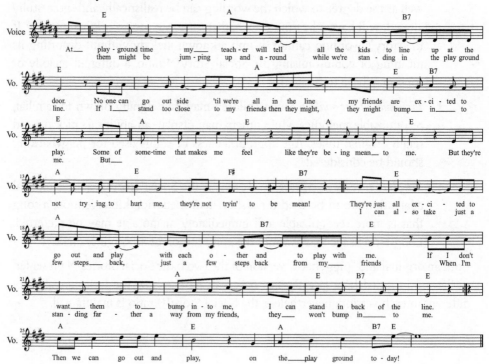

Copyright © 2012 Mike D. Brownell

Figure 6.2: Song example for "Personal Space in Playground Line"—Original

Quiet Times at School

to the tune of "She'll Be Comin' 'Round the Mountain"

Adapted Lyrics: Mike D. Brownell, MME, MT-BC

American Folk Melody

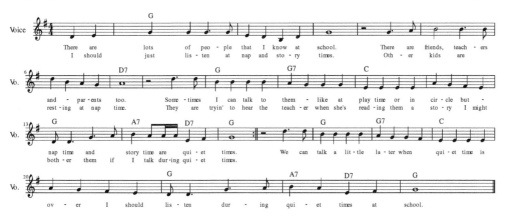

Figure 6.3: Song example for "Quiet Times at School"—"Piggyback"

Quiet Times at School

Words and Music by: Mike D. Brownell, MME, MT-BC

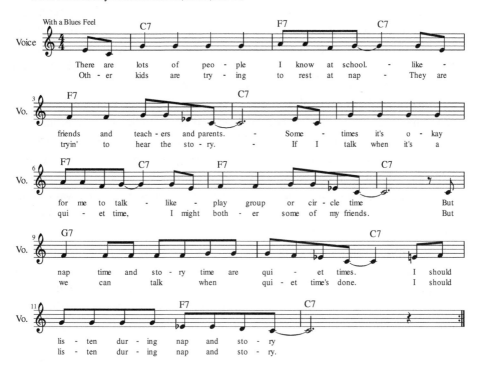

Copyright © 2012 Mike D. Brownell

Figure 6.4: Song example for "Quiet Times at School"—Original

Presentation

The same previously outlined ten-step procedure by Swaggart *et al.* (1995) can be used when incorporating a musically adapted Social Story™ and monitoring its efficacy. A printed version of the story provides a visual of the song lyrics and can be followed along, page by page, as the song is being sung. Icons, photos, or drawings should be incorporated on each page, just as they would be in a traditional Social Story™. The choice of which type of visual representation is used is dependent upon the individual child; for some, a photograph may depict an environment in an overly rigid manner while an icon conveys a more general representation. The song should be presented to the student immediately before the targeted social situation is to occur but the song and its accompanying book can be accessible all day long. Reynhout and Carter (2009) found that many educators allowed students to have access to their Social Stories™ throughout the day.

The exact method of presenting the song can be highly flexible and adaptable to the individual needs of each child. Early childhood educators, practitioners, parents, and even siblings and peers can perform the song with the child. Those comfortable with doing so can sing the song live or provide simple harmony on an accompanying instrument. Live performance has the added benefits of permitting the tempo of the song to be adapted in the moment, and allowing for pauses in the music for the student to make comments or ask questions. The child should be encouraged to actively participate rather than merely being sung to; they can sing along or independently sing the song once they become familiar with it. Children with limited or burgeoning verbal skills can be encouraged to sing selected words or phrases from the song rather than the complete lyrics. For the child participating or singing the song independently, vocal quality and musicality are not paramount. Adults singing the song need not have a flawless vocal delivery. In line with recommendations made by Kern, Wakeford, and Aldridge (2007), a positive, engaging tone of voice and facial expression should be used along with making eye contact with the student. If a live performance is selected, uniformity is recommended. If an accompanying instrument is used, it should be used every time; additionally, the song always should be sung in the same key. This consistency keeps the focus on the content of the song rather than on variability in the way it is presented.

One way to ensure homogeneity of performance is to use a recorded version of the song. This is also a helpful option for those who may not be comfortable singing live. A music therapist, music teacher, or any other musically inclined team member can produce the recording. As in live performances, musical perfection is not necessary. Efforts should be made to create a recording that is at an appropriate tempo and in which the lyrics are clearly audible. The media on which the song is recorded is open to the needs and abilities of the individual. Compact disc players and digital media devices/Mp3 players are readily available and often are familiar to children. These devices are portable, allowing children to take their song right into the environment being targeted by the Social Story™ or wherever else it may be helpful. Children can listen unobtrusively to their songs on headphones in locations where a live performance may be disruptive.

Conclusion

Setting Social Stories™—a frequently used and well-vetted intervention—to music provides young learners with ASD with yet another avenue to access pertinent social information. The musical aspect of this adaptation may allow a more engaging, interactive experience while also serving as a mnemonic device. Just as Social Stories™ can be created by parents and professionals alike, so, too, can a musical version be fashioned by anyone regardless of musical training. However, those who are not sure how to apply music to a Social Story™ may consult with a certified music therapist.

LEARNING QUESTIONS

1. What is the basic function of a Social Story™?

2. Describe the four main sentence types used in Social Stories™.

3. What is the basic Social Story™ ratio?

4. What are some considerations when deciding between an original or "piggyback" melody?

5. Who can sing the adapted songs with the child?

6. In what ways must the preferences of the child be taken into consideration?

7. What are some different ways that the songs can be presented to the child?

References

Ali, S., and Frederickson, N. (2006). Investigating the evidence base of Social Stories™. *Educational Psychology in Practice, 22*, 355–377.

Barry, L.M., and Burlew, S.B. (2004). Using Social Stories™ to teach choice and play skills to children with autism. *Focus on Autism and Other Developmental Disabilities, 19*, 45–51.

Blackstock, E.G. (1978). Cerebral asymmetry and the development of early infantile autism. *Journal of Autism and Childhood Schizophrenia, 8*, 339–353.

Bledsoe, R., Myles, B.S., and Simpson, R.L. (2003). Use of a Social Story™ intervention to improve mealtime skills of an adolescent with Asperger syndrome. *Autism, 7*, 289–295.

Brownell, M.D. (2002). Musically adapted Social Stories™ to modify behaviors in students with autism: Four case studies. *Journal of Music Therapy, 39,* 117–144.

Buday, E.M. (1995). The effects of signed and spoken words taught with music on sign and speech imitation by children with autism. *Journal of Music Therapy, 32,* 189–202.

Crozier, S., and Tincani, M.J. (2005). Using a modified Social Story™ to decrease disruptive behavior of a child with autism. *Focus on Autism and Other Developmental Disabilities, 20,* 150–157.

Gfeller, K.E. (1983). Musical mnemonics as an aid to retention with normal and learning disabled students. *Journal of Music Therapy, 20,* 179–189.

Grandin, T. (1995). The learning style of people with autism: An autobiography. In K. Quill (Ed.) *Teaching Children with Autism: Strategies to Enhance Communication and Socialization.* New York: Delmar.

Gray, C.A. (1994). *The New Social Story™ Book.* Arlington, TX: Future Horizons.

Gray, C.A. (1997). Your concerns result in a new Social Story™ ratio: A close look at directive sentences. *Access Express, 4(3),* 4–5.

Gray, C.A. (1998). Social Stories™ and comic book conversations with students with Asperger syndrome and high-functioning autism. In E. Schopler, G.V. Mesibov, and L.J. Kunce (Eds.) *Asperger Syndrome or High-Functioning Autism?* New York: Plenum Press.

Gray, C.A., and Garrand, J. (1993). Social Stories™: Improving responses of individuals with autism with accurate social information. *Focus on Autistic Behavior, 8,* 1–10.

Hagiwara, T., and Myles, B.S. (1999). A multimedia Social Story™ intervention: Teaching skills to children with autism. *Focus on Autism and Other Developmental Disabilities, 14,* 82–91.

Heaton, P. (2003). Pitch memory, labeling and disembedding in autism. *Journal of Child Psychology and Psychiatry and Allied Disciplines, 44(4),* 543–551.

Heaton, P. (2005). Interval and contour processing in autism. *Journal of Autism and Developmental Disorders, 25(6),* 787–793.

Heaton, P., Williams, K., Cummins, O., and Happe, F.G.E. (2007). Beyond perception: Musical representation and on-line processing in autism. *Journal of Autism and Developmental Disorders, 27(7),* 1355–1360.

Hinze, R.M., Larkin, C.A., and Stanton, G.M. (2008). The effect of music on enhancing the learning process of emotion identification in children with autism spectrum disorder. Unpublished master's thesis, State University of New York, New York.

Ivey, M., Heflin, J., and Alberto, P. (2004). The use of Social Stories™ to promote independent behaviors in novel events for children with PDD-NOS. *Focus on Autism and Other Developmental Disabilities, 19(3),* 164–176.

Jellison, J.A., and Miller, N.I. (1982). Recall of digit and word sequences by musicians and nonmusicians as a function of spoken and sung input and task. *Journal of Music Therapy, 19,* 102–113.

Kanner, L. (1943). Early infantile autism. *Journal of Pediatrics, 25,* 211–217.

Katagiri, J. (2009). The effect of background music and song texts on the emotional understanding of children with autism. *Journal of Music Therapy, 46,* 15–31.

Kern, P., Wakeford, L., and Aldridge, D. (2007). Improving the performance of a young child with autism during self-care tasks using embedded song interventions: A case study. *Music Therapy Perspectives, 25,* 43–51.

Kern, P., Wolery, M., and Aldridge, D. (2007). Use of songs to promote independence in morning greeting routines for young children with autism. *Journal of Autism and Developmental Disorders, 37,* 1264–1271.

Kolko, D.J., Anderson, L., and Campbell, M. (1980). Sensory preference and over-selective responding in autistic children. *Journal of Autism and Developmental Disorders, 10,* 259–271.

Kuttler, S., Myles, B.S., and Carlson, J.K. (1998). The use of Social Stories™ to reduce precursors to tantrum behavior in a student with autism. *Focus on Autism and Other Developmental Disabilities, 13,* 176–182.

Lorimer, P.A., Simpson, R.L., Myles, B.S., and Ganz, J.B. (2002). The use of Social Stories™ as a preventative behavioral intervention in a home setting with a child with autism. *Journal of Positive Behavior Interventions, 2002, 4 (1),* 53–60.

Norris, C., and Dattilo, J. (1999). Evaluating effects of a Social Story™ intervention on a young girl with autism. *Focus on Autism and Other Developmental Disabilities, 14,* 180–186.

Pasiali, V. (2004). The use of prescriptive therapeutic songs in a home-based environment to promote socials skills acquisition by children with autism: Three case studies. *Music Therapy Perspectives, 22,* 11–20.

Reynhout, G., and Carter, M. (2009). The use of Social Stories™ by teachers and their perceived efficacy. *Research in Autism Spectrum Disorders, 3,* 232–251.

Sansosti, F.J., and Powell-Smith, K.A. (2008). Using computer-presented Social Stories™ and video models to increase the social communication skills of children with high-functioning autism spectrum disorders. *Journal of Positive Behavior Interventions, 10,* 162–178.

Scattone, D., Wilczynski, S.M., Edwards, R.P., Rabain, B. (2002). Decreasing disruptive behaviors of children with autism using Social Stories™. *Journal of Autism and Developmental Disorders, 32,* 535–543.

Sherwin, A.C. (1953). Reactions to music of autistic (schizophrenic) children. *American Journal of Psychiatry, 109,* 823–831.

Soenksen, D., and Alper, S. (2006). Teaching a young child to appropriately gain attention of peers using a Social Story™ intervention. *Focus on Autism and Other Developmental Disabilities,21,* 36–44.

Swaggart, B.L., Gagnon, E., Bock, S.J., Earles, T.L., *et al.* (1995). Using Social Stories™ to teach social and behavioral skills to children with autism. *Focus on Autistic Behavior, 10(1),* 1–16.

Thaut, M.H. (1987). Visual versus auditory (musical) stimulus preferences in autistic children: A pilot study. *Journal of Autism and Developmental Disorders, 17,* 425–432.

Thaut, M.H. (1988). Measuring musical responsiveness in autistic children: A comparative analysis of improvised musical tone sequences of autistic, normal, and mentally retarded individuals. *Journal of Autism and Developmental Disorders, 18,* 561–571.

Thiemann, K.S., and Goldstein, H. (2001). Social Stories™, written text cues, and video feedback: Effects on social communication of children with autism. *Journal of Applied Behavior Analysis, 34,* 425–446.

Toplis, R., and Hadwin, J.A. (2006). Using Social Stories™ to change problematic lunchtime behaviour in school. *Educational Psychology in Practice, 22,* 53–67.

Wimpory, D., Chadwick, P., and Nash, S. (1995). Brief report. Musical interaction therapy for children with autism: An evaluative case study and two-year follow-up. *Journal of Autism and Developmental Disorders, 25,* 541–552.

Wolfe, D., and Horn, C. (1993). Use of melodies as a structural prompt for learning and retention of sequential verbal information by preschool students. *Journal of Music Therapy, 30,* 100–118.

Zimbelman, M., Paschal, A., Hawley, S.R., Molgaard, C.A., and St. Romain, T. (2007). Addressing physical inactivity among developmentally disabled students through visual schedules and Social Stories™. *Research in Developmental Disabilities, 28,* 386–396.

Ziv, N., and Goshen, M. (2006). The effect of "sad" and "happy" background music on the interpretation of a story in 5 to 6-year-old children. *British Journal of Music Education, 23,* 303–314.

Chapter 7

Nordoff-Robbins Music Therapy

An Expressive and Dynamic Approach for Young Children on the Autism Spectrum

Nina Guerrero, M.A., MT-BC, LCAT
Alan Turry, D.A., MT-BC, LCAT
NORDOFF-ROBBINS CENTER FOR MUSIC THERAPY
STEINHARDT SCHOOL OF CULTURE, EDUCATION,
AND HUMAN DEVELOPMENT
NEW YORK UNIVERSITY
NEW YORK, NY

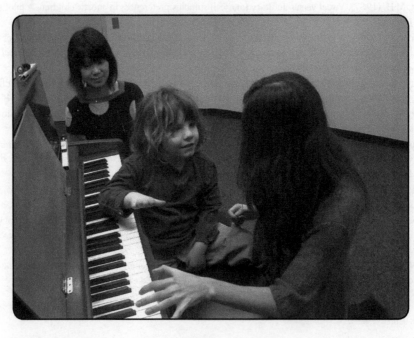

Collaborative improvisation allows the therapist to respond to subtle cues in children's expression and activity, and cultivates their spontaneity, flexibility, and initiative; through this creative partnership, the therapeutic relationship develops and developmental goals are continually addressed.
(Nina Guerrero and Alan Turry)

Paul Nordoff, American pianist and composer, and Clive Robbins, British special educator, were true pioneers in working with young children with autism spectrum disorders (ASD). Their collaboration began in 1959 at the Sunfield Children's Home in Worcestershire, United Kingdom. Together they plumbed the depth and breadth, the strength and intensity of clinical possibilities in the human response to music, establishing dynamic therapeutic relationships through musical exchange. The Nordoff-Robbins approach has expanded internationally into a wide range of settings and populations, maintaining its ongoing commitment to children with ASD. This chapter explores the use of Nordoff-Robbins music therapy to enhance the development of young children with ASD, particularly in the domains of communication and social interaction. It includes the principles and process of therapy, a brief case vignette, and a snapshot of a community-based research project.

Principles of Nordoff-Robbins music therapy
The music child

Central to the Nordoff-Robbins approach is the concept of the *music child*: "The individualized musicality inborn in every child," which reflects both "the universality of human musical sensitivity—the heritage of complex and subtle sensitivity to the ordering and relationship of tonal and rhythmic movement"—and the "uniquely personal significance of each child's musical responsiveness" (Nordoff and Robbins, 2007, p. 3). According to Nordoff and Robbins (2007), in the music child resides the healthy core potential for growth and development that exists within all human beings, adults as well as children, irrespective of disabilities.

Musical interactions as the essence of therapy

Nordoff-Robbins music therapy addresses therapeutic goals via in-depth utilization of the structural and expressive elements of both improvised and precomposed music. Musical interactions between child, therapist, and co-therapist, or among children in a group, constitute the essence of the therapy. "Change is accomplished in and through musical processes and transfers from these into the life of the client outside the therapy room" (Turry and Marcus, 2003, p. 199; Trevarthen *et al.*, 1998). Children are engaged in interactive music-making (using a variety of percussive and melodic instruments, vocalization, expressive movement, and dramatic play) to stimulate and develop self-awareness, self-regulation, communication, creative expression, and relationship. Specialized techniques of clinical improvisation enable therapists to individualize interventions to build upon each child's unique strengths while addressing his or her social, emotional, cognitive, and physical needs. Key aspects of children's self-presentation are reflected by the therapist's music, drawing them into increasingly reciprocal musical interaction. Collaborative improvisation allows the therapist to respond to subtle cues in children's expression and activity, and cultivates their spontaneity, flexibility, and initiative. Through this creative partnership, the therapeutic relationship develops and developmental goals are continually addressed (Nordoff and Robbins, 2007).

This approach seeks to cultivate children's intrinsic desire to engage with others (Aigen, 1998; Nordoff and Robbins, 2007), strengthening their motivation toward positive activity and broadening their range of expression through engaging them in a creative process (Turry and Marcus, 2003). Sessions are offered in both individual and small-group format; groups often integrate children on the autism spectrum with children who have various other needs or disabilities.

Developing communication and social interaction through shared music-making

Nordoff-Robbins music therapy draws upon expressive qualities, dynamic form, and capacity for dialogue inherent in music to address communication and social interaction issues of children with ASD (Trevarthen, 1999; Wigram and Gold, 2006), deeply exploring the communicative potential of music and seeking to activate the universal human capacities for musical perception and response that are uniquely manifested in each client (Aigen, 1998; Nordoff and Robbins, 2007; Robbins, 1993). Engagement through music may build non-verbal interactive skills that are required for effective communication, and support the emergence of functional verbal skills (Kim, Wigram, and Gold, 2009; Trevarthen et al., 1998).

Nordoff-Robbins music therapy for children with ASD emphasizes interactive elements of communication (e.g., turn-taking, call and response, and reciprocal exchange). In both precomposed songs and improvisation, musical structure is designed to leave space for the child's contributions such as playing short phrases followed by pauses (i.e., to evoke the child's attention and response). Children are encouraged to develop skills in both responding to and initiating musical and verbal communication. Improvisation promotes spontaneity and playful exchange, and motivates communication by allowing children to explore and express their interests (Nordoff and Robbins, 2007); the therapist can immediately respond to a child's verbal or musical expression, placing it in a meaningful context. Although the therapist's music is spontaneously improvised, it is clearly structured by (a) a defined key, (b) a melodic idea that is repeated, and (c) phrasing that creates a meter. Noting the child's body language, facial expressions, movements, and vocalizations, the therapist attempts to match the child's emotional state and temperament and create a musical portrait of the child.

Three related aspects of communicative interaction are evident in clinical improvisation: *social reciprocity*, *mirroring (or imitation)*; and *emotional attunement and shared attention*.

SOCIAL RECIPROCITY

Social reciprocity is a vital force in shaping young children's development of perceptual, expressive, affective, cognitive, and motor functioning, and may be considered the "foundation of human communication" (Wigram and Gold, 2006, p. 536). While children with ASD may be significantly limited in their verbal skills and also in non-verbal elements of communication involved in social reciprocity (e.g., speech prosody, pragmatics, eye contact, facial expression), their innate musicality may remain relatively intact; engagement through music may thus be a basis for their development of relationships and communication (Lim, 2010; Silverman, 2008; Trevarthen *et al.*, 1998; Wigram and Gold, 2006).

The "protoconversation" of infant and caregiver is a richly musical exchange characterized by mutually responsive shifts in rhythm, phrasing, melody, and dynamics (Trevarthen, 1980). However, for young children with ASD and their parents, this exchange often does not develop spontaneously. Music therapy interventions may include coaching parents as well as providing opportunities for children with ASD to practice and experience such musical reciprocity (see Chapter 13 for additional information). Collaborative improvisation may offer an opportunity to perceive and respond to the expressive qualities of each other's instrument-playing, vocalization, or movement. Music-making allows for meaningful interpersonal response through both simultaneous and sequential participation (i.e., playing or singing together with others or taking turns). Communication typically emerges in early development as caregivers make their actions contingent upon the infant's spontaneous facial expressions, movements, and sounds, thus giving these responses meaning. The infant is able to exercise this newfound meaning "by repeating a movement, gesture or sound which 'caused' an adult response" (Stern, 1990, p. 45). In musical improvisation, similarly, the therapist creates music that is contingent upon the client's spontaneous acts, placing these acts within a framework of musical exchange. It is the growing perception of contingency between one's own expressive acts and others'—of reciprocal influence between them—that renders these acts communicative. For children with ASD, the motivation to repeat or to be reciprocal could be the enticement of novel sounds or other stimuli. Over time, the improvisation of music with dynamically varying patterns may evoke attention, create awareness of others, and draw children with ASD into shared expressive activity.

MIRRORING (OR IMITATION)

The reciprocal understanding essential to communication depends upon individuals' implicit ability to imitate or "mirror" each other's actions and expression (Trevarthen, 2005). As described by Rizzolatti, Fogassi, and Gallese (2006, p. 61), mirroring involves direct comprehension, in which "no previous agreement between individuals—on arbitrary symbols, for instance—is needed for them to understand each other. The accord is inherent in the neural organization of both people," permitting them "to connect wordlessly." Typically, even newborns can instinctively mirror or imitate simple facial expressions, such as sticking out the tongue. The absence of such responses is often evident in young children with ASD (National Institue of Health [NIH], 2011). Various neuroscientists have located neurological mechanisms for the mirroring of gestures, language, and emotions, which they have termed the mirror neuron system (MNS). Investigators note that this system may be compromised in individuals with ASD (Hadjikhani, 2007; Ramachandran and Oberman, 2006; Rizzolatti, Fogassi, and Gallese, 2006). Hadjikhani (2007) argues that early therapeutic intervention to enhance mirror neuron capabilities for young children with ASD might be more productive than later attempts to focus on more complex behaviors that become consequences of unaddressed mirror neuron deficits. Shared music-making may provide a means to cultivate experiences of synchrony and reciprocity through mirroring (Koelsch, 2009; Overy and Molnar-Szakacs, 2009; Wan *et al.*, 2010).

EMOTIONAL ATTUNEMENT AND SHARED ATTENTION

Like preverbal parent–infant interaction, communication through musical interaction entails emotional attunement. A prerequisite to attunement is shared attention. Behavioral intervention targeting shared attention may enhance social initiative, imitation, and spontaneous speech in children with ASD (Whalen, Schreibman, and Ingersoll, 2006). In Nordoff-Robbins music therapy, shared attention may begin with the therapist's sensitive, moment-to-moment musical responses to shifts in the child's attention and interest. As the child becomes increasingly aware of the therapist's presence, he may begin to seek shared attention with the therapist in music-making. The process of attunement involves interpretive reflection rather than simple imitation. For example, a mother may show she understands her infant by responding with actions that are different from his but share common qualities; her actions are not copies of his, but "translations" that demonstrate he has made sense to her. As Benjamin (1988) argues, the experience of attunement requires mutual recognition. The understanding of this response may be lacking in young children with ASD.

Interactive music-making such as interpretive reflection may help to provide various avenues leading to attunement. In Nordoff-Robbins clinical improvisation, the therapist's music-making does not mimic the child's, but rather communicates a response by using the various musical elements (e.g., rhythm, tempo, dynamics, melody, harmony, and timbre) to reflect qualities of the child's expression. The therapist's creative flexibility of response is conducive to the child's emerging awareness of the therapist as a separate being with whom he can communicate and interact. The child is drawn into an experience of mutual listening. Perceiving that the therapist's music is related to his own but is independently unfolding, the child may be drawn to create variation in his own playing and singing, and to anticipate the therapist's response (Pavlicevic, 1997).

Clinical process

Assessment and treatment plan

In the Nordoff-Robbins approach, specific goals for each child are identified at the outset of therapy through an assessment process consisting of an intake session with the child and an interview with his or her parents or caregivers. The *Individualized Family Services Plan* or *Individualized Education Program* and evaluations by other therapy providers are reviewed. Parents also complete a developmental questionnaire, the *Vineland Adaptive Behavior Scales, Second Edition* (Vineland-II) (Sparrow, Balla, and Cicchetti, 2005).

Session format

Weekly 30-minute sessions are led by a team of two therapists: The primary therapist creates the musical framework for the session on piano or guitar, while the co-therapist supports the child's musical activity and interaction. Table 7.1 outlines a typical format for individual sessions with a child with ASD. Video examples of Nordoff-Robbins music therapy sessions can be reviewed at the First Signs ASD Video Glossary (see www.firstsigns.org/asd_video_glossary/asdvg_about.htm).

Evaluation

Since the earliest work of Paul Nordoff and Clive Robbins, session recording and analysis have been standard practice within this approach. With parents' written consent, every therapy session is videotaped and analyzed to prepare for forthcoming sessions and review the course of therapy over time. Detailed clinical notes (an "index" based on videotape review of each session) are compiled; indexing may include detailed transcription of therapists' and clients' music-making. In addition, the *Music Therapy Communication* and *Social Interaction* scale (MTCSI) (Hummel-Rossi et al., 2008) is used to rate selected sessions from the beginning, middle, and end of each clinical year for each client. The MTCSI was developed at the Nordoff-Robbins Center to code social and communicative behaviors observed in music therapy sessions, particularly in children with ASD. This instrument has yet to be validated, but promising correlations with the Vineland-II have been found in a pilot study described in the following research snapshot. Through both indexing and coding, therapists closely study session recordings: Musical and clinical developments are noted, and clients' goals and objectives are continually re-assessed. Over the course of therapy, progress toward goals and objectives is also evaluated through periodic re-administration of the Vineland-II, and consultation with parents, teachers, and other therapy providers.

Table 7.1 Session format: Typical steps of an individual Nordoff-Robbins Music Therapy session for a child with ASD	
Steps	**Content**
1	The primary therapist plays music on the piano or guitar as the co-therapist leads the child into the room. A melodic theme, often with words of greeting sung by the therapists, signifies the beginning of the session. The child is invited to join in through singing or instrument-playing. This greeting song is often improvised at first, and then re-introduced and developed in subsequent sessions. The music typically reflects the energy and temperament with which the child presents herself. By utilizing music from the very beginning moments of the session, the therapist attempts to create an environment of playful exploration for the child in which new ways of communicating and interacting are possible.
2	Next, the therapist creates different types of musical forms and assesses the child's responses, searching for aspects of the child's potential that are not readily apparent. Music is improvised to elicit and sustain positive responses and interaction, allowing the therapist to immediately pursue different clinical alternatives in response to the child's needs. The therapist's music can invite, challenge, soothe, or stimulate. As qualities of the music mirror qualities of the child's presence and actions, the child may come to identify with and take an interest in the music. The music may follow the starting and stopping of a child's running around the room, sparking the child's awareness of the therapist. The child may begin to move, vocalize, or play an instrument in a more purposeful manner that is responsive to the therapist's music. The child may offer musical initiatives that appear to seek a response from the therapist. Ultimately, the therapist aims to bring the child into a shared, communicative musical experience.
3	A precomposed piece of music may be presented, based on the child's interests and capacities. The Nordoff-Robbins repertoire of compositions addresses a variety of therapeutic goals. Compositions may feature a call-and-response or turn-taking form that can enhance communication and social interaction.
4	The session typically closes with a good-bye song, which, like the greeting song, may originate in an improvisation. The farewell song often triggers renewed communication and interaction, and may serve to review the session's events and generate anticipation for the next session.

Clinical vignette

Devon was almost four years old when he was diagnosed with ASD. His mother sadly reported that he seemed to be developing normally until the age of 18 months. At that time, she noticed he was not making good eye contact. He became less interested in relating to others. His mother observed sadly that "He stopped trying to communicate. He just lost interest." Devon was often unhappy and frustrated at home, and had difficulty sleeping.

Devon's music therapy experiences are depicted in Table 7.2 via descriptions of selected music therapy sessions, his greeting song (see Figure 7.1), comments related to his behavior, interactions with the therapists, and reflections on various aspects of the Nordoff-Robbins process.

Devon's Music Day

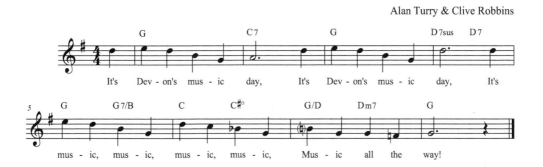

Alan Turry & Clive Robbins

Copyright © 1992 Alan Turry and Clive Robbins

Figure 7.1: Greeting song—"Devon's Music Day"

Research snapshot

Background

A pilot study examined the effects of Nordoff-Robbins music therapy on the development of communication and social interaction skills in young children with a variety of developmental delays. Since children with ASD demonstrate deficiencies in one or both of these areas, special attention was given to those participants with ASD.

Nordoff and Robbins (1965, 1968) based their early writings on descriptions, reflections, and case studies that shaped their therapeutic methodology. Some quantitative investigations of music therapy for children with ASD have been limited by small samples and have focused on narrowly defined target behaviors, using prescriptive short-term behavioral interventions (Accordino, Comer, and Heller, 2007; Wigram and Gold, 2006). There remains a need for experimental studies "examining interventions which are closer to clinical practice" (Wigram and Gold, 2006, p. 540), and exploring in greater depth the effects of music therapy in such domains as communication and social interaction.

Table 7.2 Case vignette: Nordoff-Robbins music therapy Sessions with Devon

Session	Case description	Comments
1	Shortly after being diagnosed, Devon began music therapy sessions. A gently repeated descending musical motif in the high register, improvised by the primary therapist, grabbed his attention. Though holding a toy, he immediately approached the instruments in the room—a drum, cymbal, and pentatonic xylimba—and took the mallets to join in music-making.	Therapy can build upon Devon's significant positive attributes: 1. A natural curiosity 2. Readiness to join in music-making.
	Devon began to play the drum. His playing was a bit fragmented and he moved from the drum to beat on the floor; yet Devon's *music child* was evident in his intrinsic musical sensitivity and responsiveness. He explored the instruments by playing different tempi and moving from instrument to instrument to experience their distinctive sounds. He took the mallets and played on the floor with one hand while scrubbing with the other, then resumed drumming and maintained the basic beat of the music in synchrony with the piano.	Playing the basic beat—a foundational experience that allows him to feel connected to another person and grounded in the music (Nordoff and Robbins, 2007).
	As Devon's playing increased in tempo and intensity, the therapist responded by incorporating his dynamics while creating a melodic idea and harmonic progression that enhanced the overall musical experience. The therapist anticipated the pattern that Devon was developing—rapidly playing all the notes on the xylimba, and then moving to the drum and cymbal. The therapist created a phrase that led to a cadence. As he played the final chord, Devon struck the cymbal once with great emphasis. After playing the cymbal punctuation, Devon lifted his arms over his head as if to say, "I did it—look at me!" Though his mother described him as an often unhappy and frustrated child, Devon was having a joyful and fulfilling experience. The therapist continued to play, as if to say, "Yes, that's great, but let's keep going. Let's sustain this moment of pleasure and contact." Devon seemed completely at home in this improvisational situation. Rather than appearing challenged, he seemed to enjoy the process of relating to another person through music.	*Aesthetic shaping*—the aesthetic qualities of the music motivate the child to listen and participate more fully (Turry and Marcus, 2003). The therapist is simultaneously supporting and leading the child by improvising a musical form that calls for a certain musical response. This is a seminal experience sought by the therapist, yet it is created through moment-to-moment response to the child. • Simultaneous punctuation accentuates the feeling of mutual awareness and communication. • Pause: Silence creates suspense, preceded by a diminished instead of the expected tonic chord. This evokes a sense that the music is not finished. • Musical encounters create partnership and joint attention, generating momentum, energy, and excitement. By using music to support the child's current activity while stimulating his further development, the therapist works at the child's *developmental threshold* (Nordoff and Robbins, 2007).

2	Devon again played the xylimba. He reversed his former way of playing to preserve the descending phrase he previously created, since the xylimba was incorrectly positioned with the low notes to his right. As he and the therapist paused together, Devon smiled, seemingly aware that the therapist was waiting for him.	
	The co-therapist sang improvisationally, "It's Devon's music day," capturing his bold celebratory attitude. This song (see Figure 7.1) became a "clinical theme," a melodic idea that embodied important emotional content and connection.	A defining principle of the Nordoff-Robbins approach: Emergence of memorable, dependable melodic forms that the client identifies with as his or her music (i.e., his "Hello" song).
	Devon's repetitive and restricted patterns of behavior surfaced as he moved away from the instruments and began to spin, perhaps having become overstimulated. The primary therapist shifted to ¾ meter, playing a gentle waltz, continuing the *Devon's Music Day* theme. Devon returned to the drum, shaking his head in small, rapid movements.	An advantage of improvised music: The therapist can immediately adjust the level of stimulation.
3–14	Devon shared his emotional struggles more directly. Once, he arrived upset; as the session unfolded, his crying came into the tonality of the music. Crying expressively on long tones and mirroring a phrase played by the primary therapist, Devon engaged with the therapists, jointly creating what may be an "emotional aria" expressing his distress. The therapists did not try to stop his crying, but provided a containing atmosphere in which he might feel accepted and nurtured.	Tonal crying is carefully evaluated by the therapist: • How does the vocalization relate to the music? • How can the therapist best support the child? Insofar as the child feels the therapist's emotional attunement, difficult emotions may be expressed through mutual musical creation.
	After this session, Devon continued to look forward to music therapy; his mother reported that it was the happiest time of his week.	
Final session and follow-up	In the fifteenth session, Devon displayed increased capability in handling instruments, freedom in making choices, and willingness to share experiences in a musical partnership. The repetition of *Devon's Music Day* over time helped him exhibit flexibility and inter-responsiveness within the music. He could play a slow steady beat in a relaxed, deliberate manner, both gently and boldly. The increased intimacy of the therapeutic relationship was vividly manifested as he and the primary therapist played the guitar and sang in close proximity to each other. Over a year after treatment termination, Devon's mother reported that he was doing well, singing all the time, more communicative with his parents, and generally much happier. She offered the following remark: "You led him, but you made him think he was leading you… He is so much more confident since music therapy—he's much more focused. This is spreading to the home. Devon's personality has blossomed, largely due to music therapy."		

Chapter 3 provides more in-depth discussion of music therapy research pertaining to young children with ASD.

The present pilot study addressed the following questions:

1. What changes in communication and social interaction behaviors may occur over time in young children with ASD receiving Nordoff-Robbins music therapy, as measured on the Vineland-II developmental questionnaire?

2. What changes in communication and social interaction behaviors may be observed over time in these children within their music therapy sessions, using the MTCSI?

3. How might changes over time in children's communication and social interaction profiles on the Vineland-II relate to changes in their MTCSI ratings?

Method

SETTING

The pilot study was conducted over the course of an academic year at *These Our Treasures School* (TOTS) in the southeast Bronx, New York. TOTS grew from a grass-roots initiative of parents in the community. It provides comprehensive early intervention services (both home- and center-based) and preschool special education to children from birth to age five with developmental disabilities. A Nordoff-Robbins music therapy program, established at TOTS in 2005, has earned the high regard of parents, staff, and administrators.

PARTICIPANTS

Participants were 36 children aged two through five years with various developmental delays; 18 were diagnosed with ASD. Approximately half of the children received music therapy in the fall semester only (the experimental group), and half in the spring semester only (the control group). This standard allocation of music therapy services at the school ensures that all students receive music therapy despite budget limitations. Children with ASD were distributed fairly evenly between the fall and spring cohorts.

RESEARCH DESIGN, DATA COLLECTION, AND PROCEDURE

Music therapy was offered in 30-minute group sessions once a week. In this quasi-experimental group design study, parents and teachers of all children in the study completed the Vineland-II at the beginning, middle, and end of the academic year. In both semesters, music therapy sessions were videotaped at the beginning, middle, and end of therapy; sessions were coded for each child using the MTCSI. Communication and social interaction were measured on the Vineland-II over the course of the fall semester for both the experimental group and the control group. Communication and social interaction scores on the MTCSI were investigated over the course of music therapy intervention. The MTCSI was cross-validated with the Vineland-II by analyzing correlations between domain scores across the two instruments.

Results

Preliminary analyses yielded the following results:

1. Significantly greater improvements over the fall semester for the experimental group than for the control group in both *Expressive Communication* and *Receptive Communication* sub-domains of the Vineland-II, taking a composite of ratings across teacher and parent questionnaires. Differences between experimental and control groups were especially pronounced for those children diagnosed with ASD.

2. Significant improvement in the MTCSI domain of *Joining In*, and improvement in *Reciprocal Verbal Communication*, for a sub-sample of 11 children in the experimental group. Especially pronounced improvement in both of these domains for the seven children with ASD in this sub-sample. The children with ASD showed a significant increase in the MTCSI domain of *Affective Response*.

3. Strong correlations between *Joining In* and *Reciprocal Verbal Communication* on the MTCSI and all Vineland domain standard scores (*Communication, Daily Living, Socialization, Motor*) as well as the Vineland Adaptive Behavior Composite. Strong correlations between *Vocalization* and *Affective Response* on the MTCSI and the *Communication* domain of the Vineland, and between *Turn-Taking* on the MTCSI and the *Socialization* domain of the Vineland.

Discussion

INTERPRETATIONS AND LIMITATIONS

These results suggest that improvements in various aspects of communication and social interaction may occur in young children with ASD over the course of Nordoff-Robbins music therapy interventions. Such improvements may be observed through close analysis of videotaped sessions using a music therapy rating scale, and may be reflected in parents' and teachers' responses to a developmental questionnaire. Multiple robust correlations between the MTCSI and the Vineland-II support the validity of the MTCSI and suggest that changes observed in music therapy generalize to other environments. Limitations include the small sample size of this pilot study and the need for validation of the MTCSI.

FUTURE DIRECTIONS

Future plans include the development of further outreach services to young children with ASD in the New York City metropolitan area, both in self-contained special education settings and in inclusion programs with typically developing peers. An inclusion-support intervention of creative music therapy could encompass a wide range of children with ASD, including children with significant verbal deficits who might not otherwise be considered candidates for inclusion.

Conclusion

This chapter has delineated ways in which the principles of Nordoff-Robbins music therapy may be utilized to work at the *developmental threshold* of young children with ASD. During sessions, music therapists flexibly adapt their clinical approach in response to evidence gathered through moment-to-moment music-making with children (i.e., evidence of their responses, their functioning, their *being*). As Nordoff and Robbins summarized:

> *The creative approach to therapy is…empirically directed. Therapists take their start from the child and determine clinical intentions… As a course of therapy evolves, goals become more clearly determined. Areas of response and interactivity become identified—although the unpredictabilities of an emergent response process will require that therapists always approach a child with an attitude of open improvisational readiness. Only in this way can therapists respond creatively to new challenges, and take up new opportunities to explore the child's capabilities and potential further. (2007, pp. 198–199)*

LEARNING QUESTIONS

1. How does the Nordoff-Robbins approach use the therapeutic potential of music to work at children's developmental threshold?

2. How do Nordoff-Robbins music therapists attempt to cultivate spontaneity, flexibility, and initiative in children with ASD?

3. What are some ways in which improvised music may be structured to elicit communicative interaction?

4. How may music therapy processes relate to the dynamics of parent–infant interaction in children with ASD?

5. Given the emphasis on improvisation in the Nordoff-Robbins approach, how can children's progress in therapy be systematically tracked?

References

Accordino, R., Comer, R., and Heller, W.B. (2007). Searching for music's potential: A critical examination of research on music therapy with individuals with autism. *Research in Autism Spectrum Disorders, 1,* 101–115.

Aigen, K. (1998). *Paths of Development in Nordoff-Robbins Music Therapy.* Gilsum, NH: Barcelona.

Benjamin, J. (1988). *The Bonds of Love.* New York: Pantheon.

Hadjikhani, N. (2007). Mirror neuron system and autism. In P.C. Carlisle (Ed.), *Progress in Autism Research.* New York: Nova Science.

Hummel-Rossi, B., Turry, A., Guerrero, N., Selim, N., *et al.* (2008). *Music Therapy Communication and Social Interaction Scale.* Unpublished instrument, Nordoff-Robbins Center for Music Therapy, New York University.

Kim, J., Wigram, T., and Gold, C. (2009). Emotional, motivational and interpersonal responsiveness of children with autism in improvisational music therapy. *Autism, 13(4),* 389–409.

Koelsch, S. (2009). A neuroscientific perspective on music therapy. *The Neurosciences and Music III— Disorders and Plasticity: Annals of the New York Academy of Sciences, 1169,* 374–384.

Lim, H.A. (2010). Effect of "Developmental Speech and Language Training Through Music" on speech production in children with autism spectrum disorders. *Journal of Music Therapy, 47(1),* 2–26.

National Institutes of Health (NIH) (2011). *A Parent's Guide to Autism Spectrum Disorder.* Washington, DC: U.S. Department of Health and Human Services.

Nordoff, P., and Robbins, C. (1965). Improvised music for autistic children. *Music Journal, 23(8),* 39–67.

Nordoff, P., and Robbins, C. (1968). Improvised music as therapy for autistic children. In E.T. Gaston (Ed.) *Music in Therapy.* New York: Macmillan.

Nordoff, P., and Robbins, C. (2007). *Creative Music Therapy: A Guide to Fostering Clinical Musicianship (Second Edition).* Gilsum, NH: Barcelona.

Overy, K., and Molnar-Szakacs, I. (2009). Being together in time: Musical experience and the mirror neuron system. *Music Perception, 26(5),* 489–504.

Pavlicevic, M. (1997). *Music Therapy in Context: Music, Meaning and Relationship.* London and Philadelphia: Jessica Kingsley Publishers.

Ramachandran, V.S., and Oberman, L.M. (2006). Broken mirrors. *Scientific American, 295(5),* 62–69.

Rizzolatti, G., Fogassi, L., and Gallese, V. (2006). Mirrors in the mind. *Scientific American, 295(5),* 54–61.

Robbins, C. (1993). The creative processes are universal. In M. Heal and T. Wigram (Eds.) *Music Therapy in Health and Education.* London and Philadelphia: Jessica Kingsley Publishers.

Silverman, M. (2008). Nonverbal communication, music therapy, and autism: A review of the literature. *Journal of Creativity in Mental Health, 3(1),* 3–19.

Sparrow, S.S., Balla, D., and Cicchetti, D. (2005). *Vineland Adaptive Behavior Scales—Second Edition.* Minneapolis, MN: Pearson Assessments.

Stern, D. (1990). *Diary of a Baby: What Your Child Sees, Feels, and Experiences.* New York: Basic Books.

Trevarthen, C. (1980). The foundations of intersubjectivity: Development of interpersonal and cooperative understanding in infants. In *The Social Foundations of Language and Thought: Essays in Honor of Jerome S. Bruner.* New York: Norton.

Trevarthen, C. (1999). Musicality and the intrinsic motive pulse: Evidence from human psychobiology and infant communication. *Musicae Scientiae,* 155–215 (special issue, 1999–2000).

Trevarthen, C. (2005). First things first: Infants make good use of the sympathetic rhythm of imitation, without reason or language. *Journal of Child Psychotherapy, 31(1),* 91–113.

Trevarthen, C., Aitken, K., Papoudi, D., and Robarts, J. (1998). *Children with Autism: Diagnosis and Intervention to Meet their Needs (Second Edition).* London and Philadelphia: Jessica Kingsley Publishers.

Turry, A., and Marcus, D. (2003). Using the Nordoff-Robbins approach to music therapy with adults diagnosed with autism. In D.J. Wiener and L.K. Oxford (Eds.) *Action Therapy with Families and Groups.* Washington, DC: American Psychological Association.

Wan, C.Y., Demaine, K., Zipse, L., Norton, A., and Schlaug, G. (2010). From music making to speaking: Engaging the mirror neuron system in autism. *Brain Research Bulletin, 82*, 161–168.

Whalen, C., Schreibman, L., and Ingersoll, B. (2006). The collateral effects of joint attention training on social initiations, positive affect, imitation, and spontaneous speech for young children with autism. *Journal of Autism and Developmental Disorders, 36*, 655–664.

Wigram, T., and Gold, C. (2006). Music therapy in the assessment and treatment of autistic spectrum disorders: Clinical application and research evidence. *Child: Care, Health and Development, 32(5),* 535–543.

Chapter 8

DIR®/Floortime™ Model

Introduction and Considerations for Improvisational Music Therapy

John A. Carpente, Ph.D., MT-BC, LCAT
THE REBECCA CENTER FOR MUSIC THERAPY AT MOLLOY COLLEGE
ROCKVILLE CENTRE, NY

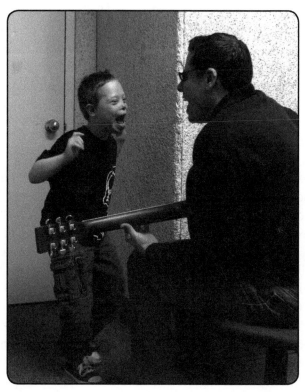

PHOTO COURTESY OF JIM PEPPLER

*The relational and aesthetic experiences intrinsic to interactive
music-making naturally give rise to affective interactions that
foster musical relatedness, reciprocity, and communication.
(John A. Carpente)*

The Developmental, Individual Difference, Relationship-based (DIR®)/Floortime™ Model, first introduced by Stanley Greenspan, is a comprehensive framework used by practitioners and parents to conduct assessments and intervention programming for children with autism spectrum disorders (ASD). This chapter provides a brief overview of the DIR®/Floortime™ Model and how it can be combined with improvisational music therapy (IMT) to facilitate healthy foundations for social-emotional development in children with ASD. A case vignette along with guidelines and considerations for music therapists, interdisciplinary team members, and parents illustrate the content of this chapter.

Introduction

The DIR®/Floortime™ Model is a developmental framework used to conceptualize and identify children's unique profiles in terms of their individual differences and functional social-emotional capacities. The model helps young children (especially those at risk for ASD) develop healthy foundations for social, emotional, and intellectual capacities, rather than simply addressing isolated skills and behaviors. Based on cognitive and developmental psychology, the model takes a comprehensive view of the child's social-emotional functioning and potential, biological processing differences, and emotional interactions with his or her caregiver (Greenspan and Wieder, 2006a, 2006b).

The DIR®/Floortime™ Model was developed in the early eighties by Stanley Greenspan who studied typical developing infants (Greenspan and Lourie, 1981; Greenspan and Shanker, 2004; Greenspan and Thorndike, 1989). His work with infants led to numerous publications which focused on child development, particularly in the areas of social emotional processes and the development of emotional intelligence, emphasizing that parental interactions are the key ingredient to a child's healthy, emotional maturation (Greenspan and Salmon, 1994; Greenspan and Shanker, 2004; Greenspan and Thorndike, 1985, 1989).

It was not until the 1990s that Greenspan introduced the DIR®/Floortime™ Model as an intervention for children with emotional and developmental challenges, including those with ASD (Greenspan, 1992; Greenspan and Wieder, 1998). The DIR®/Floortime™ Model suggests that children with ASD display difficulty in their capacity to engage in affective learning interactions due to individual differences related to the nervous system (i.e., motor-planning, sensory modulation, sequencing, sensory processing challenges) (Greenspan, 1992). Therefore, children with ASD may encounter difficulty developing the ability to engage in a continuous flow of reciprocal emotional interactions that foster symbolic and abstract thought processes (Greenspan, 2001). Research suggests that developmental relationship-based interventions, such as the DIR®/Floortime™ Model, may have beneficial treatment effects for children with ASD (Gutstein, Burgess, and Montfort, 2007; Mahoney and Perales, 2003, 2005; Rogers and DiLalla, 1991; Rogers and Lewis, 1989; Rogers et al., 2006; Solomon et al., 2007). The National Autism Center's *National Standards*

Report (2009) identifies the DIR®/Floortime™ Model as an emerging treatment for children with ASD, indicating that additional studies are needed to demonstrate consistency of the therapeutic benefits of the model. Music therapy also is identified in this way.

In 1996 Greenspan and his colleagues founded the Interdisciplinary Council on Developmental and Learning Disorders (ICDL). This non-profit organization is dedicated to the prevention, identification, and treatment of developmental and learning disorders by educating and training parents and professionals. Additional information on the DIR®/Floortime™ Model, certification training, conferences, and publications can be found on the organizational website at www.icdl.com.

What does DIR®/Floortime™ stand for?

DIR®/Floortime™ Model stands for **D**evelopmental, **I**ndividual Difference, **R**elationship-based/Floortime™ Model. The following paragraphs define each term as it applies to the model, and discuss how aspects relate to each other.

Developmental refers to a child's level within the framework of six specific levels of social-emotional developmental milestones. Each level builds upon the previous one, scaffolding to more complex, higher level capacities for expanded, creative, and reflective thought processing and the evolvement of spontaneous and empathic relationships (Greenspan, DeGangi, and Wieder, 2001; Greenspan and Thorndike, 1989). The six levels of functional emotional development are based on typical child development (Greenspan, DeGangi, and Wieder, 2001). Figure 8.1 describes each level and how it may be affected by ASD.

Individual Difference refers to how the child processes information in his or her environment (i.e., via language, motor and sensory stimuli, auditory processing, visual-spatial processing, and motor-planning). The therapist looks at each of the child's individual differences within each of the six developmental stages described in Figure 8.1 to determine how these differences may impact the child's ability to move up the developmental ladder (Greenspan and Wieder, 2005).

Relationship-based refers to the learning relationships with caregivers, therapists, and peers. All interactions and interventions are done within the context of relationships. Learning relationships are tailored to the child (while considering individual differences and developmental capacities) to maximize and foster affective and robust two-way purposeful interactions (Greenspan and Wieder, 2006a). Relationship-building represents a conduit to where learning takes place and is essential in the DIR® model.

These three components of the DIR® model complement each other by (a) identifying the developmental (social-emotional) stage in which the child currently is functioning, (b) determining what is impeding the child's development, and (c) understanding how the child relates and communicates to others (Carpente, 2011a). Each of the three components is essential in assisting the interdisciplinary intervention team to assess the child and develop an effective intervention plan.

Level 1: Shared attention and regulation occurs from age 0–3 months

The infant's ability calmly regulates while displaying emotional interest through a range of sensory experiences such as sights, sounds, and touch (Greenspan and Thorndike, 1989; Greenspan, DeGangi, and Wieder, 2001). This capacity helps the infant develop the ability to organize motor responses and integrate sensory information.

An infant at risk for ASD may show difficulty in sustaining his attention to sights or sounds, and may prefer to engage in self-stimulatory behaviors (Greenspan and Wieder, 2006b).

Level 2: Engagement and relating occurs from age 2–5 months

During this stage of development, the infant gains the ability to seek out interactions and engages intimately with his or her parents. The infant begins to understand and express a range of emotions that are supported by gestures and affect cues such as smiles and grimaces (Greenspan and Thorndike, 1989).

The infant at risk for ASD may exhibit difficulty sustaining engagement and will usually withdraw from interactions (Greenspan and Wieder, 2006b).

Level 3: Purposeful emotional interactions occur from age 4–10 months

This period signifies the child's ability to communicate through gestures in a meaningful and purposeful manner. During this developmental stage, the child forms the ability to initiate and express intentions while engaging in back-and-forth affective interactions (Greenspan and Thorndike, 1989).

A child at risk for ASD may display no interest in interacting, show very little initiative, and may engage in random or impulsive behaviors (Greenspan and Wieder, 2006b).

Level 4: Chains of back-and-forth (joint attention) emotional signaling and shared problem-solving occur from age 10–18 months

This level refers to the toddler's ability to utilize gestures in a sequential manner to communicate and solve problems through actions and word approximations (Greenspan and Shanker, 2004).

A child at risk for ASD may exhibit difficulty initiating while sustaining a continuous flow of back-and-forth interactions (Greenspan and Wieder, 2006b).

Level 5: Creating ideas occurs from age 18–30 months

During this stage, the child develops the ability to create ideas and symbols. Language skills begin to surface, and the child's ability to engage in pretend play and the capacity to differentiate between fantasy and reality emerge.

A child at risk for ASD may exhibit difficulty using words or phrases meaningfully and will repeat words that have been heard or seen (i.e., echolalia) (Greenspan and Wieder, 2006b).

Level 6: Building bridges between ideas: Logical thinking occurs at age 30–42 months

The child in this stage develops the capacity to build bridges between ideas to make logical sense of the world. The child begins to develop capacities for empathy and insight into why things occur.

A child at risk for ASD may display no words, use memorized scripts with random ideas, or use words and ideas illogically (Greenspan and Wieder, 2006b).

Figure 8.1: Six levels of development of children ages 0–42 months

Floortime™ refers to a specific technique that utilizes play (via toys, dolls, and sensory-based objects) to follow the child's lead and natural emotional interests, challenging him or her to higher levels of social, emotional, and intellectual capacities (Greenspan and Wieder, 2006a). With very young children, this playtime often takes place on the floor, eventually expanding to other venues and environments.

In the DIR®/Floortime™ Model, involvement of the family and practice in the home environment is a vital part of treatment intervention. Based on the child's unique profile, other interventions might include semi-structured problem-solving, sensory experiences, biomedical and nutritional programs, and other individual therapies (e.g., occupational therapy or speech-language therapy). Peer play may be added when the child becomes interactive (Greenspan and Wieder, n.d.).

Improvisational music therapy and DIR®/Floortime™

Improvisational music therapy

Improvisational music therapy is commonly used by Nordoff-Robbins music therapists serving young children with ASD (see Chapter 7 for more information). Clinical improvisation involves spontaneous music-making between the child and therapist; the therapist improvises music based on the child's musical and non-musical responses and reactions to the musical environment and interactions. Thus, the therapist may improvise music that supports, accompanies, and/or enhances the child's music-making process to foster musical engagement, relationship, interaction, communication, and reciprocity.

In the session, the music therapist provides various instruments that require no formal training or experience on the part of the child. The therapist improvises music (using the guitar, piano, voice, and/or percussive instruments) built around the child's musical-emotional lead. The primary role of the music therapist is to create musical experiences that deepen the child's musical involvement (Aigen, 2005b) in musical play, engaging him or her in musical-affective and reciprocal interactions (Carpente, 2011b). Improvisation techniques may include grounding, reflecting, enhancing, mirroring, imitating, synchronization, and dialoguing to engage the child (Bruscia, 1987; Nordoff and Robbins, 2007; Wigram, 2004).

Similarities and differences

The DIR®/Floortime™ technique and improvisational music therapy share several similarities. Table 8.1 outlines the most prominent ones.

When working within this combined approach, music therapists use the DIR® framework as the primary means for (a) assessing the child's strengths and needs in non-musical modes of interaction and relationship, and (b) evaluating the child's progress in these areas (Carpente, 2009, 2011a).

Clinical application

As with any music therapy intervention, improvisational music therapy follows the therapeutic process of assessment, intervention planning, intervention, evaluation, and termination. The *Individual Music-Centered Assessment Profile for Neurodevelopmental Disorders* (IMCAP-ND) was developed as a specific improvisational music therapy assessment to be used within the DIR®/Floortime™ Model (Carpente, 2011b). The IMCAP-ND is not a validated or standardized music therapy assessment tool for ASD, but is a criteria-based assessment profiling system developed by the author that provides an in-depth musical understanding of each child's ability to musically attune, engage, relate, adapt, and communicate in musical play (Carpente, 2011b). The IMCAP-ND is administered throughout the course of four to six assessment sessions. It targets six music domain areas related to the child's social-emotional responses, considering individual differences and how they impact the musical interactions. Music domain areas are evaluated by clinical observation and listening to the child's responses in play through any one or all of the four modes of musical expression (i.e., instrument play, voice, movement, gestures).

Following IMCAP-ND scoring, the music therapist collaborates with the child's parents or caregiver to develop a 13-week home-based intervention plan that includes goals and strategies. Goals are evaluated based on the criteria of the IMCAP-ND. The case scenario featured in Table 8.2 illustrates each phase of the therapeutic process of improvisational music therapy within the DIR®/Floortime™ Model.

Table 8.1 Similarities between the DIR®/Floortime™ Model and improvisational music therapy

Categories	DIR®/Floortime™ Model	Improvisational music therapy
Following the child's emotional lead	The first step in attempting to engage the child in co-active interactions; utilizing playful interactions as a means of following the child's interests and entering into his/her child's world while gauging the child's emotional state and individual differences.	The first step in seeking musical engagement; providing musical experiences that follow the child's emotional lead (e.g., through vocalizations, instruments, movement, gestures) while considering the child's individual and musical differences.
Action-based, non-directive approach	Therapist and child are involved in co-interactive experiences through play/dialogue, verbally and/or non-verbally (gestural); child plays an integral role in each interaction.	Therapist and child are co-active participants in the music-making process; the child plays an integral role in the therapeutic process and dictates the direction of the musical experiences.
Responses, reactions, and idiosyncratic behaviors are respected	Therapist joins the child's idiosyncratic behaviors (i.e., scripts, perseverative behaviors, movements) to enter into the child's world and foster relatedness and communication. The focus is not on removal of these behaviors, but on honoring and respecting them; every behavior is viewed as communicative.	Therapist musically joins or accompanies child's perserverative behaviors, improvising music based on the child's vocal, physical, and/or musical stimulatory behaviors. This may involve creating musical experiences in the tempo of the child's behaviors, other movements, and/or vocalizations; treating all behaviors as musically communicative acts and as entry points to meet the child.
Affective interactions	Therapist utilizes playful interactions while incorporating gestures, play, or pretend play to foster a continuous flow of affective back-and-forth interactions.	Therapist provides emotionally charged musical experiences to foster robust and affective musical interactions in musical play (i.e., vocalizations, instruments, movement, or gestures).
Relationship	Therapist seeks to foster a child–therapist relationship through play and dialogue (all learning occurs in and through the experience of relationships).	Therapist seeks to develop a relationship with the child in and through a range of co-active musical experiences. All musical experiences are conceptualized within the context of the relationship.

Sources: Carpente (2009, 2011b, 2012); Greenspan (1992); Greenspan and Wieder (1998, 2006a, 2006b); Nordoff and Robbins (2007).

Table 8.2 Case scenario: Improvisational music therapy with Eric based on the DIR®/Floortime™ Model	
Therapeutic process	**Case description**
Assessment	Eric is a 5-year-old boy who stopped using words at 18 months. He was diagnosed with ASD at 22 months.
	DIR Profile® (based on Greenspan's six functional emotional developmental levels as described in Figure 8.1)
	• Self-regulates (Level I) during musical interactions; becomes dysregulated when engaged for more than three measures of musical play.
	• Engages (Level II) in musical interactions; but displays difficulty sustaining engagement and maintaining two-way purposeful communication for extended periods.
	• Displays hyper-sensitivity to auditory stimuli (including music), perseverative body movements, visual-spatial process challenges, difficulty with motor-planning, sequencing, and sensory modulation.
	• Displays some capacity in problem-solving (Level IV) and may use ideas meaningfully in simple phrases (Level V).
	• Repeats memorized phrases and scripts; cannot build ideas onto these scripts (Level VI) in a relational manner.
	IMCAP-ND
	• Musically interacts primarily through movement, instrumental play, gestures, and memorized scripts, exhibiting moderate level of musical awareness to tempo, rhythm, and pitch and reflexive rather than intentional tonal vocal responses; words are often repeated scripts used when stressed or excited resulting in withdrawal from musical interactions.
	• Shows capacities for musical mutuality and relatedness, musical-affect, and musical dialoguing (Level II); constricted in range and duration.
	• Exhibits motor-planning difficulties and constant motion (moving rapidly between instruments) that interfere with musical dialoguing; vocalizes no range of affect (monotone, lacks prosody and melodic contour) and plays loudly on the drum and xylimba.
	• Has difficulty referencing the therapist during musical play (Level III); joins the tempo and melodies of therapist's music, but beats sporadically and inflexibly (Level IV), to the therapist's music (Level IV); shows limited range of musical responses (Levels IV and V); and closes circles of musical communication (i.e., completes or punctuates the endings of musical phrases) (Level IV) when prompted, but has difficulty initiating circles of musical communication.
	• Requires visual prompting, gestural cues, and verbal direction to engage in sustained musical interactions and musical adaptation (Level V), but has difficulty initiating ideas/play (Level VI).
	Music Therapy Goal Areas Based in the IMCAP-ND
	Develop the ability to:
	• increase range, sustain interaction, and initiate ideas/play/musical play (Level III: musical mutuality and relatedness)
	• socially reference and display range of affect in musical play (Level III: musical-affect)
	• open circles of musical communication while continuing to close circles in musical play (Level IV: musical dialoguing)
	• musically adapt to changes in tempo and dynamics (Level V: musical adaptation)
	• connect musical ideas with the therapist and extend the play (VI: musical inter-relatedness).

Intervention planning	*Strategies*
	• Include form, repetition, wide range of tempo, and dynamic changes in improvisation.
	• Musically follow Eric's emotional lead to foster self-regulation, engagement, and relatedness.
	• Include clear musical themes, tempo mobility (Nordoff and Robbins, 2007), high-affect, and accents on strong beats to emphasize rhythm and meter.
	• Utilize short musical phrases, repetition, and clear pauses for musical responses.
	• Use visual supports, gestural cues, verbal cues, modeling, high-affect, and hand-over-hand technique.
Intervention (Excerpts from Sessions 10 and 22)	*Session 10*
	• Eric paces while MT walks nearby, matching Eric's tempo via guitar improvisation and staccato vocalization in mixolydian mode.
	• Eric initiates singing, "Hello ____, let's play music." Music therapist (MT) replies with exaggerated high-affect, "Hello Eric, I'd love to play music. What should we play?" Eric beats on the snare drum. MT plays a variation of the theme, generating a wider range of dynamics and register.
	• MT uses gestural cues, high-affect in singing, directional pointing, and incorporates Diminished 7th chords to create tension and release when Eric beats the drum.
	• Eric recognizes the musical changes and increases the intensity of his beating. His playing is increasingly connected and flowing.
	• MT slows the music, gestures, over-emphasizes dynamic change, and incorporates a musical pause. Eric plays through the pause, extending the play by punctuating on the cymbal and socially referencing MT by smiling as he continues to play.
	• MT changes the music's intensity and dynamic range; Eric puts his hands to his ears and resumes pacing.
	• MT decreases the intensity and tempo; Eric paces more slowly.
	• MT leaves the piano, slowly walks to Eric while singing, offers him deep pressure on his arms to help him self-regulate, then leads him back into the interaction.
	Session 22
	• Eric plays the piano with MT for first time, with a driving tempo and staccato manner, initiating a lyrical idea that seems to be scripted, "Let's have some lunch."
	• MT incorporates music into the lyrical idea, models various musical expressions, then sings a related lyric, "But I just ate."
	• Eric's piano-playing becomes less detached and more melodic as MT reflects Eric's playing; musical dialogue ensues.
	• Eric increasingly interacts, initiates, and collaborates via music. Supportive interventions (e.g. gestural and hand-over-hand cues) help him continue to play.

Table continues

Table 8.2 Case scenario: Improvisational music therapy with Eric based on the DIR®/Floortime™ Model *cont.*	
Therapeutic process	**Case description**
Evaluation (following session 29)	*DIR Profile* • Improved self-regulation (Level I) and engagement in a related manner (Level II) with MT. • Increased purposeful communication (Level III), using fewer scripts and generating language appropriate to the situation. • Developed the capacity to create and build bridges between ideas, engaging in symbolic play and showing some capacity to think creatively and emotionally (Levels V and VI). *IMCAP-ND* • Increased engagement in musical mutuality and relatedness (Level II) in duration; however, tempo and dynamics range remain constricted. • Developed social reference to MT in musical play, displaying a range of affect (Level III), increased musical interaction in a relational communicative manner for extended periods, initiation in musical play with the intent to relate (Level IV), plus exhibiting capacities to open and close circles of musical communication. • Developed some capacities in the ability to create and connect musical ideas with limited range and flexibility when supported with high-affect and visual cuing. Note: Eric's parents reported that his progress in music therapy carried over into his home life in the areas of shared attention, seeking out interactions, initiating conversations, and increased frustration tolerance.
Termination	Eric's progress during individual therapy indicated that a group experience might help him incorporate and exercise his new developmental skills with his peers. Following Session 36, Eric was placed in a group with three other children.

Existing research

The literature on using music therapy in tandem with DIR®/Floortime™ is sparse. As of today, there is only one known study pertaining to combining the DIR®/Floortime™ Model with improvisational music therapy (Carpente, 2009). The study employed Nordoff-Robbins music therapy (NRMT) interventions merged within the theoretical framework of the DIR®/Floortime™ Model to ascertain if progress in musical goals paralleled progress in non-musical (DIR®) goals. Four young children with ASD received individual NRMT-based treatment that focused on musical relationship-based goals. DIR® was used as the primary means of conceptualizing and assessing the children's strengths and needs in non-musical modes of interaction and relationship.

The effects of the interventions were examined using a mixed method. For pre- and post-testing, the Functional Emotional Assessment Scale (FEAS) (Greenspan, DeGangi, and Wieder, 2001) was used to measure each child's progress in achieving goals pertinent to DIR®; musical outcomes were evaluated through the Goal Attainment Scaling (GAS) (Kiresuk, Smith, and Cardillo, 1994). Each of the four children in the study showed improvements in some of the FEAS functional emotional developmental levels (e.g., self-regulation, two-way purposeful communication), as well as in various GAS goal areas (e.g., musical attunement, musical dialoguing). However, the small number of subjects precludes accurate statistical analysis. Additional studies with larger sample sizes are still needed to determine if this treatment protocol can significantly affect developmental growth in young children with ASD.

Guidelines and considerations

It is equally important to understand both the characteristics of ASD that may impede a child's ability to engage in musical play as well as the child's musical responses upon which musical goals are based. Thus, a child who displays difficulty engaging in musical interactions may be experiencing several factors completely unrelated to music (e.g., difficulties with motor-planning, visual processing, or sensory modulation) (Carpente, 2009). As the music therapist's primary task within this model is to foster relatedness and communication, it is important to look for these qualities within children's behaviors (e.g., smiling or crying).

For music therapists

Music therapists working within this combined approach should be flexible, offering children a wide range of musical contexts while considering their unique individual and musical differences (Carpente, 2009, 2011b). Therefore, the music therapist needs to have a high level of clinical musicianship and also interpersonal skills (Carpente, 2011a). The following considerations and suggestions may help music therapists engage a child in co-active improvisational experiences.

LISTENING AND OBSERVATION

- Does the child maintain musical attunement while engaged in musical play through a range of musical experiences?

- Can the child engage in reciprocal musical relatedness for a sustained period of time, or are the musical interactions fragmented or cyclical?

- During musical play, does the child engage in a related fashion only when playing in a self-directed manner?

- Can the child adapt to the musical changes offered by the music therapist?

- Does the child display the ability to adapt to musical changes, but exhibit difficulty in initiating musical ideas during musical play?

- Does the child display the ability to direct musical interaction and initiate musical ideas, but show difficulty bridging musical ideas with the music therapist?

- Can the child engage in related musical play through a range of tempo and dynamics, or only relate when the music is played in certain tempi and/or dynamics?

MUSICAL FACILITATION

Approaching the child musically also requires following the child's emotional lead before offering musical experiences. Following the child's lead is an important principle in both the DIR®/Floortime™ Model (Greenspan, 1992) and Nordoff-Robbins music therapy (Aigen, 2005a; Nordoff and Robbins, 2007); it is the starting point for facilitating musical interactions. The following six-step process may be considered a guideline to facilitate musical interactions (Carpente, 2011b):

1. Listen to and observe the child's responses and reactions to the musical environment (Bruscia, 1987; Greenspan and Wieder, 2006b; Nordoff and Robbins, 2007).

2. Create a musical-emotional environment (Nordoff and Robbins, 2007).

3. Follow the child's musical-emotional lead (Greenspan, 1992; Nordoff and Robbins, 2007).

4. Musically synchronize with the child's instrumental music-making, vocalizations, movement, and/or gestures (Bruscia, 1987; Wigram, 2004).

5. Open a circle of musical communication within the context of the musical interaction (Bruscia, 1987; Carpente, 2009, 2011b; Greenspan, 1992).

6. Provide musical experiences within the established musical contact, helping the child expand musical interactions (Carpente, 2009, 2011b; Greenspan and Wieder, 2006a, 2006b).

For interdisciplinary collaborations

Music therapists working collaboratively with other professionals may wish to share the following ways the DIR®/Floortime™ Model can be clinically applied and experienced within music (Carpente, 2011b).

CREATING A MUSICAL ENVIRONMENT

Music therapists may support other professionals (e.g., early childhood educators, occupational therapists, speech-language pathologists, and physical therapists) working with children who have ASD by listening and observing the interaction between the child and other colleagues while creating a musical environment that enhances the experiences of their interaction (Carpente, 2012). Improvisation techniques applied by the music therapist may include reflecting, mirroring, enhancing, or exaggerating (Bruscia, 1987).

COACHING AND BEING COACHED

"Coaching is used to acknowledge and perhaps improve existing knowledge and practices, develop new skills, and promote continuous self-assessment and learning on the part of the coachee" (Shelden and Rush, 2011, p. 3). Therefore, a music therapist may coach other professionals to deepen their musical experience with children who have ASD by using music intentionally and within their scope of practice. Vice versa, a music therapist may be coached by professionals to incorporate strategies and techniques from another discipline into the context of musical experiences.

For parents

The DIR®/Floortime™ Model emphasizes the vital role of parents and other family members in children's development (Greenspan, 1992; Greenspan and Wieder, 2006a, 2006b); including parents in the therapeutic process is highly desirable. The following responses may address issues commonly expressed by parents who choose improvisational music therapy based on the DIR®/Floortime™ Model as a treatment for their children with ASD:

- *I have no music skill at all. How can I use music at home with my child?* One of the challenges parents face in providing musical experiences for their child is the lack of confidence, or sometimes fear, in attempting to sing or play music with their child (Carpente, 2012). For parents who are not trained musicians, this can be difficult; music therapists may guide them past their fears and help them experience the joy of making music through singing, instruments, or hand-clapping. The parents' role is not to play an instrument *for* the child or teach her or him to play an instrument (Carpente, 2012). The parents' role is to play music *with* the child (e.g., via a variety of instrumental or non-instrumental joint musical experiences). Parents may consult with a certified music therapist who is experienced in working with children with ASD to develop an effective home-based plan. Additional information on parent training can be found in Chapter 13.

- *When I try to engage my child in musical experiences, he withdraws from the interaction by sometimes running away, holding his ear, or engaging in self-stimulatory behaviors. What should I do?* Parents may become frustrated when they attempt to engage their child in an interactive experience and he or she withdraws from the interaction and reverts to self-stimulatory behavior. Parents may take this as a sign to alter the delivery of a musical experience (e.g., decrease or increase the tempo, adjust the dynamics, switch from singing to humming). In addition, the parent might examine how the child is processing information during musical play and try to determine which other supports the child may need to enhance the learning experience (e.g., visual support) (Carpente, 2012).

- *I'm trying to teach my child how to play or beat a drum; she seems uninterested. What should I do?* Again, the goal is not to teach the child to play an instrument or sing a song, but rather to engage the child in relational musical experiences that foster affective reciprocal musical interactions. For example, if the child beats the drum once and then walks away, the parent's task is to quickly make this response interactive. Therefore, there is no right or wrong way to play an instrument when applying the combined treatment approach (Carpente, 2012).

Conclusion

There are several similarities between the DIR®/Floortime™ Model and improvisational music therapy; the two approaches seem to complement each other well. Although research supporting the effectiveness of this combined approach is limited, children with ASD and their parents may gain unique benefits from the musical interactions and developmental growth within. Music therapists working within this therapeutic framework are advised to seek training in the DIR®/Floortime™ Model while fostering strong clinical musicianship and therapeutic skills. As this combined approach is utilized by more clinicians and becomes the subject of additional research study, more parents may recognize that this developmental-based relationship intervention may provide an appropriate treatment option for their children with ASD.

Learning questions

1. What do the letters in DIR®/Floortime™ Model stand for?

2. Name the six levels of development within the DIR®/Floortime™ Model.

3. In what ways are the DIR®/Floortime™ Model and improvisational music therapy similar?

4. The National Autism Center's *National Standards Report* (2009) identified both the DIR®/Floortime™ Model and music therapy as an _____ treatment for children with ASD.

5. How can the DIR® framework be utilized in improvisational music therapy for children with ASD?

6. How might a music therapist use improvisational techniques to engage a child with ASD?

7. What should music therapists consider when working within this combined approach?

References

Aigen, K. (2005a). *Music Centered Music Therapy*. Gilsum, NH: Barcelona Publishers.

Aigen, K. (2005b). *Being in Music: Foundations of Nordoff-Robbins Music Therapy*. Gilsum, NH: Barcelona Publishers.

Bruscia, K. (1987). *Improvisation Models of Music Therapy*. Springfield, IL: Charles C. Thomas Publications.

Carpente, J. (2009). Contributions of Nordoff-Robbins music therapy within the developmental, individual differences, relationship (DIR)-based model in the treatment of children with autism: Four case Studies. Unpublished Doctoral Dissertation, Temple University. Ann Arbor: ProQuest/UMI, Publication Number AAT 3359621.

Carpente, J. (2011a). Addressing core features of autism: Integrating Nordoff-Robbins Music Therapy within the Developmental, Individual-Difference, Relationship-based (DIR®)/Floortime™ Model. In A. Meadows (Ed.) *Developments in Music Therapy Practice: Case Study Perspectives*. Gilsum, NH: Barcelona Publishers.

Carpente, J. (2011b). *The Individual Music-centered Assessment Profile for Neurodevelopmental Disorders (IMCAP-ND®) for Children, Adolescents, and Adults: A Clinical Manual*. Unpublished manuscript.

Carpente, J. (2012). *Developmental Music Health: Orchestrating Affective Relationships in Musical-Play for Parents and Professionals*. Unpublished manual.

Greenspan, S.I. (1992). *Infancy and Early Childhood: The Practice of Clinical Assessment and Intervention with Emotional and Developmental Challenges*. Madison, CT: International Universities Press.

Greenspan, S.I. (2001). Role of emotions in the core deficits in autism and in the development of intelligence and social skills. *Journal of Developmental and Learning Disorders, 5*, 1–46.

Greenspan, S.I., and Lourie, R.S. (1981). Developmental structuralist approach to the classification of adaptive and pathologic personality organizations: Infancy and early childhood. *American Journal of Psychiatry, 138*, 725–735.

Greenspan, S.I., and Salmon, J. (1994). *Play Ground Politics: Understanding the Emotional Life of Your School-Age Child.* New York: Da Capo Lifelong Books.

Greenspan, S.I., and Shanker, S.G. (2004). *The First Idea: How Symbols, Language, and Intelligence Evolved from our Primate Ancestors to Modern Humans.* New York: Da Capo Lifelong Books.

Greenspan, S.I., and Thorndike, N. (1985). *First Feelings: Milestones in the Emotional Development of Your Baby and Child.* New York: Penguin Publishers.

Greenspan, S.I., and Thorndike, N. (1989). *The Essential Partnership: How Parents and Children can meet the Emotional Challenges of Infancy and Childhood.* New York: Viking Penguin.

Greenspan, S., and Wieder, S. (n.d.) What is the DIR®/Floortime™? Retrieved from www.icdl.com/dirFloortime/overview/documents/WhatisDIR.pdf.

Greenspan, S.I., and Wieder, S. (1998). *The Child with Special Needs: Encouraging Intellectual and Emotional Growth.* New York: Da Capo Lifelong Books.

Greenspan, S.I., and Wieder, S. (2005). Can children with autism master the core deficits and become empathetic, creative and reflective? A ten to fifteen follow-up of a sub-group of children with autism spectrum disorders (ASD) who received a comprehensive developmental, individual-differences, relationship-based (DIR) approach. *The Journal of Developmental and Learning Disorders, 9*, 1–29.

Greenspan, S.I., and Wieder, S. (2006a) *Engaging Autism: Using the Floortime Approach to Help Children Relate, Communicate, and Think.* New York: Da Capo Lifelong Books.

Greenspan, S.I., and Wieder, S. (2006b) *Infant and Early Childhood Mental Health: A Comprehensive Developmental Approach to Assessment and Intervention.* Washington, DC: American Psychiatric Association.

Greenspan, S.I., DeGangi, G., and Wieder, S. (2001). *The Functional Emotional Assessment Scale (FEAS) for Infancy and Early Childhood: Clinical and Research Applications.* Bethesda, MD: Interdisciplinary Council on Developmental and Learning Disorders.

Gutstein, S.E., Burgess, A.F., and Montfort, K. (2007). Evaluation of the relationship development intervention program. *Autism, 11*, 397–411.

Kiresuk, T.J., Smith, A., and Cardillo, J. (1994). *Goal Attainment Scaling: Applications, Theory and Measurement.* Hillsdale, NJ: Lawrence Erlbaum Associates, Inc., Publishers.

Mahoney, G., and Perales, F. (2003). Using relationship-focused intervention to enhance the social-emotional functioning of young children with autism spectrum disorders. *Topics in Early Childhood Special Education, 23(2)*, 77–89.

Mahoney, G., and Perales, F. (2005). Relationship focused early intervention with children with pervasive developmental disorders and other disabilities: A comparative study. *JDBP: Journal of Developmental and Behavioral Pediatrics, 26(2)*, 77–85.

National Autism Center (NAC) (2009). *National Standards Report.* The National Standards Project—Addressing the need for evidence-based practice guidelines for autism spectrum disorders. Randolph, MA: NAC.

Nordoff, P., and Robbins, C. (2007). *Creative Music Therapy: A Guide to Fostering Clinical Musicianship.* Gilsum, NH: Barcelona Publishers.

Rogers, S.J., and Lewis, H. (1989). An effective day treatment model for young children with pervasive developmental disorders. *Journal of the American Academy of Child and Adolescent Psychiatry, 28(2)*, 207–214.

Rogers, S.J., and DiLalla, D.L. (1991). A comparative study of the effects of a developmentally based instructional model on young children with autism and young children with other disorders of behavior and development. *Topics in Early Childhood Special Education, 11*, 29–47.

Rogers, S.J., Hayden, D., Hepburn, S., Charlifue-Smith, R., Hall, T., and Hayes, A. (2006). Teaching young nonverbal children with autism useful speech: A pilot study of the Denver model and PROMPT interventions. *Journal of Autism and Developmental Disorders, 36*, 1007–1024.

Shelden, D.D., and Rush, M.L. (2011). *The Early Childhood Coaching Handbook*. Baltimore, MD: Paul H. Brookes Publishing Co., Inc.

Solomon, R., Necheles, J., Ferch, C., and Bruckman, D. (2007). Pilot study of a parent training program for young children with autism: The play project home consultation program. *Autism, 11(3)*, 205–224.

Wigram, T. (2004). *Improvisation: Methods and Techniques for Music Therapy Clinicians, Educators and Students*. London and Philadelphia: Jessica Kingsley Publishers.

Chapter 9

Strategies and Techniques

Making it Happen for Young Children
with Autism Spectrum Disorders

Marcia Humpal, M.Ed., MT-BC
OLMSTED FALLS, OH

Petra Kern, Ph.D., MT-DMtG, MT-BC, MTA
MUSIC THERAPY CONSULTING
SANTA BARBARA, CA

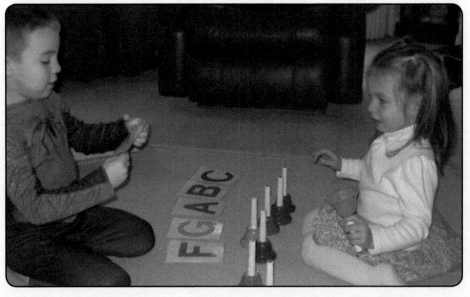

*Instructional strategies and music therapy techniques should complement
the unique learning style of each child with autism spectrum disorders.
(Marcia Humpal and Petra Kern)*

Music therapy service delivery to young children with autism spectrum disorders (ASD) and their families takes many forms. It may support comprehensive treatment models and focused interventions, address multiple goals and objectives, include individuals and groups, and be provided in various settings. Therefore, the way music therapists determine what strategies and techniques to employ will vary accordingly, always being guided by the interests, strengths, and needs of the individual child and the family's priorities. This chapter focuses on instructional strategies used in evidence-based practice and music therapy techniques that are applied when providing music therapy interventions for young children with ASD. Topics such as structure and routines, prompting, planning for transitions, organizing the environment, giving additional response time as well as peer involvement are addressed. Examples and tips from parents, professionals, and individuals with ASD accompany this chapter.

How do children with ASD learn?[1]
Developmentally appropriate practice
Developmentally appropriate practice supports the concept of play-based learning for all children for self-regulation as well as promoting language, cognition, and social competence. Young children's learning and development typically follow specific sequences, with higher level skills and knowledge building on those already acquired; however, learning and development evolve at varying and often uneven rates (Copple and Bredekamp, 2009; Sandall, Schwartz, and Joseph, 2001). These rates may be inconsistent in one area of functioning, but on target or even advanced in another area (NAEYC, 2009).

For children with ASD, play skill development often does not follow the typical continuum; these children may display atypical development in social, communication, and behavioral areas (Barton et al., 2011; National Institute of Mental Health, 2011). Traditional developmental teaching strategies (e.g., verbal instruction, imitation of teachers and peers, and independent learning) depend largely on a child's internal motivation to learn. Therefore, these instructional strategies might not be effective tools for learning in children with ASD (National Research Council [NRC], 2001). Hence, the developmental approach needs to be modified or combined with other instructional strategies to ensure that the educational goals of children with ASD are met (NPDC on ASD, 2008; Sandall, McLean, and Smith, 2000; Wolery, 1994). In Temple Grandin's (an adult with ASD) words, "Young children with autism spectrum disorders do not learn by listening to and watching others as do typical children. They need to be specifically taught things that others seem to learn by osmosis" (Grandin, 2011, p. 21).

---

1   Information presented under this section is originally from Kern (2004) and has been
    updated to reflect more current substantiating research.

Strategies for supporting social development

According to the NRC (2001), instructional strategies used to improve social skills in children with ASD fall into three categories:

1. *Adult-directed instruction* of specific goals of social skills (e.g., joint attention, response by gaze, imitation, turn-taking, and initiating social interactions).

2. *Child-centered approach*, in which adults follow the child's lead, encourage and sustain interactions, scaffold to higher levels, and extend the duration of interaction.

3. *Peer-mediated strategies*, in which typically developing peers prompt and maintain social engagement.

Common evidence-based interventions and instructional strategies used to increase social interaction in children with ASD include *Applied Behavior Analysis* (ABA) using reinforcement, prompting, time delay, and task analysis; *Joint Attention Interventions*; *Social Stories™*; and *Peer-Mediated Instruction and Intervention* (National Autism Center [NAC], 2009), among others identified as "emerging practices."

Strategies for supporting language and communication development

Frequently applied evidence-based interventions and instructional strategies as identified by the NAC (2009) for supporting language and communication development in children with ASD include *Applied Behavior Analysis* (ABA), *Verbal Behaviour* (VA), *Video Modeling*, *Naturalistic Teaching Strategies*, and *Augmentative and Alternative Communication* (AAC). These vary greatly along the continuum of behavioral to developmental approaches. Because the child's lack of motivation to use language and communication is often an issue, strategies to increase language and communication in children with ASD must capitalize on their natural desires and preferences within their environment. Frequently, the environment is arranged to provide opportunities for communication; adults immediately reward, imitate, and expand upon the child's smallest attempt to communicate (Dawson and Osterling, 1997).

Augmentative and Alternative Communication (AAC) is likely to be introduced if a child with ASD demonstrates non-functional language, has limited verbal communication skills, or has difficulty with language comprehension (Drager, Light, and Fink, 2009). AAC strategies use assistive devices, such as visual communication symbols (pictures, written words, objects), visual schedules, displays on communication boards, voice output devices with digitized speech, and sign language, in place of or in combination with verbal language (Sigafoos and Drasgow, 2001). The most widely applied symbolic communication system is the Picture Exchange Communication System (PECS) (Frost and Bondy, 2002), which capitalizes on the strong visual processing of many children with ASD. Technological advances (e.g., specific language and communication apps for children with ASD) have made AAC resources much more accessible and prolific (see Chapter 15).

Strategies for preventing challenging behaviors

One of the most stressful issues faced by parents and professionals might be the challenging behaviors of children with ASD. Previously thought to be a typical part of the stages of development in young children, challenging behaviors in young children with ASD may actually result in major barriers to social opportunities, community participation, and even successful inclusion (Dunlap and Strain, 2009).

Challenging behaviors may fall under three descriptive categories: (1) *destructive* (i.e., exemplified by acts of aggression, self-injurious behavior, or property destruction), (2) *disruptive* (i.e., loud and long tantrums, repetitive noises, running, or any other behavior that greatly disturbs others or the ongoing routine of the setting), or (3) *irritating/interfering* (i.e., "self-stimulatory" or stereotypic behaviors, perserverative actions and speech) (Dunlap and Strain, 2009; NRC, 2001).

The following interventions and strategies listed by the NAC (2009) as being evidence-based may prevent challenging behaviors: schedules using words, pictures, objects or photographs; self-management strategies such as checklists, visual prompts, and tokens, as well as structured teaching with rules and routines; planning for transitions; and structured learning environments. While positive behavior supports and a multi-tiered, hierarchal framework of prevention and intervention have shown promise, no single strategy has proved effective in preventing challenging behaviors in all children with ASD (Dunlap and Strain, 2009).

Interventions to prevent or reduce challenging behaviors vary from discrete trial and naturalistic behavior approaches (e.g., Pivotal Response Training and incidental teaching) to developmental approaches (i.e., those that recognize the needs of highly structured environments, adult attention, and consistency). McGee, Morrier, and Daly (2001) suggest that "increased fun decreases problem behaviors" (p. 176). This statement indicates that providing highly preferred play materials or topic areas as well as choices regarding preferred activities may boost the child's interest and engagement. Structured teaching and highly structured environments can also prevent challenging behaviors, because structure adds to the child's understanding of the classroom routines and activities (Mesibov, Shea, and Schopler, 2005).

The wide range of learning styles and individual differences within children with ASD requires that instructional strategies be tailored to each child's individual interests, abilities, and needs. The remainder of this chapter will address the following core instructional strategies as they apply to music therapy practice. Some of these instructional strategies have developed into focused interventions and are identified as being evidence-based (marked with *) by the National Professional Development Center on ASD (NPDC on ASD, n.d.) and National Autism Center (NAC, 2009):

- establishing structure, predictability, and routines
- using verbal, gestural, model, physical, and visual prompts*
- planning for transitions
- organizing the learning environment*

- giving additional response time and opportunities to repeat

- including active involvement of peers.*

Figure 9.1 introduces music therapy techniques used in early childhood settings. Additional information that follows will explain how these techniques apply to music therapy interventions for young children with ASD.

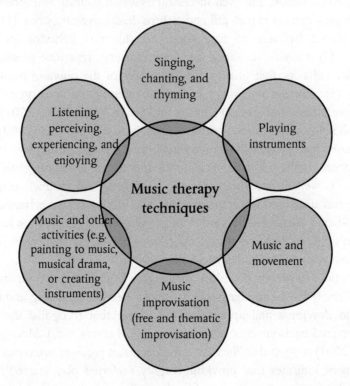

Source: Adapted from Kern, P. (2008a). Common Techniques. SOS Early Childhood. Paper presented with Marcia Humpal at the 10th Anniversary Conference of AMTA, St. Louis, MO, USA, November 2008.

Figure 9.1: Music therapy techniques used with young children with ASD

Embedding instructional strategies in music therapy practice

When working with young children with ASD and their families, music therapists should implement and embed instructional strategies identified for a particular child in a manner that is consistent with that of other intervention team members. This will increase the probability of skill generalization across situations and persons and provide the child with ASD with multiple opportunities to learn through repetition (Hatton, Shaw, and Cox, 2008).

Parents and other interdisciplinary team members may consider combining instructional strategies with music therapy techniques. Music motivates children with ASD to naturally participate in learning (Walworth, 2010). The elements of music (i.e., rhythm, melody, harmony, dynamics, duration, pitch, and timbre) provide a variety of stimulation for learning and development for all young children. By engaging in singing, playing instruments, moving to music, or listening to music, children with ASD can join their typically developing peers and siblings in activities that may be of interest to each of them.

Establishing structure, predictability, and routines

DESCRIPTION

Structure, predictability, and routines are essential aspects of any instruction for young children with ASD (Dawson and Osterling, 1997). Especially when teaching new skills, providing clear structure and establishing predictable routines may help children anticipate and understand what is to come next (NAC, 2009). *Structured teaching* (i.e., visually based approach to creating structured environments), meaningful and functional *rules and routines* (i.e., clearly defined rules and daily routines), and other organization tools may reduce confusion and promote understanding, participation, and on-task behavior of young children with ASD (Mesibov, Shea, and Schopler, 2005; Tien and Lee, 2007). For more information on *structured teaching* and *rules and routines*, visit the Autism Internet Module at www.autisminternetmodules.org.

Structure, predictability, and routines can be easily embedded in music therapy sessions. Early childhood music therapy sessions often follow a specific sequence of events, have established rules related to music-making and listening, and include activities that make expectations clear. For example, in a study by Kern, Wolery, and Aldridge (2007), a greeting song structured and prompted the expectation of a five-step morning greeting routine for two children with ASD, promoting their independence during the morning arrival time at their preschool program. It should be noted that not only meaningful and functional rules and routines but also the form (i.e., measures, repetition, meter) and progression (i.e., rhythm, duration, melody, harmony) of the music itself provide structure and predictability.

MAKING IT HAPPEN

For establishing structure, predictability, and routines, the following recommendations adopted from Mesibov, Shea, and Schopler (2005) should be considered in music therapy practice:

- Provide music therapy services at the same time every day/week, same location, and with a similar set-up of the environment (e.g., Tuesdays at 9:15 a.m. during circle time).

- Be consistent with session activities and routines (e.g., use the same greeting song followed by a constant routine of music therapy techniques).

- Establish rules for the music therapy session (e.g., when to play an instrument, be quiet, choose an instrument, or return it to the music bag).

- Use music with a clear form (e.g., ABA), simple scales (e.g., pentatonic), and chord progressions (e.g., three-chord progression) that lead to a resolution.

- Use songs with clear lyrics (i.e., that prompt the expectation and next step).

- Include props (e.g., puppets, scarves, books), which may make expectations more obvious and keep children engaged.

- Embed picture cards (e.g., indicating "time to listen") and visual schedules (e.g., representations of each music activity) to express expectations and prompt subsequent steps.

Case example

Four-year-old Oliver who has ASD attends preschool with his typically developing peers; a music therapist leads music circle time with the group once per week.

After gathering the children in a circle, she always sings the same hello song to greet each by name. A picture schedule prompts Oliver to the second activity, which is playing drums. The music therapist reminds all children of previously established rules. They are to play the instrument when she says "One, two, ready to go!" while conducting with hand gestures; and they should stop when she says "One, two, three, and stop!" while making one final drumbeat. For the next activity, Oliver chooses *Chicka, Chicka, Boom, Boom* (Martin and Archambault, 1989) from three picture cards representing songs. The group speaks rhythmically together while holding up the accompanying letter from the alphabet. When it is time for the final activity, the music therapist brings out a glockenspiel, with bars arranged in a C pentatonic scale. Together, they sing the "Good-bye" song (see song transcript in Figure 9.2), while each child gets a turn to play the instrument.

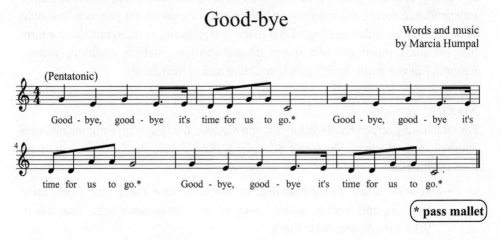

Good-bye

Words and music
by Marcia Humpal

(Pentatonic)

Good - bye, good - bye it's time for us to go.* Good - bye, good - bye it's

time for us to go.* Good - bye, good - bye it's time for us to go.*

(* **pass mallet**)

Figure 9.2: Song—"Good-bye"

Using verbal, gestural, model, physical, and visual prompts

DESCRIPTION

According to Neitzel and Wolery (2009a), prompting procedures are usually given by adults or peers to a child with ASD to support the learning of a specific skill. Practitioners typically apply prompting procedures in a systematic manner (i.e., least-to-most prompts, simultaneous prompting, graduated guidance) and choose prompts from the following categories: *verbal prompts* (i.e., verbal statement), *gestural prompts* (i.e., movement that cues a particular behavior or skill), *model prompts* (i.e., demonstration of the target skill or behavior), *physical prompts* (i.e., touching the child to cue the target skill), and *visual prompts* (i.e., providing pictures, photos, or objects cueing the event). For more information on *prompting*, visit the Autism Internet Module on this evidence-based focused intervention at www.autisminternetmodules. org.

Musical events can be combined with a variety of prompts. In a study by Kern, Wolery, and Aldridge (2007), a child with ASD was prompted to greet his peers during the morning arrival time at his preschool by a laminated stick figure waving "hello" during the singing of a greeting song. Furman (2001) recommended using pictures representing elements of an action song to prompt children with ASD about sequential information. Technology has opened other appealing avenues for prompting. For example, apps such as *Tap to Talk* can be applied as visual and verbal prompts for making instrument choices (see Chapter 15).

MAKING IT HAPPEN

When using *prompting*, Wolery (1994) and Neitzel and Wolery (2009a) recommend considering the following:

- Apply prompts that interdisciplinary team members use effectively with the target child, always providing the least amount of assistance necessary.

- Use prompts immediately before or as the child performs the target skill.

- Provide short, concise verbal prompts (e.g., "Your turn. Play the drum."), give clear gestural prompts (e.g., conduct to cue playing an instrument), perform simple model prompts (e.g., spin around to music), give easy physical prompts (e.g., take the child's hand and shake the tambourine), and use clear visual prompts (e.g., picture schedule of upcoming musical experiences).

- Provide positive reinforcement for the child.

- Fade prompting gradually to promote the child's independence.

CASE EXAMPLE

It's Kevin's turn to play the tambourine during a mother-child music therapy group session. However, the two-year-old boy with ASD does not know what to do with the musical instrument. His mother first uses a gestural prompt by raising her arms up in the air and shaking her hands while singing the "Tambourine Song" along with the music therapist (see song transcript in Figure 9.3). When Kevin still does not respond, she physically prompts him by taking his hand and shaking the tambourine up in the air with him until it's time to stop.

Tambourine Song

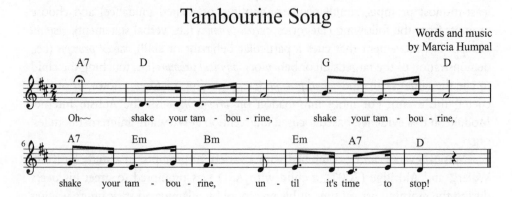

Words and music
by Marcia Humpal

Copyright © 2011 Marcia Humpal

Figure 9.3: Song—"Tambourine Song"

Planning for transitions

DESCRIPTION
Each day is filled with many transitions. Transitioning between events, locations, and people can be challenging and produce anxiety in young children with ASD (Hemmeter *et al.*, 2008; Wolery, Anthony, and Heckathorn, 1998). Core strategies can help children with ASD successfully manage transitions. Examples of these strategies include the use of structure and routines (Marcus, Schopler, and Lord, 2001) and visual cued instruction (Quill, 2000).

Songs and sound cues can signal transitions and prepare the child for what is coming next (Kern, 2008b). Results of three case examples from a pilot study conducted by Register and Humpal (2007) indicated that transition songs encourage children to respond more quickly to directives, elicit a greater level of calmness among children during times of transition, and facilitate a sense of group cohesiveness. Furthermore, transition songs and sound cues were well received by teachers as a way to manage the classroom.

MAKING IT HAPPEN
When creating and applying transition songs Humpal and Register (2004) and Kern (2008b) make the following suggestions:

- Compose songs to address specific target situations (that can be sung by various individuals across multiple settings), using original music or a familiar melody.

- Write lyrics that repeat the central message several times.

- Transcribe the lyrics with the tune noted and post it near the location the transition occurs (e.g., on the counter above the sink for a hand-washing song).

- Sing directly and repeatedly to the child and model the task at hand until the transition is completed.

- Provide a minimum level of prompting (e.g., picture symbol) until the child learns what is expected from him or her during the specific transition.

- Make the transition seamless (i.e., move immediately onto the next activity or arrive at the appropriate location as soon as the transition song ends).

- Use the same transition song across different environments and situations and with different facilitators beyond the music therapy session.

CASE EXAMPLE

Justin, a three-year-old boy with ASD, arrives at his preschool classroom. The music therapist hands a picture of his coat hanging on a hook. Initially she takes his hand, guides him to the coat rack, and sings, "Take off your coat and hang it up, take off your coat and hang it up, take off your coat and hang it up, then you can go play" (see song transcript in Figure 9.4). After Justin hangs up his coat, the music therapist immediately takes the coat picture, substitutes it with another that represents the next activity, and begins singing about this next event on his classroom schedule.

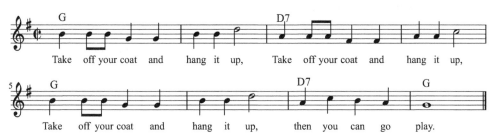

Take Off Your Coat
to the tune of "Skip to My Lou"

Adapted by Marcia Humpal   American folk melody

Copyright © 1996 Marcia Humpal

Figure 9.4: Song—"Take Off Your Coat"

Organizing the learning environment

DESCRIPTION

Young children with ASD are frequently overwhelmed by the multiple stimuli in an environment. Because they are distracted or disturbed, they may exhibit difficulty learning, completing tasks, or participating in activities (NPDC on ASD, 2008). Well-organized and structured environments can support their learning (Mesibov, Shea, and Schopler, 2005). Prominent strategies used to optimize learning environments for individuals with ASD are *environmental organization* (i.e., defined spaces) *utilizing visual schedules* (i.e., objects, pictures, or written instructions outlining a sequence of events), and *developing visual work/activity systems* (i.e., a child's visual "to do" list within a given timeframe) (Carnahan *et al.*, 2011; Mesibov, Shea, and Schopler, 2005; NPDC on ASD, 2008). For more information on *structured work systems and activity organization*, visit the Autism Internet Module on this evidence-based focused intervention at www.autisminternetmodules.org.

Defined music areas can be created in the family's home, preschool classrooms, and outdoor environments (Cryer, Harms, and Riley, 2003; Kern and Wakeford, 2007). In a study, Kern and Aldridge (2006) created an outdoor music center (i.e., Music Hut) to facilitate the involvement of four children with ASD in meaningful play and peer interactions during playground time in an inclusive preschool. In a clinical article, Furman (2001) described using a visual schedule to guide children with ASD through each activity of a music therapy session. Additionally, structured work systems in use by the child with ASD can be embedded into small-group music therapy activities.

MAKING IT HAPPEN

To organize the learning environment, the following recommendations adopted from the NPDC on ASD (2008) should be considered in music therapy practice:

- Define the music area by arranging furniture or materials (e.g., shelves with music instruments) into a designated space (e.g., corner of a preschool classroom with few distractions).

- Mark a spot within this space to indicate where children should sit (e.g., carpet squares, bean bags, pillows) and make sure that all children can see the facilitator.

- Adapt the physical structure to the individual child's needs (e.g., a quiet music listening area).

- Organize and label the music instruments and props clearly (e.g., containers with different types of musical instruments identified with photographs and word labels).

- Embed visual supports and schedules meeting the demands of the particular activity (e.g., picture symbols representing songs or each step of a session plan).

- Support the child's work/activity system (e.g., child's checklist indicating the activity/task, frequency counts, accomplishment, and next step).

CASE EXAMPLE

Fifteen minutes before the music therapy session, the music therapist transforms the circle time area into a music space for Jack, a five-year-old boy who has ASD, and his typically developing peers. Colorful pillows mark a spot for each child, while all music instruments are labeled and organized in containers placed in a music cart she brings with her. For this session, she has prepared a visual schedule for Jack on her iPad (i.e., *First Ten Visual Schedule app*) providing a picture for each session activity (i.e., gathering activity; greeting song; dancing; singing; playing instruments; listening to music; and good-bye song). As the group of children gathers, the music therapist and Jack look at the schedule. He checkmarks the picture to indicate that the first activity has been accomplished; the music therapist immediately shows him the next picture that prompts him to the next activity, the greeting song.

Giving additional response time and opportunities to repeat

DESCRIPTION

Compared to their typically developing peers, children with disabilities, especially those with ASD, may need additional time and multiple repetitions to learn a variety of single behavior or multiple-step skills (Wolery, 1994). One effective and efficient strategy for applying new skills across the day, settings, activities, and situations is *time delay*, a prompt-fading procedure (i.e., mostly model prompts) that includes a cue, child response, and feedback. Specific *time delay* procedures that may be effective for use with young children with ASD when focusing on language/communication, academic, and social/play skills are *constant time delay* (i.e., a prompt is delayed for a fixed number of seconds; e.g., four seconds at a time), and *progressive time delay* (i.e., prompt interval is gradually increased; e.g., from one to six seconds) (Neitzel and Wolery, 2009b). For more information on *time delay*, visit the Autism Internet Module on this evidence-based focused intervention at www.autisminternetmodules.org.

Additional response time and opportunities for repetition can naturally be built into music. For example, a music rest (i.e., an interval of silence in a musical piece) can be used for a *constant time delay* (e.g., four rest beats for four seconds) or a *progressive time delay* (e.g., number of rest beats increases from one to four). Sounds and sequences are often repeated in music (as indicated by a repeat sign or *da capo*), which can be utilized to give children with ASD multiple opportunities for repetition within one musical piece. Furthermore, intentionally prepared musical material can be easily implemented by parents, peers, and practitioners across disciplines, settings, activities, and situations.

MAKING IT HAPPEN

When using *time delay*, Wolery (1994) and Neitzel and Wolery (2009b) suggest the following steps:

- Identify the target skill to be learned (e.g., taking turns playing an instrument).

- Assess the child's current skills (e.g., can the child attend, wait, or imitate playing an instrument?—all prerequisites for applying time delay).

- Select the target stimulus and cue (e.g., present the instrument and sing "Your turn to play the [*name of instrument*]").

- Identify activities and times for teaching (e.g., taking turns in playing three instruments within the context of circle music time and at home).

- Select the controlling prompt (e.g., hit the gong—fixed zero-second delay).

- Determine response interval (e.g., constant time delay—four seconds).

- Identify reinforcers (e.g., applause from adults and peers).

CASE EXAMPLE

A goal for Fabian, a five-year-old boy with ASD, is to take turns during group activities with peers. During his group music therapy session, he cannot wait to play the gong, his favorite instrument. While his peers are patiently waiting for their turn to play, he gets out of his seat and excitedly jumps up and down. The music therapist sings and signs the "Please Wait" song (Kern and Snell, 2007), which reminds him to wait in his seat. When it is Fabian's turn to play, the music therapist presents the gong (target cue) to him while singing, "It's Fabian's time to play…" She immediately hits the gong (controlling prompt). She repeats her singing, "It's Fabian's turn to play…," pausing four seconds (constant time delay) for Fabian to respond. After he hits the gong (correct response), the music therapist says, "You took your turn playing the gong!" His peers join her in rewarding Fabian with a big round of applause (positive feedback). During this session, the music therapist gives Fabian several more opportunities to take turns playing the gong and other instruments. She encourages peers, classroom teachers, and parents to apply the same procedure when playing instruments with Fabian throughout the day and in different environments (e.g., on the playground, at a play group, or at home).

Active involvement of peers

DESCRIPTION

Learning occurs within a social context, and in children's natural environment, therefore, peers of young children with ASD can play an important role in promoting their acquisition of skills. In a *peer-mediated instruction and intervention* process, peers are systematically taught how to engage with children with ASD to improve targeted skills. Involving peers in this manner is an effective way to address communication/

language, and social skill development with children with ASD (DiSalvo and Oswald, 2002; NAC, 2009; Neitzel, 2008). For more information on *peer-mediated instruction and intervention*, visit the Autism Internet Module on this evidence-based focused intervention at www.autisminternetmodules.org.

Music therapy services in early childhood settings are often provided in small-group sessions that include typically developing peers. Designing interventions that involve systematic support from peers has long been documented in early childhood music therapy inclusion programming (Hughes *et al.*, 1990; Humpal, 1991). Kern and Aldridge (2006) employed peer-mediated instruction as part of a song intervention study to increase the interactions and meaningful play of three children with ASD on an inclusive preschool playground. Fidelity ratings demonstrated that peers implemented most parts of the five-step intervention procedures correctly.

MAKING IT HAPPEN

For implementing peer-mediated instructions and interventions in music therapy practice the following recommendations adopted from Neitzel (2008) should be considered:

- Design a simple music intervention that supports a specific learning goal of the target child with ASD.

- Prepare the procedure and corresponding materials.

- Select peers who (a) are interested in music-making, (b) demonstrate social competencies and strong language skills, (c) have a positive relationship with the child with ASD, (d) are able to follow directions, (e) can attend to a task for an adequate amount of time, (f) are motivated to participate, and (g) are available on a regular basis.

- Educate peers about differences and similarities, and explain how this will apply when making music with the target child with ASD (e.g., instead of simply passing a drumstick, place it in the child's hand and say "Your turn to play the drum").

- Introduce the specific music intervention to the child with ASD and peers by modeling each step of the procedure, giving each child the opportunity to practice, and provide support for completing the task correctly.

- Provide prompts and reinforcement as necessary until peers are proficient in applying the music activity, then fade any additional support.

- Observe the target child's progress and provide positive feedback as well as motivation for peers to continue.

CASE EXAMPLE

Three-year-old Aliyah who has ASD likes to sing and spin around; however, she does not respond when her peers invite her to dance with them. Instead, she runs away, disappointing her peers who really like her. Aliyah's music therapist is working with her to increase peer interactions. She explains to the peers that Aliyah may not understand what they want from her. Perhaps it would be best to take her hand and show her how to spin around together. While she is demonstrating this to the peers, the music therapist teaches them the song, "All I really like to do, is to have a dance with you (…). Round and round and round we go, sometimes fast and sometimes slow." Aliyah observes the little group with excitement. Together, they once more invite her to join the dancing, but this time they take her hand and say "Come dance with us." The music therapist supports the children by singing the song and encouraging the peers to dance. After three sessions, the children know the song; they independently do the dance routine with Aliyah. She obviously enjoys the experience and smiles as she sings along with her peers.

Conclusion

This chapter examined instructional strategies and related music therapy techniques that have been successfully used with young children with ASD. Determining effective strategies and techniques requires an understanding of developmentally appropriate practice and must be guided by the child's unique learning style, strengths, and specific needs. Not all strategies will be effective for all children with ASD. Because children with ASD are considerably challenged in transferring and adapting learned skills from one context to another (NAC, 2009), generalization will not naturally occur and needs to be explicitly learned through planning and programming (Mesibov, Shea, and Schopler, 2005). However, many of the described instructional strategies outlined in this chapter can support the functional use of newly learned skills across children's naturally occurring activities and routines when intentionally applied. Professionals and parents may gain additional knowledge from their daily experiences with individuals with ASD and also learn from individuals with ASD who share their insights in speaking and writing. Figure 9.5 reflects these thoughts and summarizes some of the more prominent tips to consider and remember when working with young children with ASD.

Remember

- Accept the child unconditionally.
- Focus on what children can do rather than on what they cannot do.
- Provide focused as well as challenging activities at the appropriate developmental level.
- Include activities that include typically developing peers.
- Work with the family and the professional team to ensure continuity.
- If a child has an outburst, think about what happened immediately prior to it or what the child might be trying to communicate via the behavior.
- Include visual cues and provide demonstrations that the child can see.
- Avoid using long sentences or explanations—show, then tell.
- Be aware of possible hyper-sensitivity to loud sounds, aversion to textures, or reactions to fluorescent lights and arrange the environment accordingly (e.g., let the child sit or play in a different area of the room).
- Make alternate forms of communication available (e.g., pictures; augmentative communication devices; cue cards).
- Provide structure, predictability, and a regular routine.
- Be consistent.
- Give advance notice of change to help the child transition.
- Recognize and utilize the child's interests or special objects.
- Make time for fun activities.

Sources: Adamek and Darrow (2005); Grandin (2002); National Institute of Mental Health (2011); Santomauro (2011); Willis (2009).

Figure 9.5: Tips from parents, professionals, and individuals with ASD

LEARNING QUESTIONS

1. In which way do children with ASD learn differently than typically developing children?

2. Name at least two strategies that can support social development, communication, and language skills, and prevent challenging behaviors of children with ASD.

3. What music therapy techniques are typically used in early childhood settings and with children with ASD?

4. What six core instructional strategies for children with ASD are introduced in this chapter?

5. How can a music therapy session be structured to provide predictable routines?

6. Give an example of how verbal, gestural, model, physical, and visual prompts can be combined with musical events.

7. What should be considered when creating and using transition songs with young children who have ASD?

8. Discuss how the three prominent strategies used to optimize the learning environment for individuals with ASD may apply to music therapy practice.

9. Give an example of how time delay can be applied in music therapy sessions.

10. What are considerations for planning peer-mediated music therapy interventions?

References

Adamek, M., and Darrow, A. (2005). *Music in Special Education.* Silver Spring, MD: AMTA.

Barton, E.E., Reichow, B., Wolery, M., and Chen, C.-I. (2011). We can all participate! Adapting circle time for children with autism. *Young Exceptional Children, 14(2),* 2–21.

Carnahan, C., Harte, H., Schumacher Dyke, K., Hume, K., and Borders, K. (2011). Structured work systems: Supporting meaningful engagement in preschool settings for children with autism spectrum disorders. *Young Exceptional Children, 14(1),* 2–16.

Copple, C., and Bredekamp, S. (2009). *Developmentally Appropriate Practice in Early Childhood Programs Serving Children from Birth Through Age 8 (Third Edition).* Washington, DC: NAEYC.

Cryer, D., Harms, T., and Riley, C. (2003). *Early Childhood Environments Rating Scales—Revised.* New York: Teachers College, Columbia University.

Dawson, G., and Osterling, J. (1997). Early intervention in autism. In M.J. Guralnick (Ed.) *The Effectiveness of Early Intervention.* Baltimore, MD: Paul H. Brookes Publishing Co.

DiSalvo, C.A., and Oswald, D.P. (2002). Peer-mediated interventions to increase the social interaction of children with autism: Consideration of peer expectancies. *Focus on Autism and Other Developmental Disorders, 17(4),* 198–207.

Drager, K.D.R., Light, J.C., and Fink, E.H. (2009). Using AAC technologies to build social interaction with young children with autism spectrum disorders. In P. Mirenda and T. Iacono (Eds.) *Autism Spectrum Disorders and AAC.* Baltimore, MD: Paul H. Brookes Publishing Co.

Dunlap, G., and Strain, P. (2009). Preventing challenging behavior: A model for young children with autism spectrum disorder. TACSEI teleconference, 2 November. Retrieved from www.challengingbehavior.org/explore/webinars/11.2.2009_tacsei_presentation_teleconference.htm.

Frost, L., and Bondy, A. (2002). *PECS: The Picture Exchange Communication System Training Manual (Second Edition).* Cherry Hill, NJ: Pyramid Educational Consultants, Inc.

Furman, A. (2001). Young children with autism spectrum disorder. *Early Childhood Connections, 7(2),* 43–49.

Grandin, T. (2002). Teaching tips for children and adults with autism. Autism is treatable page. Autism Research Institute. Retrieved from www.autism.com/ind_teaching_tips.asp.

Grandin, T. (2011). *The way I see it. A personal look at autism & Asperger's.* Arlington, TX: Future Horizons.

Gray, C., and Garand, J. (1993). Social Stories™: Improving responses of students with autism with accurate social information. *Focus on Autistic Behavior, 8,* 1–10.

Hatton, D., Shaw, E., and Cox, A.W. (2008). Guiding principles for interventions and education. In A. Cox, D. Hatton, G.A. Williams, and R.E. Pretzel (Eds.) *Foundations of Autism Spectrum Disorders: An Online Course* (Session 4). Chapel Hill, NC: National Professional Development Center on Autism Spectrum Disorders, FPG Child Development Institute, the University of North Carolina.

Hemmeter, M.L., Ostrosky, M.M., Artman, K.M., and Kinder, K.A. (2008). Moving right along… Planning transitions to prevent challenging behavior. *Young Children, 63(3),* 18–25.

Hughes, J., Robbins, B., McKenzie, B., and Robb, S. (1990). Integrating exceptional and nonexceptional young children through music play: A pilot program. *Music Therapy Perspectives, 8,* 52–56.

Humpal, M. (1991). The effects of an integrated early childhood music program on social interaction among children with handicaps and their typical peers. *Journal of Music Therapy, 28(3),* 161–177.

Humpal, M. and Register, D. (2004). Tips for tuneful transitions. Paper presented at the 6th annual AMTA conference, Austin, TX, November.

Kern, P. (2004). *Using a Music Therapy Collaborative Consultative Approach for the Inclusion of Young Children with Autism in a Childcare Program.* Unpublished doctoral dissertation, University of Witten-Herdecke, Germany.

Kern, P. (2008a). Common Techniques. SOS Early Childhood. Paper presented with Marcia Humpal at the 10th Anniversary Conference of AMTA, St. Louis, MO, USA, November 2008.

Kern, P. (2008b). Singing our way through the day: Using music with young children during daily routines. *Children and Families, 22(2),* 50–56.

Kern, P., and Aldridge, D. (2006). Using embedded music therapy interventions to support outdoor play of young children with autism in an inclusive community-based child care program. *Journal of Music Therapy, 43(4),* 270–294.

Kern, P., and Snell, A.M. (2007). *Songbook Vol. I: Songs and Laughter on the Playground.* Santa Barbara, CA: De La Vista Publisher.

Kern, P., and Wakeford, L. (2007). Supporting outdoor play for young children: The zone model of playground supervision. *Young Children, 62(2),* 12–16.

Kern, P., Wolery, M., and Aldridge, D. (2007). Use of songs to promote independence in morning greeting routines for young children with autism. *Journal of Autism and Developmental Disorders, 37(7),* 1264–1271.

Marcus, L., Schopler, E., and Lord, C. (2001). TEACCH Services for preschool children. In J.S. Handelman and S.L. Harris (Eds.) *Preschool Education Programs for Childrenm with Autism (Second Edition).* Autsin, TX: Pro-Ed.

Martin, B., and Archambault, J. (1989). *Chicka, Chicka, Boom, Boom.* New York, London, Toronto, Sydney, and Singapore: Aladdin Paperbacks.

McGee, G.G., Morrier, M.J., and Daly, T. (2001). The Walden early childhood programs. In J.S. Handelman and S.L. Harris (Eds.) *Preschool Education Programs for Children with Autism (Second Edition)*. Austin, TX: Pro-Ed.

Mesibov, G.B., Shea, V., and Schopler, E. (2005). *The TEACCH Approach to Autism Spectrum Disorders*. New York: Plenum Press.

NAEYC (2009). Position statement. *Developmentally Appropriate Practice in Early Childhood Programs Serving Children from Birth through Age 8*. Washington, DC: NAEYC.

National Autism Center (NAC) (2009). *National Standards Report*. The National Standards Project— Addressing the need for evidence-based practice guidelines for autism spectrum disorders. Randolph, MA: NAC.

National Institute of Mental Health (2011). *Early Intervention: A Parent's Guide to Autism Spectrum Disorder*. Bethesda, MD: National Institute of Mental Health.

National Professional Development Center on Autism Spectrum Disorders (NPDC on ASD) (n.d.) Home. Retrieved from http://autismpdc.fpg.unc.edu.

National Professional Development Center on Autism Spectrum Disorders (NPDC on ASD) (2008). Session 6: Instructional strategies and learning environments. In *Foundations of Autism Spectrum Disorders: An Online Course*. Chapel Hill, NC: FPG Child Development Institute, the University of North Carolina.

National Research Council (NRC) (2001). *Educating Children with Autism*. Washington, DC: The National Academies Press.

Neitzel, J. (2008). *Steps for Implementation: PMII for Early Childhood*. Chapel Hill, NC: National Professional Development Center on Autism Spectrum Disorders, FPG Child Development Institute, the University of North Carolina.

Neitzel, J., and Wolery, M. (2009a). Overview of Prompting. Chapel Hill, NC: The National Professional Development Center on Autism Spectrum Disorders, FPG Child Development Institute, the University of North Carolina.

Neitzel, J., and Wolery, M. (2009b). *Steps for Implementation: Time Delay*. Chapel Hill, NC: The National Professional Development Center on Autism Spectrum Disorders, FPG Child Development Institute, the University of North Carolina.

Quill, K.A. (2000). *Do–Watch–Listen–Say: Social Communication Intervention for Children with Autism*. Baltimore, MD: Paul H. Brookes Publishing Co.

Register, D., and Humpal, M. (2007). Using musical transitions in early childhood classrooms: Three case examples. *Music Therapy Perspectives, 25(1)*, 25–31.

Sandall, S., McLean, M.E., and Smith, B.J. (2000). *DEC: Recommended Practices in Early Intervention/Early Childhood Special Education*. Longmont, CO: Sopris West.

Sandall, S., Schwartz, I., and Joseph, G. (2001). A building blocks model for effective instruction in inclusive early childhood settings. *Young Exceptional Children, 4(3)*, 3–9.

Santomauro, J. (2011). *Autism All-Stars: How We Use Our Autism and Asperger Traits to Shine in Life*. London and Philadelphia: Jessica Kingsley Publishers.

Sigafoos, J., and Drasgow, E. (2001). Conditional use of aided and unaided AAC: A review and clinical case demonstration. *Focus on Autism and Other Developmental Disabilities, 16(3)*, 152–161.

Tien, K.C., and Lee, H.J. (2007). Structure/modifications. In S. Henry and B.S. Myles (Eds.) *The Comprehensive Autism Planning System (CAPS) for Individuals with Asperger Syndrome, Autism, and Related Disabilities: Integrating Best Practice Throughout the Student's Day*. Shawnee Mission, KS: Autism Asperger Publishing Company.

Walworth, D. (2010). Incorporating music into daily routines: Family education and integration. *imagine 1*, (1), 28–31.

Willis, C. (2009). Young children with autism spectrum disorder: Strategies that work. *Young Children, 64 (1)*, 81–89.

Wolery, M. (1994). Instructional strategies for teaching young children with special needs. In M. Wolery and J. Wilbers (Ed.) *Including Children with Special Needs in Early Childhood Programs*. Washington, DC: National Association for the Education of Young Children.

Wolery, M., Anthony, L., and Heckathorn, J. (1998). Transition-based teaching: Effects on transitions, teachers' behavior, and children's learning. *Journal of Early Intervention, 21(20)*, 117–131.

PART 4

Collaboration and Consultation

Chapter 10

Collaborative Consultation

Embedding Music Therapy Interventions for Young Children with Autism Spectrum Disorders in Inclusive Preschool Settings

Petra Kern, Ph.D., MT-DMtG, MT-BC, MTA
MUSIC THERAPY CONSULTING
SANTA BARBARA, CA

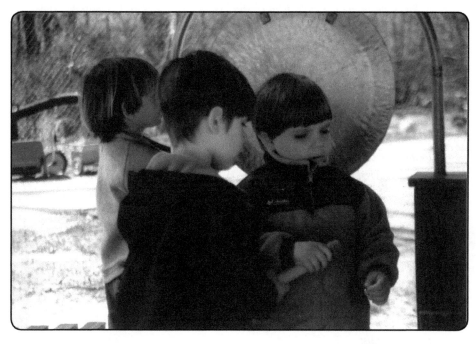

PHOTO COURTESY OF PETRA KERN

Music is a natural way for children to explore the world
around them and to interact within a social environment.
(Petra Kern)

This chapter introduces music therapy as an intervention option for young children with autism spectrum disorders (ASD) enrolled in inclusive childcare programs. A case scenario illustrates a step-by-step music therapy intervention process, which can be embedded in the child's daily activities and routines. The roles of interdisciplinary team members in the intervention process and current practice and research information from the field of music therapy are also described.

Case vignette
Scenario 1: Child performance and referral

> Megan and Kaila are teaching at an inclusive community-based childcare program in the United States. Enrolled in their class are 12 children (ages three to four), including one child with cerebral palsy, one with Down Syndrome, and Justin, a four-year-old European-American boy with ASD. Justin is functioning on the Childhood ASD Rating Scale (CARS) in the mild to moderate range on the autism spectrum. Since joining the classroom two months ago, Justin has bonded with the classroom teachers, but has made insufficient progress in interacting with peers and communicating with others. He prefers being alone and often engages in repetitive behaviors such as spinning in circles. Megan and Kaila are continuously looking for strategies and intervention options that could be beneficial for Justin to improve his skills. Megan observed that Justin hums many children's songs to himself and responds positively to music. Whenever music is involved in classroom activities, Justin is very attentive and motivated to participate, and he seems to stay engaged with tasks for a longer time. Justin's parents also noticed that listening to familiar children's songs comforts him. Watching Sesame Street's™ music program helps him learn about colors, numbers, and letters. Dancing to music makes him laugh. During the next interdisciplinary team meeting, Justin's mom talks about his affinity for music and asks if a music intervention could support his learning. The occupational therapist suggests consulting with Emma, a music therapist with whom she has worked before. Justin's mom asks Megan if she would contact the music therapist.

Justin's difficulty in communicating and interacting with others as well as his repetitive behaviors are typical characteristics of ASD, which is generally evident before age three (American Psychiatric Association [APA], 2000; Centers for Disease Control and Prevention [CDC], 2012). Although not included in the diagnostic criteria, Justin's heightened interest and positive response to music is often seen in children with ASD, as noted in testimonies from parents and teachers as well as in self-reports from individuals with ASD. Turnbull (2010), for instance, says during a Division of Early Childhood (DEC) webinar, "This is Jay at his fortieth birthday party doing what he loved so much…a love that started in early childhood, which is music." Grandin (n.d.), herself diagnosed with ASD, reports that during elementary school she had difficulty with speech production, but "Singing, however, was easy." And Williams (1996) describes having "memory for long strings of patterns" such as music patterns, and remembers the emotional impact music had when she was playing piano as a teenager with ASD.

Moreover, the growing research literature on the musical responsiveness and aptitudes of individuals with ASD provides scientific evidence for anecdotal reports (e.g., Applebaum *et al.*, 1979; Heaton, 2003; Heaton, Hermelin, and Pring, 1998; Thaut, 1987). At present, there is no scientific explanation for the interest and aptitude in music that children with ASD may demonstrate. It should be noted, however, that not all children with ASD show interest and aptitude in music, and some may even display unusual or negative responses to certain sounds due to sensory processing issues (Ermer and Dunn, 1998).

Given that music can function as a primary motivator or positive reinforcement technique for learning in children with ASD (Koegel, Rincover, and Engel, 1982), music therapy might be an appropriate intervention option. Most young children like to sing, chant, rhyme, dance, or listen to music in their daily lives; therefore, music may provide natural learning opportunities for all children and can encourage or facilitate inclusion of children with ASD (Kern, 2008).

In the United States, children with ASD enrolled in educational settings are typically referred to music therapy by parents and/or interdisciplinary team members as part of the child's Individualized Education Program (IEP) if:

- additional support is necessary to achieve the child's learning goals based on slow or insufficient progress, interfering behaviors, or limited number of instructional approaches/interventions to which the child has been responsive

- music is a documented learning modality of the child; that is, the child shows positive response to sound and music (e.g., significant changes in attention, motivation, ability to stay on task during music activities), is capable of grasping new information and concepts through music (e.g., memorizing a sequence of steps through songs), and/or demonstrates unique difference in his/her abilities (e.g., communicative responses, academic and motor functioning, emotional and social engagement)

- there is evidence that the child's IEP goal areas can be functionally supported by a music therapy intervention.

(King and Coleman, 2006; Lazar, 2007; Snell, 2002)

Some music therapists provide a referral form to IEP teams for determining if the child qualifies for a comprehensive music therapy assessment. When considering music therapy services for children with ASD, parents, classroom teachers, and specialists may want to ask the questions outlined in Table 10.1.

Table 10.1 Questions for considering music therapy as an intervention option for ASD
Ten questions to ask a music therapist
1. Are you a board-certified music therapist?
2. When would it be appropriate to refer a child with ASD for music therapy?
3. Which research outcomes support the benefits of music therapy interventions for children with ASD?
4. How can a music therapy assessment contribute to the child's IEP?
5. Which strategies, techniques, and materials will you use with children with ASD?
6. Can current music options offered to the child be applied more intentionally?
7. How can a music therapy intervention be implemented in daily activities and routines?
8. Which service delivery model would be appropriate?
9. What would in-service and/or staff training look like?
10. What are the reimbursement options for early childhood music therapy services?

Scenario 2: Initial interview and assessment

Justin's teacher Megan contacts the music therapist Emma to find out more about music therapy and to see if music therapy interventions would be beneficial for improving Justin's functional skills during daily activities and routines. At the initial contact, Emma listens to Megan's request and answers her questions. Then Emma asks Megan about Justin's strengths and needs, his musical responsiveness, preferences, and aptitude, his current IEP goals, instructional strategies in use, the services already provided, as well as the family's preferences and values. After talking with Emma, Megan is convinced that music could be a beneficial learning tool for Justin. Therefore, she arranges an onsite visit with Emma. During her visit, Emma asks if she may review Justin's records with his parents' permission. Then, she participates in the classroom activities and routines while observing Justin's behavior in different situations and across settings. She also engages Justin in music-making during free play to learn more about his current level of functioning in all developmental areas. During circle time, Emma asks Megan to include typical music activities. On the playground, Emma invites a group of children to explore musical instruments she brought with her. As she and the children start improvising on the drums and making up a song, Emma notices that Justin stays in close proximity to the group. She models singing in a toy microphone and offers Justin a turn. He imitates vowels while rhythmically jumping up and down to the group's drumming. After briefly reflecting with Megan on her observations,

Emma agrees to work on an assessment report and make suggestions during the forthcoming interdisciplinary team meeting.

Seeking more information about music therapy, Megan and Justin's mom would probably discover the following definition: "Music Therapy is the clinical and evidence-based use of music interventions to accomplish individualized goals within a therapeutic relationship by a credentialed professional who has completed an approved music therapy program" (AMTA, n.d.). Additional answers to frequently asked questions may be found at the website of the World Federation of Music Therapy (WFMT) at www.wfmt.info. Music therapy is an allied health profession similar to speech-language pathology, physical therapy, and occupational therapy. Among the four general treatment options available for children with ASD (i.e., *Behavior and Communication Approaches, Dietary Approaches, Medication,* and *Complementary and Alternative Medicine*) (CDC, 2012), music therapy typically falls under "*Complementary and Alternative Medicine.*"

Music therapy interventions offer age and developmentally appropriate learning opportunities to improve core skills and independent functioning of children with ASD in daily life (Kern, Wakeford, and Aldridge, 2007; Kern, Wolery, and Aldridge, 2007). Music intervention can be embedded in the child's natural environment such as the home or childcare program's playground, and may be adapted to the individual's needs (Kern and Aldridge, 2006). Music therapy sessions provide familiarity, consistency, structure, and predictability, which all support the learning style of children with ASD (Kern, 2008).

As a member of an interdisciplinary team or contracting partner, music therapists work in close collaboration with parents, early childhood educators, and other specialists to maximize children's learning. Music therapists working in early childhood settings may (a) suggest curriculum modifications and adaptations, (b) assist in designing embedded learning opportunities, or (c) provide direct music therapy services.

Music therapy services may be reimbursed by the childcare program's operation funds, private grants, or as a related service under federal laws such as the Individuals with Disabilities Education Act (IDEA) in the U.S. (Schwartz, 2006). According to a policy clarification statement from the United States Department of Education, direct or consultative music therapy services can be included on a child's IEP if the IEP team determines this service is necessary for the achievement of the child's educational program (U.S. Department of Education, 2010).

In order to understand and address the individual needs of a child with ASD and to determine the eligibility for music therapy services, music therapists conduct an assessment. Parts of the assessment process are (a) reviewing of medical and educational records, (b) surveying/interviewing family and staff involved with the child, (c) observing the child in different contexts, and (d) evaluating the child in his/her natural environment (King and Coleman, 2006; Lazar, 2007; Snell, 2002).

During the direct assessment, the music therapist engages the child with ASD in music listening, improvisation, singing, and movement to assess his or her musical skills (i.e., musical responsiveness, preferences, and aptitude) and non-musical skills (i.e., communication, academic, motor, emotional, and social skills) in his or her natural environment. Music therapists may apply unique music therapy assessment tools and checklists designed for use with children of varying disabilities, including ASD (e.g., Carpente, 2011; Hummel-Rossi *et al.*, 2008; King and Coleman, 2006; Lazar, 2007; Snell, 2002), or the assessment procedures utilized by the childcare program. In order to meet the constantly changing needs of young children with ASD, music therapists engage in ongoing assessment and follow-ups throughout the intervention process. The music therapy assessment is one component of an evaluation process that assists the interdisciplinary team in finding the most appropriate intervention options and supports for children with ASD.

Scenario 3: Decision-making and intervention planning

The music therapist Emma meets with Justin's interdisciplinary team, including Justin's mom, the early childhood educators Megan and Kaila, the occupational therapist, the speech-language pathologist, the physical therapist, and the special educator. Emma refers to the assessment report and summarizes what she had observed in each skill area by giving examples and explaining the baseline data she has collected on Justin's behavior. The interdisciplinary team confirms her observations and asks how a music therapy intervention could provide learning opportunities for improving Justin's IEP-related skills. Emma suggests that Justin's peer interaction and expressive communication targeted goals could be addressed via music therapy. She gives examples of how music can support social and communication skills in children with ASD and provides evidence from peer-reviewed research literature. Additionally, she informs the team about possible service delivery models and how strategies already in use with Justin can be included in the music therapy intervention. Following the five-step decision-making process of evidence-based practice in early childhood (i.e., pose the question, find the best available research evidence, appraise the evidence quality and relevance, integrate research with value and wisdom, and evaluate), the team comes to the conclusion that an embedded music therapy intervention may be highly beneficial for Justin. The team asks Emma to prepare the music intervention, including specific strategies and supports, and to suggest how it can be easily implemented and evaluated by the classroom teachers throughout the childcare day.

As in Justin's case, each child with ASD has unique strengths and weaknesses. Therefore, educational and therapeutic interventions must be individualized to the child's individual needs and abilities (National Research Council [NRC], 2001). Based on the assessment results, the music therapist suggests which goal areas may be addressed effectively through a music therapy intervention. Goal areas typically targeted by music therapists working with individuals on the ASD spectrum may fall under the three developmental domain areas outlined in the SCERTS® Model: social communication, emotional regulation, and transactional support, as well as corresponding sub-domains of these areas (Walworth, Register, and Engel, 2009).

The results of a Cochrane review (Gold, Wigram, and Elefant, 2006), a meta-analysis (Whipple, 2004), and more recent scientific literature indicate that there is an emerging body of evidence supporting the effectiveness of music therapy as an intervention for individuals on the autism spectrum. However, many of the previously published studies do not meet the scientific rigor proposed by experts in the field of ASD (Reichow, Volkmar, and Cicchetti, 2008) and the Council for Exceptional Children (2006). Music therapy interventions for individuals on the autism spectrum most likely fall under the *Promising Practice* level of evidence-based practice (Kern, 2010; Umbarger, 2007) or *Emerging Practice* (National Autism Center [NAC], 2009).

According to the most recent meta-analysis conducted by Whipple (see Chapter 3) music intervention studies which meet rigorous study criteria (i.e., NAC, 2009; Reichow, Volkmar, and Cicchetti, 2008) are reported to be valid for young children with ASD in developing communication, interpersonal, personal responsibility, and play skills. However, ultimately, the intervention team must weigh the research evidence against (a) professional expertise and experience, (b) family values, beliefs, and priorities, and (c) various local and contextual factors, while keeping the child's characteristics and preferences in mind, in order to decide if music therapy would be the best intervention option for the particular child with ASD (Buysse *et al.*, 2006).

When a music therapy intervention is deemed appropriate, the team collaboratively develops functional goals and objectives that are specific, measurable, attainable, realistic, and have a timeframe (King and Coleman, 2006). In collaboration with the team, the music therapist develops a written *Intervention Plan* that may include the information outlined in Table 10.2. The content therein can easily be transferred to the childcare program's existing planning and documentation forms such as an activity matrix (e.g., Schwartz, 2010) or a consultation form (e.g., Buysse and Wesley, 2005). When providing direct services, the music therapist prepares a *Session Plan* for each session that includes various opportunities for the child with ASD to practice the targeted skills. In the *Progress Notes*, the music therapist documents the child's performance, adaptations, and the next steps.

Table 10.2 Content of a music therapy intervention plan for a child with ASD	
Elements	**Description**
Short client description	Child's demographics, records, strengths, and needs.
Intervention goals and objectives	Functional and measurable goals that can be addressed by a music therapy intervention.
Model of service delivery	Individual pull-out, small group pull-out, one-to-one in class, group activity, individual during routines, or consultation and assigned roles of the team members.
Location and length of the intervention	Individualized and depends on service delivery model provided.
Modification of the environment/materials	Change of the acoustics; selection, adaptation, and arrangement of musical materials; application of assistive technology.
Function of music	Cue an activity or event; prompt a sequence or steps; stimulate learning in developmental domains; distract from undesired behavior; reinforce positive behavior; and/or create a stimulating or relaxing environment.
Music therapy techniques	Music listening, singing, chanting, rhyming, instrument play, music and movement, music improvisation, or music combined with other creative activities (e.g., painting to music).
Population specific strategies (i.e., ASD)	Provide structure, predictability, and routines; use verbal, gestural, model, physical, and visual prompts; plan for transitions; organize the learning environment; present concrete tasks and break them down to smaller parts; extend response time and opportunities for repetition; include peer and adult support; utilize generalization.
Data collection/ measurement procedure	Method of collecting baseline and intervention data, including recording forms and other means of evidence of the child's progress (e.g., audio or video recordings).

Sources: Humpal and Colwell (2006); Kern (2008); Lazar (2007); McWilliam (1996); Snell (2002).

Scenario 4: Staff training and continuous support

During the next visit, Emma discusses the objectives, strategies, and the music intervention procedure with the interdisciplinary team. After Justin's mom gives permission and the team reaches consensus on the intervention details, Emma trains the staff on how to use a song she has selected for Justin (see Figure 10.1). In alignment with Justin's IEP goals and short-term objectives, the song offers Justin the following three learning opportunities: (a) to enhance interest in and awareness of others, (b) to increase imitation of peers, and (c) to improve expressive communication. In order to make Justin feel more comfortable with the new song, Emma included the American Sign Language signs for "you" and "I" that he already knows. When Emma models the music intervention during circle time, she invites all the children to imitate and practice the signs while singing the first part of the song. Then, she gathers everyone around a large drum and hands out drumsticks while singing "one, two, three, four, take your stick" and asks the children to play after her as the words of the song indicate. Next, she picks Justin as a play partner and repeats the song with him, while his teacher Megan prompts him physically to play his part when it is his turn. The other children suggest trying out the shakers with the song, and each of them finds a partner with whom to sing and play. Megan supports Justin in pointing out a peer while singing "you and I" and imitating the motor actions of his partner who plays the shaker. As soon as Justin is familiar with the song and routine, Emma recommends pausing at the end of each song line to let Justin fill in the missing word, then in the future extending to accommodate filling in complete phrases.

Additionally, Emma suggests applying the song to other situations during the day. For instance, a hand-washing routine could be composed by altering the lyrics: "You and I, we wash our hands…one, two, three, four, turn the water on and wet your hands…get the soap…rub your hand…rinse your hands…turn the water off…dry your hands…all done now…job well done." Emma recommends combining the song with picture symbols following the sequence of steps involved in hand-washing. To ensure consistency and generalization across settings, she sends a note and a recording of the song to Justin's parents and encourages them to use the song at home. Because the melody of the song follows the speech-language rhythm of the words, it can also be spoken instead of sung, and eventually faded out completely.

You and I!

Words and music
by Petra Kern

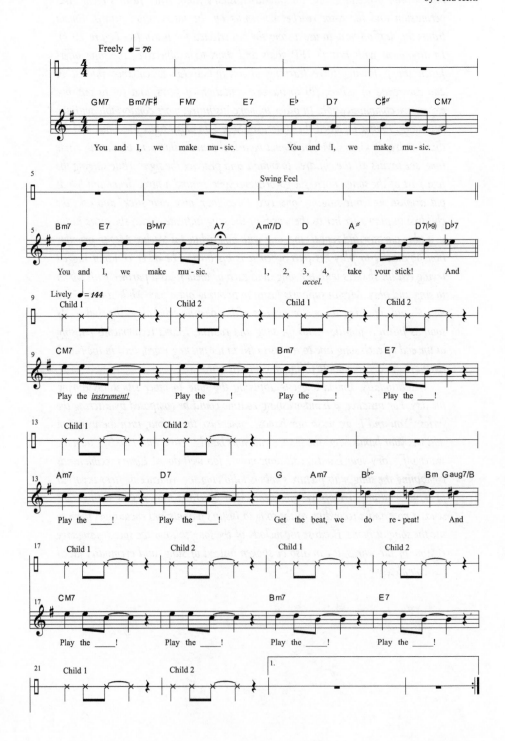

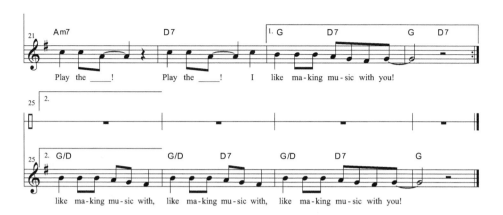

Note: *Repeat for additional instruments. Use sign language for "you," "I," and "music."*

Copyright © 2002 Petra Kern

Source: *Kern, P., and Snell, A.M. (2007). Songbook Vol. I: Songs and Laughter on the Playground. Santa Barbara, CA: De La Vista Publisher. Reprinted with permission.*

Figure 10.1: *Intervention song—"You and I"*

> To evaluate Justin's performance, Emma prepared an observational recording form, which utilizes frequency counts of Justin's behavior over a three-month period. The classroom teachers agree to collect data related to the following short-term objectives listed on Justin's IEP:
>
> 1. Justin will point out a peer to play with two out of three times during the song activity with minimal physical prompting by adults.
>
> 2. Justin will take turns and imitate a peer's motor action five out of eight opportunities provided by the song with minimal physical prompting by adults.
>
> 3. Justin will correctly fill in half of the song lyrics with three or fewer verbal promptings by adults.
>
> After the classroom teachers feel confident in applying the song and collecting performance data, Emma offers her continued support via video conferencing, email, and additional onsite visits. Two weeks later, Megan makes use of this offer as Justin continuously plays the drum during the song without waiting for his turn to imitate. Megan records the challenging situation with her iPad and sends it to Emma for review. Emma responds the following day and suggests using only one drumstick, clarifying that the children should play one after another. Emma also checks in with Megan about Justin's overall performance data and encourages her to continue with the adaptations.

Contemporary service delivery for children with ASD is based on an integrated therapy model—specialized therapies are embedded in the child's daily routines and activities (NRC, 2001). Within the continuum of service delivery models (i.e., individual pull-out, small group pull-out, one-to-one in class, group activity, individual during routines, or consultation), the collaborative consultative approach is seen as the most integrated and desirable model as it attends to values such as normalization, continuity, maintenance, and generalization (McWilliam, 1996). When choosing a collaborative consultative service delivery model such as in Justin's case, the early childhood educators, parents, and specialists engage equally in defining the problem, identifying the goals, and planning the intervention. The music therapy consultant conducts the assessment, provides training on the use of the music therapy strategies and techniques, supports the teacher during the implementation, and follows up with teachers and parents (Buysse and Wesley, 2005).

Music therapists working in educational settings frequently use embedded intervention strategies as well as collaborative and consultative approaches when serving young children with ASD (Register, 2002; Snell, 2002). A series of single-case experimental studies conducted by Kern and colleagues demonstrated that a collaborative consultative approach can be effective in enabling early childhood educators to implement music therapy interventions successfully. Through individualized song interventions, children with ASD acquired new skills and improved in deficit areas such as transitioning from home to school (Kern, Wolery, and Aldridge, 2007), following multiple-step tasks during classroom routines (Kern, Wakeford, and Aldridge, 2007), and peer interaction on a childcare playground (Kern and Aldridge, 2006). In fact, the song "You and I," introduced in the case vignette, was written for one of the four participants in the playground interaction study.

Scenario 5: Final evaluation and termination

Three months after the implementation of the plan, Justin's performance data indicates that he made great progress and accomplished the set objectives. Megan invites Emma for a final classroom visit to share and celebrate Justin's achievements with his mom and the entire class. Emma is pleased with Justin's progress and with the early childhood educator's persistence and accuracy in implementing the music intervention. She joins all the children in singing Justin's song "You and I" during circle time and everyone applauds after Justin plays his drum part. Emma records the song and sends it back as an mp3 file to the class with a hip underlying rhythm loop from GarageBand™. After listening to the audio file, the children in Megan and Kaila's class enthusiastically suggest recording all their favorite songs. Megan decides to create a song playlist, which she uploads on the classroom's website so that parents and extended family members can access it. The playlist description includes comments from the children and features "Justin on drums." Justin's mom is proud of her son and happy that he is seen as a child who likes to make music, just like everyone else in the class.

Finally, the team holds a summary conference to reflect on Justin's skill improvements and to discuss if additional goal areas should be addressed through a music therapy intervention. Emma asks for feedback on her consultative services and agrees to send a final report.

If the child with ASD has successfully reached the objectives, as Justin's classroom teacher documented, the music therapy intervention can be terminated. Other reasons for termination of a music therapy intervention may be that (a) the data does not indicate improvements after intervention modification or within the established timeframe, (b) the child responds negatively to the intervention (e.g., overstimulation), or (c) the parents decide to discontinue the service (Gfeller and Davis, 2008).

After the intervention team decides that the music therapy service will be terminated, the music therapist prepares a *Final Evaluation*, including a summary of the child's progress made in quantifiable terms, a discussion of the factors contributing or encumbering the child's progress, referral to other services, and practical recommendations for future work with the child. The intervention team may also discuss follow-up services or if additional music therapy services might be beneficial for the child in other goal areas to support the child's educational program (Gfeller and Davis, 2008).

Singing a song and creating an individualized song playlist as Megan did in the case vignette are great ways to celebrate and remember the child's progress. Placing a copy of the music in the child's profile or portfolio also supports evidence of improvement. Acknowledging and celebrating the child's success and achievement concludes the music therapy intervention.

Conclusion

Music therapy is a viable treatment option for young children with ASD that can build on musical preferences and aptitudes, create meaningful context for learning, and support engagement in social and daily life tasks. Music therapy interventions may be particularly effective when implemented in children's natural environments through a systematic process of collaborating and consulting with others. Music therapists can train and empower family members, early childhood education staff, and peers to apply music-based interventions for skill development in children with ASD within daily activities and routines. Working together may assure normalization, continuity, and generalization of skills of children with ASD. Continued sharing of expertise and further research collaborations between early childhood education staff and music therapists may support the attainment of the ultimate goal of improving the lives of young children with ASD and their families.

LEARNING QUESTIONS

1. Why should music be considered as an intervention option for children with ASD?

2. When is a referral to music therapy appropriate?

3. How does a music therapist engage a child with ASD during the assessment process?

4. What content may be included in an Individualized Intervention Program for a child with ASD?

5. How can music therapy interventions be embedded in a child's natural environment?

6. Which role do interdisciplinary team members play in implementing the music therapy intervention for a child with ASD enrolled in an inclusive childcare program?

7. When can a music therapy intervention be terminated?

References

American Music Therapy Association (AMTA) (n.d.) What is the profession of music therapy? Retrieved from www.musictherapy.org.

American Psychiatric Association (APA) (2000). *Diagnostic and Statistical Manual of Mental Disorders (Fourth Edition). Text Revision.* Washington, DC: APA.

Applebaum, E., Egel, A.L., Koegel, R.L., and Imhoff, B. (1979). Measuring musical abilities of autistic children. *Journal of ASD and Developmental Disorders, 9(3),* 279–285.

Buysse, V., and Wesley, P. (2005). *Consultation in Early Childhood Settings.* Baltimore, MD: Paul H. Brookes Publishing Co.

Buysse, V., Wesley, P.W., Snyder, P., and Winton, P. (2006). Evidence-based practice: What does it really mean for the early childhood field? *Young Exceptional Children, 9(4),* 2–11.

Carpente, J. (2011). *The Individual Music-Centered Assessment Profile for Neurodevelopmental Disorders (IMCAP-ND) for Children, Adolescents, and Adults: A Clinical Manual.* Unpublished manual.

Centers for Disease Control and Prevention (CDC) (2010). Autism spectrum disorders (ASDs). Retrieved from www.cdc.gov/ncbddd/autism/index.html.

Council for Exceptional Children (2006). *CEC Evidence-Based Professional Practice Proposal.* Arlington, VA: Professional Standards and Practice Committee.

Ermer, J., and Dunn, W. (1998). The sensory profile: A discriminate analysis of children with and without disabilities. *Journal of Occupational Therapy, 52,* 283–290.

Gfeller, K.E., and Davis, W.B. (2008). The music therapy treatment process. In W.B. Davis, K.E. Gfeller, and M.H. Thaut (Eds.) *An Introduction to Music Therapy Theory and Practice (Third Edition).* Silver Spring, MD: The American Music Therapy Association, Inc.

Gold, C., Wigram, T., and Elefant, C. (2006). Music therapy for autistic spectrum disorder. *Cochrane Database of Systematic Reviews,* 2006, Issue 2. Art. No.: CD004381. doi:10.1002/14651858. CD004381.pub2.

Grandin, T. (n.d.) An inside view of ASD. Retrieved from www.autism.com/index.php/advocacy-grandin.

Heaton, P. (2003). Pitch memory, labelling and disembedding in ASD. *Journal of Child Psychiatry and Psychology, 44(4),* 543–551.

Heaton, P., Hermelin, B., and Pring, L. (1998). ASD and pitch processing: A precursor for savant musical ability? *Music Perception, 15(3),* 291–305.

Hummel-Rossi, B., Turry, A., Guerrero, N., and Selim, N. (2008). *Music Therapy Communication and Social Interaction Scale—Group.* Unpublished instrument, Nordoff-Robbins Center for Music Therapy, New York University.

Humpal, M., and Colwell, C. (Eds.) (2006). *Effective Clinical Practice in Music Therapy: Early Childhood and School Age Educational Settings—Using Music to Maximize Learning* [Monograph]. Silver Spring, MD: The American Music Therapy Association, Inc.

Kern, P. (2008). Singing our way through the day: Using music with young children during daily routines. *Children and Families, 22(2),* 50–56.

Kern, P. (2010). Evidence-based practice in early childhood music therapy: A decision-making process. *Music Therapy Perspectives, 28(2),* 116–123.

Kern, P., and Aldridge, D. (2006). Using embedded music therapy interventions to support outdoor play of young children with ASD in an inclusive community-based childcare program. *Journal of Music Therapy, 43(4),* 270–294.

Kern, P., and Snell, A.M. (2007). *Songbook Vol. I: Songs and Laughter on the Playground.* Santa Barbara, CA: De La Vista Publisher.

Kern, P., Wakeford, L., and Aldridge, D. (2007). Improving the performance of a young child with ASD during self-care tasks using embedded song interventions: A case study. *Music Therapy Perspectives, 25(1),* 43–51.

Kern, P., Wolery, M., and Aldridge, D. (2007). Use of songs to promote independence in morning greeting routines for young children with ASD. *Journal of Autism and Developmental Disorders, 37,* 1264–1271.

King, B., and Coleman, K.A. (2006). Development of a special education music therapy process. In M.E. Humpal and C. Colwell (Eds.) *Best Practices in Music Therapy Monograph: Early Childhood and School Age.* Silver Spring, MD: The American Music Therapy Association, Inc.

Koegel, R.L., Rincover, A., and Engel, A.L. (1982). *Educating and Understanding Autistic Children.* San Diego, CA: College Hill.

Lazar, M. (2007). (November) When is music therapy necessary? Determining eligibility through the IEP. In P. Kern and M. Lazar (Co-Chairs) *The ASD Agenda: An Evidence-Based Approach to Music Therapy.* Institute conducted at the meeting of the American Music Therapy Association, Louisville, KY.

McWilliam, R.A. (Ed.) (1996). *Rethinking Pull-Out Services in Early Intervention: A Professional Resource.* Baltimore, MD: Paul H. Brookes Publishing Co.

National Autism Center (NAC) (2009). *National Standards Report.* The National Standards Project— Addressing the need for evidence-based practice guidelines for autism spectrum disorders. Randolph, MA: NAC.

National Research Council (NRC) (2001). *Educating Children with ASD.* Committee on Educational Interventions for Children with ASD. C. Lord and J.P. McGee (Eds.) Division of Behavioral and Social Science and Education. Washington, DC: National Academy Press.

Register, D. (2002). Collaboration and consultation: A survey of board certified music therapists. *Journal of Music Therapy, 39(4),* 305–321.

Reichow, B., Volkmar, F.R., and Cicchetti, D.V. (2008). Development of the evaluation method for evaluating and determining evidence-based practice in ASD. *Journal of Autism and Developmental Disorders, 38,* 1311–1319.

Schwartz, E.K. (2006). Eligibility and legal aspects. In M. Humpal and C. Colwell (Eds.) *Effective Clinical Practice in Music Therapy: Early Childhood and School Age Educational Settings—Using Music to Maximize Learning* [Monograph]. Silver Spring, MD: The American Music Therapy Association, Inc.

Schwartz, I. (2010). Using building blocks to promote learning in inclusive settings. DEC teleconference 4 February. Retrieved from www.dec-sped.org/uploads/docs/professionals/mono11_teleconference/02_04_10_Call_Recording.wav.

Snell, A.M. (2002). Music therapy for learners with ASD in a public school setting. In B.L. Wilson (Ed.) *Models of Music Therapy Interventions in School Settings (Second Edition)*. Silver Spring, MD: The American Music Therapy Association, Inc.

Thaut, M. (1987). Visual versus auditory (musical) stimulus preferences in autistic children: A pilot study. *Journal of ASD and Developmental Disorders, 17(3)*, 425–432.

Turnbull, A. (2010). Quality inclusive services in a diverse society. DEC teleconference 4 February. Retrieved from www.dec-sped.org/uploads/docs/professionals/mono11_teleconference/02_04_10_Call_Recording.wav.

Umbarger, G.T. (2007). State of the evidence regarding complementary and alternative medical treatments for autism spectrum disorder. *Education and Training in Developmental Disabilities, 42(2)*, 437–447.

U.S. Department of Education (2010). Questions and answers on Individualized Education Programs (IEPs), evaluations and reevaluations. Retrieved from http://idea.ed.gov/explore/view/p/%2Croot%2Cdynamic%2CQaCorner%2C3%2C.

Walworth, D.D., Register, D., and Engel, J.N. (2009). Using the SCERTS model assessment tool to identify music therapy goals for clients with autism spectrum disorder. *Journal of Music Therapy, 46(3)*, 204–216.

Whipple, J. (2004). Music in intervention for children and adolescents with ASD: Meta-analysis. *Journal of Music Therapy, 41(2)*, 90–106.

Williams, D. (1996). *ASD: An Inside-Out Approach*. London and Philadelphia: Jessica Kingsley Publishers.

World Federation of Music Therapy (WFMT) (2011). FAQ music therapy: what is music therapy? Retrieved from www.wfmt.info/WFMT/FAQ_Music_Therapy.html.

Chapter 11

Communication and Language Development

Implications for Music Therapy and Autism Spectrum Disorders

Hayoung A. Lim, Ph.D., MT-BC
SAM HOUSTON STATE UNIVERSITY
HUNTSVILLE, TX

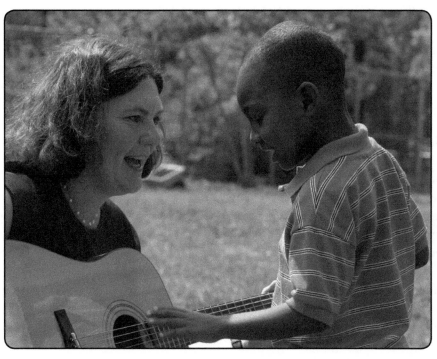

PHOTO COURTESY OF DON TRULL

*Children with autism spectrum disorders can perceive and
produce functional language embedded in music; the effect
of music on language development might be explained by the
inherent structure of music stimuli and the intact capacity of
pattern perception and production within this population.
(Hayoung A. Lim)*

Communicating with others in daily life situations is often challenging for young children with autism spectrum disorders (ASD). Impairments in communication and language development is one of three core characteristics defining ASD. Therefore, practitioners and parents must be able to recognize the signs and know about evidence-based interventions to support improving everyday communication in young children with ASD. The purpose of this chapter is to discuss social communication and speech and language impairments in young children with ASD and to apply evidence-based practice to support communication through music therapy interventions.

Social communication and speech-language features in young children with ASD

Background

The diagnostic schemes and description of the underlying deficits in ASD have evolved and changed since Leo Kanner's first description of infantile autism in 1943 (Prizant and Wetherby, 2005). Difficulty in the development of communication and language is the one criterion for diagnosis that has remained constant (American Psychiatric Association [APA], 2000). Speech and language impairments specifically have been regarded as one of the most significant deficits in ASD (Lord and Paul, 1997; Rapin and Dunn, 2003). Most parents of children with ASD initially become concerned that something is not quite right in their child's development when early delay or regression occurs in the development of communication and speech (Lord and Paul, 1997). Social communication ability is the key for success in everyday activities for children with ASD. It refers to using language (e.g., syntax, semantics, pragmatics) in social situations. Speech-language development stands for verbal means of communicating (e.g., articulation, fluency) and using a set of socially shared rules to communicate (e.g., word meanings, how to change words or put words together) (Prizant and Wetherby, 2005). Effective interventions to improve communication and speech-language skills are a high treatment priority for children with ASD. As a foundation for the understanding of the remainder of this chapter, Table 11.1 provides a glossary of communication plus speech and language-related terms.

Table 11.1 Glossary of basic communication and speech-language terms related to ASD	
Terminology	**Description**
Echolalia	Repetition of utterance with similar intonation of words or phrases that someone else has said.
Prosody	Variation of tone used when speaking (i.e., intonation) and vocal stress, which is the relative emphasis given to certain syllables in a word. The elements of prosody are derived from the acoustics of speech; they include the pitch accent on stressed syllables, loudness (i.e., dynamic accent), and full vowel length (i.e., duration) of sound production.
Phonology	Phonological processing skills include the ability to recognize and produce rhyming words or patterns of alliteration, segmenting or breaking apart words into syllables/sounds, identify where a specific sound occurs in a word, and blend sounds into words.
Syntax	Rules and principles that govern the formation of grammatical sentences and phrases from words.
Semantics	Meanings that are encoded in language.
Pragmatics	Communicative functions, in conversation and discourse, which require individuals to take successive turns in adopting the roles of speaker and listener. Pragmatics are directly involved in speaking with coherence, relevance, sequential organization, and a correct timeframe within the given context.
Lexical growth	Development in language in terms of its vocabulary, including its words and expressions.
Mand	Verbal operant of independent requesting for items.
Tact	Verbal operant of labeling or describing.
Echoic operant	Verbal operant of vocal imitation.
Intraverbal operant	Verbal operant of social interaction or conversation.

Sources: Autism Speaks (2012). Glossary of terms. Retrieved from www.autismspeaks.org/what-autism/ video-glossary/glossary-terms; Children Speech Care Center (2002). Glossary of speech-language related terms. Retrieved from www.childspeak.net/glossary.html.

Social communication development

Children with ASD rarely engage in play with their siblings or peers. They only communicate sporadically in social situations, indicating difficulties acquiring skills pertaining to the structure of language (e.g., using signs, words, sentences) and communication necessary for social exchange (e.g., greeting, commenting, sharing affect, seeking information). Furthermore, these children seem less motivated to interact with persons of any age (Kaiser, Nietfeld, and Roberts, 2010).

Communication difficulties vary, depending upon the intellectual and social development of the individual with ASD. Those who can speak often say things that have no content or information (Paul and Sutherland, 2005). Others may use prefabricated phrases such as "My name is John" to start a conversation, even when speaking with friends or family. Still others may repeat learned scripts such as those heard while watching videos or television commercials. Some individuals with higher intelligence may be able to speak in depth about topics that interest them (e.g., cars, cartoon characters, or dinosaurs) but are unable to engage in an interactive conversation on these same topics. Many children with ASD are often unable to use gestures either as a primary means of communication (as in sign language) or to assist verbal communication (e.g., pointing, showing) (Kaiser, Nietfeld, and Roberts, 2010). The lack of using non-verbal interaction including gestures and joint attention and the absence of social exchange (i.e., turn-taking, attention to the other's focus of attention) indicate impairments in social communication even before spoken language emerges (Kaiser, Nietfeld, and Roberts, 2010).

Speech-language development

Many studies which focused on the language of verbal children with ASD identified aberrant speech features such as unusual word choice, pronoun reversal, echolalia, incoherent discourse, unresponsiveness to questions, aberrant prosody, and lack of drive to communicate (Rapin and Dunn, 2003). Table 11.2 provides a summary of speech-language development in children with ASD compared to other disabilities or typically developing children.

The particular speech and language deficits might be explained by abnormal auditory cortical processing in individuals with ASD, perhaps due to problems or deficits in the neural mechanisms for the perception and production of sounds. The most prominent research findings on speech-language deficits related to the neural mechanisms for ASD address:

- a persistent abnormality in the secondary auditory cortex (i.e., auditory associative area) in children with ASD (Rapin and Dunn, 2003)

- less activation of the left hemisphere temporal word-processing network in adults with ASD than in typical comparison participants (Boddaert et al., 2003)

- abnormal cortical activities in children with ASD, similar to those previously described in adults with ASD (Boddaert *et al.*, 2004).

A dysfunction of left-speech-related cortical areas could be the origin of the language developmental impairments observed in individuals with ASD. A number of studies about speech and language development indicate that children with ASD can still learn language and develop their communication skills through speech despite these possible brain dysfunctions. Researchers suggest focusing on the children's sparse capacity for language development and exploring ways to facilitate their functional speech (Lim, 2010a; Lord and Paul, 1997; Prizant and Wetherby, 2005).

Table 11.2 Summary of speech-language features of young children with ASD	
Comparison to other disabilities or typical development	**Speech-language features**
Differences	Production and comprehension of speech is more severely compromised in children with ASD than in children with other developmental disorders (Lord and Paul, 1997).
	Children with ASD exhibit more severe comprehension and pragmatic deficits than children with developmental language disorders (Rapin and Dunn, 2003).
	The language disorders of children with ASD include universally impaired pragmatics, including problems with conversational use of language, and comprehension of discourse (Rapin and Dunn, 2003).
	Children with ASD have a prevalence of higher order processing disorders (e.g., lexical or syntactic impairments) and impaired semantic classification of words (Tager-Flusberg, 1997, 2003).
	Children with ASD have semantic word retrieval deficits due to impaired comprehension and formulating of discourse (Rapin and Dunn, 2003).
	Many children with ASD are quite devoid of speech affect or prosody (Tager-Flusberg, 1997).
	In spite of these deficits, more than half of all children with ASD show an intact ability to perceive and produce speech sounds, and do develop some level of functional speech (Lim, 2010a; Paul and Sutherland, 2005; Schuler, 1995; Tager-Flusberg, 1997).

Table continues

Table 11.2 Summary of speech-language features of young children with ASD *cont.*	
Comparison to other disabilities or typical development	Speech-language features
Differences *cont.*	Children with ASD who do develop some functional language have relatively little difficulty acquiring the formal, rule-governed components of language, such as phonology and syntax. In contrast, certain pragmatic aspects of language, those that entail an understanding of others' thoughts or emotions, are specifically and uniquely impaired in individuals with ASD (Tager-Flusberg, 1997)
Similarities	Children with ASD exhibit much greater similarity to other children without ASD than do children with many other types of disabilities, acquiring computational and semantic aspects of language and learning grammatical structures in the same order as their typically developing peers. However, their rate of growth is often slower (Tager-Flusberg *et al.*, 1990; Tager-Flusberg and Calkins, 1990).
	Children with ASD and children who are typically developing assign words to the same conceptual categories (Lord and Paul, 1997; Paul and Sutherland, 2005).
	High-functioning children with ASD use semantic groupings (e.g., bird, boat, food) to categorize and to retrieve words in ways that are very similar to those used by children without ASD (Boucher, 1988; Lord and Paul, 1997; Minshew and Goldstein, 1993; Tager-Flusberg, 1985).
	Children with ASD demonstrate grammatical development in ways that are similar to those of children who are typically developing (Tager-Flusberg and Calkins, 1990).
	Lexical growth (i.e., vocabulary learning) and semantic representations of children with ASD may show a developmental pattern similar to that of children who are typically developing (Tager-Flusberg, 1985; 1986).
	The development of word usage is similar to yet slower than that of children without ASD (Travis and Sigman, 2001).

Incorporating music into communication and language development with children with ASD

Similarities between speech-language patterns and music

Speech-language patterns of children with ASD are characterized by repetition of unanalyzed forms that may be non-communicative or may be used as a means to express communicative intent (Prizant *et al.*, 1997). One of the most salient examples is echolalia, the repetition of utterance with similar intonation of words or phrases that someone else has said (Prizant *et al.*, 1997). Such expressive patterns in ASD may reflect Gestalt language acquisition indicating an inability to analyze or segment others' utterances and recognize their internal structure or processing. Gestalt language acquisition in children with ASD may be explained by the perception and production of patterns in their speech (Lim, 2009, 2010a). Collectively, children with ASD appear to have intact pattern perception and production ability. They also tend to follow the Gestalt style of language acquisition, which is based on pattern perception.

Similarly, expressive musical elements and thus musical behaviors (e.g., listening, performing, composing) require pattern perception and production. Music is composed of many separate yet interconnected components such as pitch, melody, rhythm, harmony, form, timbre, and dynamics. These elements typically are arranged in patterns and perceived as "music." This musical pattern perception is commonly ruled by Gestalt laws of perception (Radocy and Boyle, 2003). Gestalt psychology emphasizes the importance of figure-ground relationships in perceptual pattern organization and has proposed a number of organizational principles including proximity, similarity, common direction, simplicity, and closure (Eysenck, 2001). Similar perceptual processes are at work when perceiving organized patterns in music (Eysenck, 2001; Lim, 2009; Lipscomb, 1996; Radocy and Boyle, 2003). Researchers in music therapy have reported that children with ASD may respond favorably and appropriately to musical sounds as the possible result of intact musical pattern perception and production (Lim, 2010a; Thaut, 1999). Children with ASD may recognize emotional expression in music at a simple level by the intact perception of melody patterns in music, such as a key or melodic mode (Heaton, Hermelin, and Pring, 1999). They may perceive and produce well-organized melodic and rhythmic musical patterns (Lim, 2010a). Therefore, following patterns in music may facilitate the Gestalt style of language acquisition and consequently speech-language development in children with ASD (Lim, 2011).

Research outcomes

A study by Lim (2010a) examined the effect of developmental speech-language training through music (DSLM) on the speech production of 50 children with ASD. Participants in music training watched a music video containing six songs and pictures of 36 target words; those in speech training watched a speech video containing six stories and pictures, and those in the control condition received no treatment. Music training was effective for enhancing the children's speech production (i.e., semantics, phonology, pragmatics, and prosody). Children with ASD appeared to perceive important linguistic information embedded in music stimuli, organized by principles of pattern perception; they were able to produce the words as functional speech. Music's effect on speech production might be explained by the inherent structure of music stimuli and the intact capacity of pattern perception and production in children with ASD. Furthermore, age-appropriate and carefully designed music interventions have been used as a consistent and reliable way to facilitate speech and language as well as develop communication skills (Lim, 2010a; Prizant and Wetherby, 2005; Sundberg and Partington, 1998; Whipple, 2004).

A new speech pattern embedded in a song that is not too familiar and not too complex may capture the best perceptual capacity in children with ASD, and presentation of corresponding visual materials (e.g., pictures, photos, and real objects) may facilitate the perceptual mechanisms. The following case vignette, which describes using both an original and familiar tune, illustrates this premise:

> A five-year-old boy with ASD was receiving music therapy services to address communication difficulties; the child could not speak a single word. The music therapist attempted to engage the child by singing an originally composed song, using pictures to reinforce the meaning. The child intensely looked at the mouth of the music therapist as well as at the pictures. However, when the music therapist sang well-known songs such as "Twinkle, Twinkle, Little Star" and "Old MacDonald," the child turned his head away.

Using Applied Behavior Analysis (ABA) Verbal Behavior (VB) in music therapy

The principles and techniques of Applied Behavior Analysis (ABA) are frequently used with children with ASD as an effective treatment for skill improvement (Sturmey and Fitzer, 2007). See Chapter 5 for more detailed information.

Based on the principles of ABA, the intent of the Verbal Behavior (VB) approach is to help children with ASD learn functional language (Barbera, 2007; Sturmey and Fitzer, 2007); language is seen as a behavior that can be shaped and reinforced. Careful attention is paid not only to what a child is saying but also to why he or she is using the language (Barbera, 2007).

Pairing components of music with the ABA VB method may be used as successfully as ABA VB speech training to enhance the functional verbal production in children with ASD. A study by Lim and Draper (2011) compared a common form of ABA VB approach using musical components with the ABA VB method as part of developmental speech-language training in the speech production of 22 preschoolers with ASD. Participants were randomly assigned a set of target words for each of the three training conditions: music incorporated ABA VB, speech ABA VB, and no-training. Results indicated that both music and speech trainings were effective for production of the four ABA verbal operants: Mand, Tact, Echoic, and Intraverbal (see Table 11.1 for definitions).

The structure and curriculum of the ABA VB training method can be carefully designed to utilize various combinations of musical sounds. Pairing target verbal instructions/prompts with singing seems to establish effective antecedent variables and automatic reinforcement, and may increase the frequency of the target verbal operant production in children with ASD. Participating in music training might be a positive reinforcement for continuing production of the verbal operants in children with ASD (Lim, 2009; Lim and Draper, 2011).

Use of music can make an integrative bridge between naturalistic approaches (i.e., milieu teaching) and the didactic ABA VB approaches. Systemically designed music activities may establish reinforcement and preferred experiences for the children (Lim and Draper, 2011). Music time provided in the classrooms of children with ASD may provide the necessary structure for the language training. Various musical instruments and favorite songs can be used as motivational variables and natural reinforcers. An active music-making experience with instruments and songs may increase spontaneous communication with adults and peers (Lim, 2010b). Additionally, group music experiences in the child's natural environment may provide multiple opportunities to practice social communication skills such as greeting others, singing along, or sharing ideas (Kern, Wolery, and Aldridge, 2007; Lim, 2010b). Music-based interventions prepared by certified music therapists and facilitated by parents or caregivers in the child's home can also provide opportunities for practicing functional communication and generalization of skills.

Using Aided Augmentative and Alternative Communication (AAC) in music therapy

Aided Augmentative and Alternative Communication (AAC) is frequently used to support communication of individuals with ASD who have no or limited language. Such tools offer children with ASD ways to make their wants and needs known. AAC offers a means to communicate, but it is not intended to replace actual speech. Augmenting input is useful for reception and also for pairing speech with modeling expressive language. Music therapists report using AAC to increase receptive communication, especially via use of picture schedules (Gadberry, 2011). AAC may be categorized into three levels. *Low tech AAC* involves using signs, pictures, photographs, and objects to aid communication. For example, the child with ASD may be given a small toy stop sign to use for indicating when to stop the music (Wellman, 2010). *Light tech AAC* refers to devices such as switches that may be activated by touch but are not computer-based. Output may be recorded and easily changed, making their use extremely versatile within actual sessions. *High tech AAC* incorporates a computer component. SLTs or SLPs should be consulted prior to using AAC devices to learn how they work and also because of their complexity and the ever-changing possibilities for their use (Gaberry, 2012).

Collaborating with speech-language pathologists

The communication support needed by children with ASD is varied and complex, requiring collaboration from many disciplines. Speech/language therapists and pathologists (SLTs/SLPs), special educators, and music therapists who address speech-language goals and training for children with ASD must combine specialized knowledge of communication with specific knowledge of ASD to provide effective collaboration (Diehl, 2003). The SLP's role is to serve as a member of a collaborative team in (1) identifying patterns of strengths and challenges in communication and (2) providing social, behavioral, and communication supports in school/community and other therapy settings (Diehl, 2003). The selection of materials and interventions based on scientific evidence and a more systematic implementation of a speech/language training tool through music may produce more consistent procedures and outcomes indicated by the collaborating practice with SLPs and other professionals (Geist *et al.*, 2008).

Music therapists should embed the SLT's/SLP's current curriculum or training module being used with the child with ASD into their music therapy interventions. Target words and/or sentences for language assessment and training need to be carefully determined. Therefore, it is advisable to consult with an SLT or SLP when applying music to speech-language training interventions. For a comprehensive evaluation of the progress of the child's speech-language development, the music therapist should consistently monitor and refer to the client's progress and/or treatment outcome from the child's speech therapy.

One of the greatest benefits of a music therapist-led speech-language training intervention is the opportunity to provide quality musical materials. If the music therapy intervention for speech and language development is presented with carefully arranged or composed songs and well-facilitated musical experiences, the therapeutic effects of the intervention may be enhanced. Because of the skill sets needed many SLTs/SLPs who are not musically inclined tend to avoid using music in their practices. However, recorded music with the same quality can be used in speech-language training for children with ASD. SLTs and/or SLPs who would like to incorporate musical experiences in their sessions might consult with music therapists and ask them to record musical materials that could be used in therapy. In addition, music therapists could ask the SLPs where music might be able to enhance specific goals and/or objectives, then consult the procedure of treatment planning and provide the musical materials based on a spirit of collaboration.

Applying key principles of social communication and speech-language development to music therapy practice

Carefully designed age-appropriate music interventions can provide a rich opportunity for productive experiences for young children with communication impairments (Geist *et al.*, 2008; Lim, 2010a). When using music in speech and language training for children with ASD, music therapists may want to adhere to the following guidelines:

- Recognize the importance and effectiveness of music for children's learning, development, and socio-cultural participation.

- Consider each child's unique interests, musical preference, developmental levels, and learning style (making adaptations as necessary).

- Identify the function of musical stimuli and analyze each child's musical responses.

- Identify and select musical stimuli or musical experiences which are intrinsically motivating for the child and can provide effective ways to repeatedly practice targeted goals.

- Create and support opportunities that include typically developing peers as musical partners.

- Be open and creative to reach each child's full potential for the music-making experience.

Table 11.3 provides a selection of theoretical implications and corresponding clinical applications for using music in speech and language training for children with ASD.

Table 11.3 Examples of clinical applications in music therapy

Statement from the research literature	Application in music therapy
Children with ASD have an intact ability to imitate a basic level of gestures and procedures (Charman and Baron-Cohen, 1994).	Implement imitation-based activities (e.g., vocal imitation) by including gestures or visual prompts along with the musical stimuli. When working with young children with autism, use single-step cues, but know that most can follow simple two-step cues.
Prefabricated routines refer to memorized whole utterances or phrases, which a speaker may use without any knowledge of their internal structure (Prizant, 1983).	Use memorized utterances to increase the functional phrasing of young children. Use phrases such as "I want _____." Or "This is a _____." Understand that utterances are predominantly echolalic but may fulfill a conversational need of the child.
Modeling language in a context of active involvement and in synchrony with relevant action patterns is a powerful teaching strategy (Lim, 2010b).	Begin to practice language skills using active child involvement. For example, ask a question in a song that affords a specific response (e.g., "How are you today?"). When working on language goals, make sure that the examples are clearly articulated and concrete (i.e., not abstract or figurative).
A simple verbal phrase repeated to a rhythmic pattern might sustain the child's attention and interest (Berger, 2002).	Add a steady rhythm to a short phrase by clapping, playing on a hand drum, or using a metronome. This rhythm may help the child focus and increase clarity of speech.
An intervention should include appropriate contexts containing communicative exchanges and activities of high motivation and interest (Prizant et al., 1997).	Design interventions for social communication to engage the child with ASD and match language he or she naturally uses. For example, hang an instrument in a tree on the playground; the child must then ask for adult support to reach and play the desired object.
Children with ASD tend to sustain their attention as well as perceive and produce more linguistic information when target words are embedded in simple and repetitive combinations of musical patterns that are symmetrical and parallel in form (Lim, 2009, 2010a).	Choose songs that are lively and active for working on language-related goals with children who have ASD. Selected songs should be simple and repetitive as more repetitions offer more opportunities for the child to hear and learn the words.

Conclusion

Music can be an effective tool in communication and language development for children with ASD. Well-designed and implemented musical experience can improve communication skills and facilitate speech-language development in young children with ASD. Children with ASD often respond attentively to music stimuli, and may perceive important linguistic information embedded in the music stimuli. As a result, children with ASD may develop enhanced receptive language skills, produce functional vocabulary words and sentences, and experience improved communication, conversations, and interactions with others.

LEARNING QUESTIONS

1. How do the speech-language features of young children with ASD differ from those of children with other types of developmental disorders or children who are developing typically?

2. Describe three research-based clinical music therapy applications appropriate for use in speech-language training for children with ASD.

3. How can music be incorporated in ABA VB training for children with ASD?

4. What is the perceptual commonality between music and speech?

5. How does the Gestalt style of language acquisition relate to speech and language development in children with ASD?

6. What are pragmatics and how is echolalia defined?

7. How may collaboration between music therapists and speech/ language therapists and pathologists be beneficial to each?

References

American Psychiatric Association (APA) (2000). *Diagnostic and Statistical Manual of Mental Disorders (Fourth Edition). Text Revision.* Washington, DC: APA.

Autism Speaks (2012). Glossary of terms. Retrieved from www.autismspeaks.org/what-autism/video-glossary/glossary-terms.

Barbera, M.L. (2007). *The Verbal Behaviour Approach.* London and Philadelphia: Jessica Kingsley Publishers.

Berger, D.S. (2002). *Music Therapy, Sensory Integration and the Autistic Child.* London and Philadelphia: Jessica Kingsley Publishers.

Boddaert, N., Chabane, N., Belin, P., Bourgeois, M., *et al.* (2003). Perception of complex sounds: Abnormal pattern of cortical activation in autism. *American Journal of Psychiatry, 161,* 2057–2060.

Boddaert, N., Chabane, N., Belin, P., Bourgeois, M., *et al.* (2004). Perception of complex sounds in autism: Abnormal auditory cortical processing in children. *American Journal of Psychiatry, 161,* 2117–2120.

Boucher, J. (1988). Word fluency in high-functioning autistic children. *Journal of Autism and Developmental Disorders, 18,* 637–645.

Charman, T., and Baron-Cohen, S. (1994). Another look at imitation in autism. *Development and Psychopathology, 6,* 403–413.

Children Speech Care Center (2002). Glossary of speech-language related terms. Retrieved from www. childspeech.net/ glossary.html.

Diehl, S.F. (2003). The SLP's role in collaborative assessment and intervention for children with ASD. *Topics in Language Disorders, 23(2),* 95–115.

Eysenck, M.W. (2001). *Principles of Cognitive Psychology (Second Edition).* Philadelphia, PA: Psychology Press Ltd.

Gadberry, A. (2011). A survey of the use of aided Augmentative and Alternative Communication during music therapy sessions with persons with autism spectrum disorders. *Journal of Music Therapy, 48(1),* 74–89.

Gadberry, A. (2012). Utilizing Augmentative and Alternative Communication in music therapy sessions. *imagine, 3(1),* 44–45.

Geist, K., McCarthy, J., Rogers-Smith, A., and Porter, J. (2008). Integrating music therapy services and speech language service for children with severe communication impairments: A co-treatment model. *Journal of Instructional Psychology, 35(4),* 311–316.

Heaton, P., Hermelin, B., and Pring, L. (1999). Can children with autistic spectrum disorder perceive affect in music? An experimental investigation. *Psychological Medicine, 29,* 1405–1410.

Kaiser, A.P., Nietfeld, J.P., and Roberts, M.Y. (2010). Applying evidence-based practice to support communication with children who have autism spectrum disorders. In H. Schertz, C. Wong, and S. Odom (Eds.) *Young Exceptional Children Monograph Series 12.* Missoula, MT: DEC.

Kern, P., Wolery, M., and Aldridge, D. (2007). Use of songs to promote independence in morning greeting routines for young children with autism. *Journal of Autism and Developmental Disorders, 37,* 1264–1271.

Lim, H.A. (2009). Use of music to improve speech production in children with autism spectrum disorders: Theoretical orientation. *Music Therapy Perspectives, 27(2),* 103–114.

Lim, H.A. (2010a). Effect of "Developmental Speech and Language Training through Music" on speech production in children with autism spectrum disorders. *Journal of Music Therapy, 47(1),* 3–25.

Lim, H.A. (2010b). Use of music in Applied Behaviour Analysis Verbal Behaviour approach for children with autism spectrum disorders. *Music Therapy Perspectives, 28(2),* 95–105.

Lim, H.A. (2011). *Developmental Speech-Language Training Through Music for Children with Autism Spectrum Disorders.* London and Philadelphia: Jessica Kingsley Publishers.

Lim, H.A., and Draper, E. (2011). The effects of music therapy incorporated with Applied Behavior Analysis Verbal Behavior approach for children with autism spectrum disorders. *Journal of Music Therapy, 48(4),* 532–550.

Lipscomb, S.D. (1996). The cognitive organization of musical sound. In D.A. Hodges (Ed.) *Handbook of Music Psychology (Second Edition).* San Antonio, TX: IMR Press.

Lord, C., and Paul, R. (1997). Language and communication in autism. In D. Cohen and F. Volkmar (Eds.) *Handbook of Autism and Pervasive Developmental Disorders.* New York: John Wiley and Sons, Inc.

Minshew, N.J., and Goldstein, G. (1993). Is autism an amnesic disorder? Evidence from the California Verbal Learning Test. *Neuropsychology, 7,* 209–216.

Paul, R., and Sutherland, D. (2005). Enhancing early language in children with autism spectrum disorders. In F. Volkmar, R. Paul, A., Klin, and D. Cohen (Eds.) *Handbook of Autism and Pervasive Developmental Disorders.* New York: John Wiley and Sons, Inc.

Prizant, B.M. (1983). Language acquisition and communicative behaviour in autism: Toward an understanding of the "whole" of it. *Journal of Speech and Hearing Disorders, 48,* 296–307.

Prizant, B.M., and Wetherby, A.M. (2005). Critical issues in enhancing communication abilities for persons with autism spectrum disorders. In F. Volkmar, R. Paul, A., Klin, and D. Cohen (Eds.) *Handbook of Autism and Pervasive Developmental Disorders.* New York: John Wiley and Sons, Inc.

Prizant, B.M., Schuler, A.L., Wetherby, A.M., and Rydell, P. (1997). Enhancing language and communication development: Language approaches. In D. Cohen and F. Volkmar (Eds.) *Handbook of Autism and Pervasive Developmental Disorders.* New York: John Wiley and Sons, Inc.

Radocy, R.E., and Boyle, J.D. (2003). *Psychological Foundation of Musical Behavior (Fourth Edition).* Springfield, IL: Charles C. Thomas Publisher, Ltd.

Rapin, I., and Dunn, M. (2003). Update of the language disorders of individuals on the autistic spectrum. *Brain and Development, 25,* 166–172.

Schuler, A.L. (1995). Thinking in autism: Differences in learning and development. In K. Quill (Ed.) *Teaching Children with Autism: Methods to Enhance Communication and Socialization.* Albany, NY: Delmar.

Sturmey, P., and Fitzer, A. (2007). *Autism Spectrum Disorders: Applied Behavior Analysis, Evidence, and Practice.* Austin, TX: Pro-Ed, Inc.

Sundberg, M.L., and Partington, J.W. (1998). *Teaching Language to Children with Autism or Other Developmental Disabilities.* Pleasant Hill, CA: Behavior Analysts, Inc.

Tager-Flusberg, H. (1985). The conceptual basis for referential word meaning in children with autism. *Child Development, 56,* 1167–1178.

Tager-Flushberg, H. (1986). Constraints on the representation of work meaning: Evidence from autistic and mentally retarded children. In S.A. Kucsaj and M. Barrett (Eds.) *The Development of Word Meaning.* New York: Springer-Verlag.

Tager-Flusberg, H. (1997). Perspectives on language and communication in autism. In D. Cohen and F. Volkmar (Eds.) *Handbook of Autism and Pervasive Developmental Disorders.* New York: John Wiley and Sons, Inc.

Tager-Flusberg, H. (2003). Language impairment in children with complex neurodevelopmental disorders: The case of autism. In Y. Levy and J. Schaeffer (Eds.) *Language Competence Across Population: Toward a Definition of Specific Language Impairment.* Mahwah, NJ: Lawrence Erlbaum Associates.

Tager-Flusberg, H., and Calkins, S. (1990). Does imitation facilitate the acquisition of grammar? Evidence from a study of autistic, Down Syndrome and normal children. *Journal of Child Language, 17,* 591–606.

Tager-Flusberg, H., Calkins, S., Nolin, T., Baumberger, T., Anderson, M., and Chadwick-Dias, A. (1990). A longitudinal study of language acquisition in autistic and Down Syndrome children. *Journal of Autism and Developmental Disorders, 20,* 1–21.

Thaut, M.H. (1999). Music therapy with autistic children. In W. Davis, K. Gfeller, and M. Thaut (Eds.) *An Introduction to Music Therapy: Theory and Practice.* New York: McGraw-Hill.

Travis, L., and Sigman, M. (2001). Links between social understanding and social behavior in verbally able children with autism. *Journal of Autism and Developmental Disorders, 31,* 119–130.

Wellman, R. (2012). Augmentative Communication and Assistive Technology in early childhood music therapy. *imagine, 1(1),* 58–59.

Whipple, J. (2004). Music in intervention for children and adolescents with autism: A meta-analysis. *Journal of Music Therapy, 41(2),* 90–106.

Chapter 12

Sensory Processing in Children with Autism Spectrum Disorders

Applications for Music Therapy Practice

Linn Wakeford, M.S., OTR/L

University of North Carolina at Chapel Hill

Chapel Hill, NC

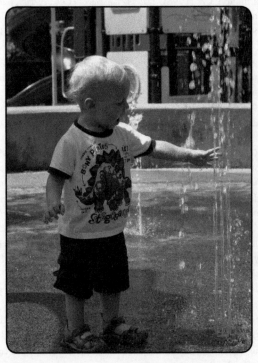

PHOTO COURTESY OF KIRSTEN BALHOFF

Everyday life is full of sensory experiences that invite us to explore and to learn. We want children with autism spectrum disorders and sensory processing differences to embrace those experiences as much as possible!
(Linn Wakeford)

Individuals diagnosed with an autism spectrum disorder (ASD) often demonstrate impairments in sensory/regulatory functioning. While atypical responses to sensation have generally been considered an associated, rather than diagnostic, feature of ASD, recent research has shown that sensory processing differences are prevalent among this population. "Hyper- or hypo-reactivity to sensory input or unusual interest in sensory aspects of environment" is now included in the proposed *DSM-V* criteria for ASD diagnosis as a symptom under *restricted/repetitive behaviors, interests, or activities* (American Psychiatric Association, 2011). Therefore, those working with young children at risk for or diagnosed with ASD must understand how sensory processing differences present themselves, as well as evidence-based methods of intervening, in order to support the participation of the child and his/her family in everyday life activities. This chapter will include a discussion of sensory features common to ASD, theoretical models, assessment, and intervention, as well as suggestions for ways in which music therapists can use an understanding of this information to enhance intervention for young children with ASD.

Sensory features

Before discussing the sensory features and processing patterns associated with ASD, there are two basic pieces of knowledge that should be introduced as a foundation for the understanding of the remainder of this chapter. The first is related to the sensory systems themselves, and the second is focused on qualities of sensation. Table 12.1 provides an overview of the sensory systems, and Table 12.2 provides information about the qualities of sensation that may need to be considered. It is also important to note that although these sensory systems and qualities of sensation are discussed individually at times, most sensory experiences that occur in "real life" are a combination of multiple sensory systems and qualities.

The sensory features associated with ASD have been characterized in various ways, but current research has led to consideration of three primary patterns of sensory processing, which include over-responsivity, under-responsivity, and sensory-seeking behaviors (Ashburner, Ziviani, and Rodger, 2008; Ben-Sasson *et al.*, 2009; Boyd *et al.*, 2010). Many children present with mixed patterns of sensory processing, i.e., over-responsiveness to one or two types of sensation, and hypo-responsiveness to another type. Over-responsivity (also called hyper-responsivity) refers to a significantly heightened and aversive response to one or more types of sensory input, such as overly sensitive responses to sound. Under-responsivity (also called hypo-responsivity) refers to the lack of or delay in an expected response to sensation (such as lack of response to a loud sound). Sensory-seeking behaviors include a variety of efforts on the part of the child to increase experiences of certain types of sensation, and these behaviors may result from being over- or under-responsive, or both. Although each child with ASD presents with individual variations in sensory processing patterns, a common mixed pattern includes over-responsivity to auditory and tactile (sound and touch) sensations, and under-responsiveness to the types of sensation most often experienced during movement (vestibular, proprioceptive, deep pressure). Over-responsivity to smell may also be present, and may have a significant effect on food choices (sometimes more so even than food textures). Furthermore, although people with ASD often possess some strengths in using visual information (Maekawa *et al.*, 2011), it is important to note that they also can be overwhelmed by visual information, especially if it is novel, plentiful, and/or presented in a social context (Chawarska and Shic, 2009). Children with ASD may need help to learn how to make sense of visual information and use it functionally (Chawarska and Shic, 2009; Dunn, Myles, and Orr, 2002).

Atypical patterns of sensory processing may result in difficulties with self-regulatory behaviors and/or praxis (i.e., the ability to plan, organize, and execute new or unfamiliar motor activities). In order to optimize intervention, music therapists can benefit from understanding the effect of sensory processing on behavior, consulting with an occupational therapist to determine a child's sensory processing patterns, and then collaborating to design interventions that address sensory processing differences, and that ultimately lead to the child's successful engagement in everyday environments and activities.

Table 12.1 Sensory systems

Sensory system	Function
Auditory	Detection of all elements of sound, including vibration.
Visual	Vision; detection of light.
Olfactory	Detection of odor; contributes to taste sensations.
Tactile	Detection of light and deep pressure touch, temperature, pain, vibration, localization of touch.
Gustatory	Taste (although the olfactory system influences this as well).
Vestibular	Movement and position of head in relationship to the rest of the body; significant connections with visual and auditory systems; contributes to development of body scheme.
Proprioceptive	Detection of traction/compression of joints and activation/relaxation of muscles; contributes significantly to development of body scheme, awareness of body in space.

Table 12.2 Qualities of sensation	
Quality	**Definitions/examples**
Intensity	The magnitude of a sensation, given its innate qualities (e.g., the loudness of sound, range of motion required to paint on large vs. small piece of paper, brightness of color, tightness of a hug).
Frequency	How often the sensation occurs (e.g., ticking of a clock, being bumped into while in line for the water fountain).
Duration	How long the sensation lasts (e.g., riding in a car to the grocery store, sensation of wet wipes on bare skin while having diaper changed).
Rhythm	The extent to which frequency and duration of sensation is predictable, repetitive, and evenly spaced in space or time (e.g., phone ring, being touched during game of tag). Rhythmical sensations are often calming, unless other qualities override this (e.g., rhythmical but loud sounds may be alerting).
Novelty	The extent to which the child is familiar with or has previously experienced the sensation. Novel sensory experiences are often alerting, and may even be aversive; familiar sensations are more easily managed.
Complexity	The extent to which the experience includes multiple sensations or multiple aspects of a single type of sensation (e.g., Gregorian chant vs. Bach chorale; going to a basketball game vs. sitting on a sofa watching it on TV).

Effects of sensory processing on behavior
Self-regulation

Self-regulation refers to one's ability to monitor and adapt to a variety of social, emotional, and sensory events in order to maintain an appropriate state of arousal (alertness), given the demands of the environment. For instance, the demands of the environment for reading in the book corner alone are much different than those for engaging on the playground, in terms of the types of sensation that need to be "managed." Evidence of self-regulation typically appears behaviorally, though in extreme instances of dysregulation, autonomic nervous system responses, such as fainting or vomiting, may also occur. Children who are over-responsive to one or more types of sensation find those sensations, or particular forms or combinations of them, painful and extremely distressing, and may find it very difficult to regulate their level of arousal in response to those sensations. They may also have prolonged responses to aversive sensory events, taking longer to recover from them than children who process those sensations in a more typical manner (Schaaf *et al.*, 2003). For instance, a child who is particularly sensitive to sound may over-react and become inconsolable when the fire alarm goes off in the childcare classroom, and may be affected by this very startling event for the rest of the day. Other children initially may be alarmed, but are fine after a few moments. Children who are over-responsive to sensation may demonstrate anxious, resistant, or avoidant behaviors, particularly when confronted with new or unfamiliar activities or environments. If they choose to participate in spite of their own concerns, these children may appear overly alert, have difficulty concentrating, and appear irritable. If made to participate, they may engage in resistant or aggressive behaviors such as tantruming, running away, hitting, biting, or yelling. Becoming withdrawn, physically retreating from an activity, or exhibiting other "shutting down" behaviors may indicate that the child has reached his or her limit in terms of meeting sensory challenges and is becoming overwhelmed.

Children who present with under-responsiveness to one or more types of sensation may appear to be withdrawn or unengaged, but this is often the result of too little sensation to be processed rather than too much. That is, these children actually need greater intensity, frequency, novelty, or complexity of some types of sensation to reach a level of alertness that allows them to participate successfully. Children with under-responsive patterns of sensory processing may initially resist efforts to engage them because they are not yet alert enough to be aware of their interest in the activity. Once more specific or enhanced cues are presented, they often will engage.

Sensory-seeking behaviors may be used by children with under- and over-responsive patterns of sensory processing as a way to regulate (raise or lower) their own arousal levels. Sensory-seeking behaviors may include fidgeting, touching, moving, using force, or vocalizing. They may be used to calm one's self (such as squeezing into a small space under a table in the book corner of the classroom), or to alert one's self (such as vocalizing loudly or crashing a toy car into the bookshelf). While self-regulation can be supported by sensory-seeking behaviors, children often need help learning how to seek needed sensory experiences in socially acceptable ways. Other factors may influence the ability of the child both to process sensory input and to regulate responses; those factors include hunger, thirst, fatigue, and overall emotional state. For instance, when a child is hungry, tired, angry, or excited, his or her ability to manage over-sensitive reactions is limited, and behaviors will probably reflect more intense responses to sensory experiences.

Mixed patterns of sensory processing are common in children with ASD and present a variety of self-regulation challenges. The child may try to manage both over- and under-responsivity to find a comfortable level of arousal/alertness. For children with ASD, the challenges presented by particular types or combinations of sensations may be even more significant when they occur in social contexts (Baranek et al., 2006; Keane, 2004). Over time, the development of more effective communication, cognitive maturing, and overall life experiences may allow the child to make positive changes in self-regulatory behaviors (Ben Itzchak and Zachor,

2011; Smith *et al.*, 2010). However, early intervention is important in addressing all features of ASD (including sensory processing), in order to support participation in daily life activities, and to support parents and other caregivers in managing difficult behaviors that may occur (Dunn, 1997; Pillay *et al.*, 2011).

Praxis

Praxis refers to the ability to plan and execute new or unfamiliar motor behaviors. It occurs in three stages: ideation, planning, and execution. Praxis requires the ability to generate an idea about what to do, mentally organize the sequence of movements, and execute the movements using the appropriate sequence, force, rate, and timing for success. For example, kicking a ball into a goal or drawing with crayons are tasks that require the child to control the force, direction, and speed of their movements, as well as imagine what a successful outcome will look like (i.e., ball in the goal or a shape on the paper). Praxis requires that one have an adequate body scheme, or sense of one's own body moving in space, to execute motor patterns successfully. Body scheme is developed based primarily on the sensations derived from movement (i.e., vestibular, proprioceptive, and tactile), although other sensory systems (e.g., visual) may contribute to the total sensorimotor feedback loop that occurs during motor activities. When children are hypo-responsive to vestibular, proprioceptive, and tactile sensations that occur during movement activities, their body scheme may be inaccurate, causing uncertainty about how their body is actually moving in space and in relationship to other objects (moving or stationary) within that environment. The end result of this hypo-responsiveness and inaccurate body scheme is that children often appear clumsy or uncoordinated. This may be evident during gross motor activities (e.g., outdoor games), manipulative activities (e.g., clothing fasteners, drawing or writing), and/or oral motor activities, such as eating or talking.

Theoretical and conceptual models guiding practice

There are a number of theories and models that can be used to guide assessment and intervention practices that address sensory features in young children with ASD. These models support a common outcome—the optimal fit among the child, his or her environment, and the routine or activity in which the child is engaged. However, the models differ in terms of what they seek to change, and how they propose making those changes. This significantly influences the course of intervention, which may be aimed at remediation, modification, or education. For instance, models that propose to change the child's intrinsic abilities to process various types of sensation as a way to create this optimal fit will support a remediative approach to intervention (i.e., focusing strategies on changing something about the child) rather than on the environment or the activity. Other theories or models may focus more on making changes in the environment or within the activity or routine itself. Several theories are described briefly below.

Ecological, transactional, and dynamic systems theories

Though modeled somewhat differently, ecological (Bronfenbrenner, 1992), transactional (Law et al., 1996), and dynamic systems (Smith and Thelen, 2003) theories all recognize an ongoing interaction among the child and his or her environment, and highlight the importance of context as an influence on performance. Each of these theories allows for a holistic view of situations made difficult due to sensory processing differences (e.g., the effect on parents, siblings, and others) and may lead to interventions that seek to change aspects of the environment (including social contexts), aspects of the task, and/or behaviors of the child to create an optimal fit and ultimately successful engagement.

Coping theory

Typically applied in situations that demand psychosocial interventions, coping theory addresses the ability of an individual to return to an emotional equilibrium after a new or challenging event has occurred, so that engagement in an activity can begin or continue (Olsen, 1999). Intervention based on this theory may support the development of the child's ability to meet challenges presented by sensory differences in a positive manner and to develop resilience in the face of those challenges (Baranek, Wakeford, and David, 2008). This intervention may make use of changes in or additions to the environment to help create the optimal fit, changing the child by adding to their repertoire of coping behaviors (i.e., teaching them new ways to behave).

Motor learning theory

Motor learning theory (Shumway-Cook and Woollacott, 2000) targets the acquisition or modification of motor skills and may be useful in addressing the needs of children who have difficulties in the area of praxis. Intervention based on motor learning theory includes frequent opportunities for practice in natural settings, provision of meaningful feedback (including enhanced sensory input), use of cognitive and/or language-based strategies, and a focus on generalization of skills (Baranek, Wakeford, and David, 2008).

Sensory integration (SI) theory

Originally developed by A. Jean Ayres beginning in the early 1960s, SI theory is based on assumptions about the ways in which sensation is processed and organized within the central nervous system, and then integrated to help produce an adaptive behavioral theory response. The SI treatment approach uses specific and intentional combinations of sensory input, implemented by a therapist in the context of the child's play, in a manner that is theorized to enhance neural processing. Enhanced neural processing is assumed to lead to more adaptive behaviors (Ayres, 1972). This remediative approach is controversial, in part because of lack of empirical support for the efficacy of the intervention, and in part because it has spurred the development of a number of sensory-based interventions that also lack a supportive body of evidence (Baranek, 2002). In general, while SI theory is a well-known and "popular" approach to treatment, evidence-based practitioners generally do not use this theory to guide their work with children with ASD.

Sensory processing theories

More contemporary theories of sensory processing, such as those described by Dunn (1997), Dunn, Saiter, and Rinner (2002), and Baranek (1998; Baranek, Reinhartsen, and Wannamaker, 2001), acknowledge the ongoing, ever-changing nature of child, environment, and activity interactions, with particular focus on the ways in which individual patterns of sensory processing influence these interactions. Interventions based on these theories lead to individualized approaches that may include adapting activities, modifying environments, encouraging child participation, and supporting parents and other caregivers, through collaboration and education. The goal of the intervention is to minimize the influence of sensory processing differences and maximize successful performance of daily life activities.

Assessment

Assessment of sensory processing patterns is based on a combination of skilled observations by an occupational therapist (OT) familiar with sensory processing, and collaborative discussion with parents and/or other caregivers who know the child well. In addition to considering the responses of the child, the OT must also consider the environment and activity in which responses occurred. Although children with ASD tend to have patterns of responses to sensation that are individually fairly consistent, a number of factors can influence those responses in particular situations. As noted, hunger, fatigue, emotional state, interest, or motivation can affect response patterns. For instance, a child may have aversive responses to the coolness of the water coming from a sprinkler and the unpredictable rate at which that happens, but be so excited about going down the slide that he sits in the path of the water. He is willing to manage the aversive sensations in order to experience the pleasurable ones. Therefore, observations should occur in more than one instance, if possible, to discern whether the child's responses reflect true patterns of sensory processing or are the result of isolated or specific circumstances. Observations should be made not only of the behavior of the child, but also of the other aspects (e.g., social, sensory, physical) of the environment and of the activities in which the child is engaged. There are also several caregiver report measures (e.g., *Infant/Toddler Sensory Profile*, Dunn, 2002; *Sensory Processing Measure*, Miller-Kuhaneck, Henry, and Glennon, 2007) that are commonly used to assist identification of a child's sensory processing patterns and differences. These assessments are completed by a parent or teacher, typically, and scored and interpreted by the OT. Results should then be discussed with parents and teachers to ascertain whether the identified patterns seem accurate for that child.

A thorough assessment process is important not only to gather information about the child's sensory processing differences, but also to ascertain when those sensory processing differences *are not* the cause of particular child behaviors. For instance, without thorough assessment, an assumption may be made that a young, non-verbal child reacts aversively to getting his hair cut because of the tactile sensations on his head and around his face. In fact, what actually bothers him is that the hairstylist unpredictably moves in front of him, blocking the video that he is watching.

Intervention

Table 12.3 outlines a number of evidence-based strategies that may be used to address the effects on everyday life that sensory processing differences create for young children with ASD. These strategies can be implemented in a manner that is congruent with family-centered practices and daily activities and routines, in natural environments. Many of these strategies have empirical support for their use to address the needs of children with ASD, and most have been tested in early childhood contexts (Wolery, 1994). However, their application specifically to children with sensory processing differences is largely untested. It is important that these strategies be individualized and that some means of data collection be included in implementation planning to regularly measure the efficacy of the strategies and satisfaction with changes in child participation.

Table 12.3 Examples of evidence-based intervention strategies to address sensory processing differences and support participation of the young child with ASD	
Strategy and reference/resource	**Potential use in addressing sensory processing differences**
Educational and Parent-Mediated Interventions Gutstein, Burgess, and Montfort, 2007; Jaegermann and Klein, 2010; Mahoney and Perales, 2003, 2005; Mahoney *et al.*, 1999	Educational interventions are aimed at helping parents (and other caregivers) understand the ways in which children process sensory information and the behavior of results of those patterns of sensory processing. This may allow parents to better understand and interpret the behaviors exhibited by their child, and lead to broader perspectives that will support intervention planning. Parent-mediated interventions that teach parents different ways to interact with their child may support the parent–child interactions that are disrupted due to sensory-related behaviors and/or parent interpretation of those behaviors.

Social Stories™/Sensory Stories Baltazar and Bax, 2004; Barry and Burlew, 2004; Case-Smith and Arbesman, 2008; Gray and Garand, 1993; Kuoch and Mirenda, 2003; Marr *et al.*, 2007	May be written specifically to help a child learn different options for behavior when confronted with unwanted sensations, or when feeling as if he/she needs more sensation.
Visual Supports Ball, 1999; Bryan and Gast, 2000; Case-Smith and Arbesman, 2008; Dettmer *et al.*, 2000; Wakeford, 2008	May help a child generate ideas for play activities, prepare for a sequence of events, make transitions more easily, and provide more predictability and control over aversive features in the environment; may take a variety of forms, including pictures (drawings or photographs) and objects, and are used to assist the child in the prediction, understanding, and response aspects of managing daily events.
Priming Dunn, Saiter, and Rinner, 2002; Koegel *et al.*, 2003	Allows a child to watch or see what will be included in an activity without any demand for actual performance. The child can then "get used to" the idea of the activity before attempting to participate. This is especially helpful for those who are over-responsive.
Video Modeling MacDonald *et al.*, 2005; Maione and Mirenda, 2006; McCoy and Hermansen, 2007; Paterson and Arco, 2007	Video modeling is the use of a video representation of a targeted behavior to teach that behavior; the representation, or model, may be provided by a peer, an adult, or edited clips of the child him/herself. The behavior may be related to social interactions, communication, daily living skills, or play. In support of those with sensory processing difficulties, it allows the child to see the activity and to have adaptive methods of managing self-regulation or praxis challenges, offering a combination of priming, modeling, and opportunities for practice.
Task Modifications Baranek, Wakeford, and David, 2008; Wakeford and Baranek, 2011	Allows for adaptations to specific aspects of an activity, so that the child can continue to participate (e.g., offering tools other than hands for "fingerpainting" for the child averse to messy hands, or using big paper taped to the wall, bright colors, and large strokes for the child who needs more intensity of sensation).

Table continues

Table 12.3 Examples of evidence-based intervention strategies to address sensory processing differences and support participation of the young child with ASD *cont.*

Strategy and reference/resource	Potential use in addressing sensory processing differences
Arrangement or Modification of Physical Environment Baranek, Wakeford, and David, 2008; Duker and Rasing, 1989; Wakeford and Baranek, 2011	Arranging aspects of the built and natural environment can allow for various types of sensory experiences, such as the placement of stepping stones beside the driveway and up to the front door of the house so that the child can jump from one to another rather than simply walking up a smooth path, or the placement of pillows and throw blankets on the sofa to allow a child to "cocoon" her/himself when sibling play gets too loud.
Modifying the Social Environment, Including Peer-Mediated Interventions Bass and Mulick, 2007; Harper, Symon, and Frea, 2007; Robertson *et al.*, 2003; Rosenberg and Boulware, 2005; Sawyer *et al.*, 2003; Wakeford and Baranek, 2011	A child with sensory hypo-responsiveness may be given several partners to dance with at the beginning of circle time while the child with hyper-responsiveness may need fewer peers (and the likelihood of noise and unexpected touch) while playing in the block area of the classroom. For a child with praxis difficulties, a specific peer can be coached to help the child generate ideas for new activities.
Providing Specific "Roles" for the Child Baranek, Wakeford, and David, 2008	Children may take on roles in the home or classroom that allow them to be a part of the community in that situation, participate with others, and have sensory needs met. For instance, a child with aversions to touch (e.g., being bumped into) who often has difficulty with transitions may help the teacher flick the light to signal the transition, or help a teacher clean up until everyone is seated at circle time. For a child with sensory-seeking behaviors, activities with more intense sensory qualities may be offered (e.g., helping move things, hand things out at circle, or going with a teacher or parent to get things that are elsewhere in the building or home).

Suggestions for music therapists

The following suggestions are examples of how a music therapist (MT) may work to address sensory processing issues in children with ASD. This list is in no way exhaustive; intervention teams that include both music therapists and occupational therapists are encouraged to consider these ideas, as well as create their own, to facilitate successful engagement for children with ASD.

- Work with the OT in the assessment process. An MT has the opportunity to observe children interacting with music in many ways; those observations can provide important information about a child's sensory preferences and processing patterns because of the multiple sensory experiences that exist within music activities.

- Analyze the instruments, the ways in which they can be used, and the total music experiences provided from a "sensory perspective." Consider the variety of sounds, textures, colors, movements, etc. that are available with each instrument or music activity. This analysis allows the MT to develop a sort of catalogue or cross-referencing system to help match musical experiences to sensory needs. Table 12.4 provides an example of this type of analysis.

- As noted by Berger (2002), the MT's most important tools include the elements of music (i.e., rhythm, melody, harmony, dynamics, timbre, and form). Consider how each of these tools is congruent with one or more of the qualities of sensation (i.e., intensity, frequency, duration, rhythm, novelty, and complexity). The MT can use that intersection of musical element and sensory quality to help design interventions that meet sensory needs.

- Avoid assumptions about the effect of music or music activities on an individual child. Although many children find a wide variety of musical experiences fun and motivating, children with ASD may have significant preferences and dislikes based on how they perceive and process those experiences. Berger (2002) relates a relevant example in which a child had relatively negative responses to many of the music activities presented in music therapy. When he discovered a large gong, he immensely enjoyed striking it, despite the intensity and duration of the sound it produced. Berger goes on to enumerate "erroneous assumptions" about music and music therapy. One of these assumptions summarizes the rest: "The person will respond to the music according to the intent of the therapist" (p. 93).

- Advocate for the use of music therapy interventions as complementary to others that may be used (i.e., as part of an intervention "package"). For instance, the combination of a uniquely composed song, a laminated picture sequence, and the use of vigorous, deep pressure touch (rather than light touch) may help both parent and child manage washing the child's hair with much more ease than would any one of those strategies alone. In fact, research has demonstrated that the use of music interventions as a means of modifying tasks in this and similar ways can be useful for children with ASD (Brownell, 2002; Kern, Wakeford, and Aldridge, 2007; Register and Humpal, 2007).

Table 12.4 Sample analyses of musical instruments and activity

Instrument	Auditory	Visual	Tactile	Proprioceptive and Vestibular (from positioning and movement of body)
Tambourine	Sound of hand or other body part on head of tambourine, sound of cymbals (may be rhythmic or arrhythmic, and can vary in volume and tempo, i.e. intensity, frequency, duration). Sound varies based on way in which instrument is contacted, such as stroking, patting, scratching the head, flicking finger against head or cymbals, etc.	Roundness, white color and smooth appearance of head, small shiny cymbals positioned along sides and close together.	Smoothness of head, ridged texture of sides created by cymbals. Holding tambourine may create light or deep pressure touch, depending on how tightly it is held. Slap of tambourine against body (will vary depending on how loudly or quickly it is played). Tactile input varies based on way in which instrument is contacted, such as stroking, patting, scratching the head, flicking finger against head or cymbals, etc.	Shaking of tambourine, movement of arm to slap it against hand or other body part, weight shift and movement of hips if played against hip or leg, etc. (all will vary with tempo, volume at which it is played, and also the position of the player, for instance standing, sitting on floor or in chair, etc.).
Recorder	Variety of tones, resonance depending on material of which recorder is made.	Smoothness of instrument, tapered end, holes, color, length, diameter.	Holding recorder in two hands, fingers covering and uncovering holes, instrument in mouth and resting on lips, air flow, mild vibration from resonance of instrument.	Posture and stability needed to be still, hold instrument over time to correct position in mouth, expansion and compression of ribcage during respiration.

Music activity (from perspective of a child in the group)			
"Sandbox Wiggles" song, accompanied by guitar, in sandbox on playground with a class of preschool children (Kern and Wakeford, 2007)	Sounds of guitar, adults/other children singing along, own voice, other children playing elsewhere on playground. Tune is rhythmical, moderate tempo; lyrics describe actions for children to make (e.g., wiggle toes in sand, pour sand into hands, clap); names of children can be inserted to individualize.	Adult fingers pressing and strumming guitar strings, shape of guitar and spatial arrangement of strings, frets, hole, etc.; watching peers move to music, watching own body movements; color, visual texture of sand; other children running in and out of visual field in background.	Palm to palm touch for clapping; sand on body parts; touching sand, possibly having other children put sand on your hands, toes, etc. or touching you with sandy fingers/hands or bumping up against you as you move to music.	Movement of body parts in response to words of song (e.g. clapping, holding scoop and pouring sand from it, toes moving in sand) and includes weight shift and postural control needed to position whole body to make these movements possible.

Source: Wakeford, L. (2010). Sensory processing: key points and ideas for application in music therapy. imagine, 1,(1) Podcast Handout, p. 4. Reprinted with permission.

- Specifically consider the ways in which music and musical elements can be applied to:
  - enhancing sensory feedback for those with praxis difficulties
  - organizing and sequencing tasks (often difficult for those who are inattentive due to too little or too much sensation)
  - maintaining focus (often difficult when there is too much or too little sensation, or when sensory-seeking behaviors prevail)
  - shifting attention from less desired or noxious sensations to those that are more pleasing or easily managed
  - transitioning from one activity to the next (often difficult if the next activity has undesirable sensory qualities or is an unknown)
  - teaching or reminding a child about coping strategies or options for behavior (e.g., musical sensory story)
  - supporting social engagement while minimizing the "sensory risks" of being engaged with another child.

- Keep in mind that the goal of intervening for sensory processing differences is to support successful participation in everyday life and in natural contexts; design intervention strategies accordingly. While music can have a variety of effects on neurological and other physical and mental processes in humans, there is currently no scientific evidence that any of those effects (or the effects of any behavioral or educational intervention purported to make changes within the central nervous system) actually lead to permanent changes in sensory processing or translate to more successful functioning in everyday life. However, there is a growing body of evidence that task adaptations, behavioral interventions, and environmental modifications can substantially increase a child's success. Music therapists can have a powerful role in making this happen.

Conclusion

Many children with ASD demonstrate patterns of sensory processing that include over-responsiveness, under-responsiveness, and sensory seeking; mixed patterns are common. The effects of sensory processing impairments include difficulty with self-regulation (e.g., achieving and maintaining the level of arousal or alertness that is required by the activity and/or environment) and praxis (the ability to plan and execute new or complex motor behaviors). There are a variety of evidence-based approaches that occupational therapists may use to address these issues; each can be complemented by music therapy interventions. To do so, the music therapist must understand the basics of sensory processing, being able to analyze and make use of the sensory features and qualities of music experiences.

LEARNING QUESTIONS

1. Name and briefly describe each of the three primary patterns of sensory processing that may be seen in children with ASD.

2. Name and briefly define each of the six qualities of sensation discussed in this chapter.

3. There are a number of factors that may influence a child's ability to respond adaptively to sensory experiences. Name and give an example of at least two of those factors.

4. Explain how a music therapist can assist the occupational therapist in determining a child's sensory processing patterns and the ways in which those patterns influence participation in everyday activities.

5. Name an instrument or music activity you often use in your practice, and analyze it from a sensory processing perspective.

6. Choose one of the intervention strategies in Table 12.3. Discuss at least two ways a music therapist could support the use of the strategy through use of musical elements or a music activity.

7. Think about a young child with ASD with whom you recently have worked. What patterns of sensory processing, and for which senses, do you think were most often used by this child? Why? How might you help support that child's participation in daily routines and activities by addressing sensory processing issues?

References

American Psychiatric Association (APA) (2011). DSM-5 Development. Available at www.dsm5.org/Pages/Default.aspx.

Ashburner, J., Ziviani, J., and Rodger, S. (2008). Sensory processing and classroom emotional, behavioral, and educational outcomes in children with autism spectrum disorder. *American Journal of Occupational Therapy, 62*, 564–573.

Ayres, A.J. (1972). *Sensory Integration and Learning Disabilities.* Los Angeles: Western Psychological Services.

Ball, D. (1999). Visual supports: Helping children with autism. *OT Practice, 4(8)*, 37–40.

Baltazar, A., and Bax, B.E. (2004). Writing social stories for the child with sensory integration dysfunction: An introductory resource and guide for therapists, teachers, and parents. *Sensory Integration Special Interest Section Quarterly, 27*, 1–3.

Baranek, G.T. (1998). Sensory processing in persons with autism and developmental disabilities: Considerations for research and clinical practice. *Sensory Integration Special Interest Section Newsletter*, American Occupational Therapy Association, June, 21(2), pp. 1–4.

Baranek, G.T. (2002). Efficacy of sensory-motor interventions for children with autism. *Journal of Autism and Developmental Disorders, 32(5)*, 397–422.

Baranek, G.T., David, F.J., Poe, M.D., Stone, W.L., and Watson, L.R. (2006). Sensory Experiences Questionnaire: Discriminating sensory features in young children with autism, developmental delays, and typical development. *Journal of Child Psychology and Psychiatry, 47*, 591–601.

Baranek, G.T., Reinhartsen, D.B., and Wannamaker, S.W. (2001). Play: Engaging children with autism. In T. Huebner (Ed.) *Autism: A Sensorimotor Approach to Management.* Philadelphia: F.A. Davis.

Baranek, G.T., Wakeford, C.L., and David, F.J. (2008). Understanding, assessing, and treating sensory-motor issues in young children with autism. In K. Chawarska, A. Klin, and F. Volkmar (Eds.) *Autism Spectrum Disorders in Infancy and Early Childhood.* New York: Guilford Press.

Barry, L.M., and Burlew, S.B. (2004). Using social stories to teach choice and play skills to children with autism. *Focus on Autism and Other Developmental Disabilities, 19*, 45–51.

Bass, J.D., and Mulick, J.A. (2007). Social play skill enhancement of children with autism using peers and siblings as therapists. *Psychology in the Schools, 44*, 727–735.

Ben Itzchak, E., and Zachor, D.A. (2011). Who benefits from early intervention in autism spectrum disorders? *Research in Autism Spectrum Disorders, 5*, 345–350.

Ben-Sasson, A., Hen, L., Fluss, R., Cermak, S.A., Engel-Yeger, B., and Gal, E. (2009). A meta-analysis of sensory modulation symptoms in individuals with autism spectrum disorders. *Journal of Autism and Developmental Disorders, 39*, 1–11.

Berger, D.S. (2002). *Music Therapy, Sensory Integration and the Autistic Child.* London and Philadelphia: Jessica Kingsley Publishers.

Boyd, B.A., Baranek, G.T., Sideris, J., Poe, M.D., *et al.* (2010). Sensory features and repetitive behaviors in children with autism and developmental delays. *Autism Research, 3*, 78–87.

Bronfenbrenner, U. (1992). Ecological Systems Theory. Reprinted from original in U. Bronfenbrenner (Ed.) *Making Human Beings Human: Bioecological Perspectives on Human Development.* Thousand Oaks, CA: Sage.

Brownell, M.D. (2002). Musically adapted social stories to modify behaviors in students with autism: Four case studies. *Journal of Music Therapy, 39(2)*, 117–144.

Bryan, L.C., and Gast, D.L. (2000). Teaching on-task and on-schedule behaviors to high-functioning children with autism via picture activity schedules. *Journal of Autism and Developmental Disorders, 30(6)*, 553–567.

Case-Smith, J., and Arbesman, M. (2008). Evidence-based review of interventions for autism used in or of relevance to occupational therapy. *American Journal of Occupational Therapy, 62*, 416–429.

Chawarska, K., and Shic, F. (2009). Looking but not seeing: Atypical visual scanning and recognition of faces in 2 and 4-year-old children with autism spectrum disorder. *Journal of Autism and Developmental Disorders, 39*, 1663–1672.

Dettmer, S., Simpson, R.L., Myles, B.S., and Ganz, J.B. (2000). The use of visual supports to facilitate transitions of students with autism. *Focus on Autism and Other Developmental Disabilities, 15*, 163–169.

Duker, P.C., and Rasing, E. (1989). Effects of redesigning the physical environment on self-stimulation and on-task behavior in three autistic-type developmentally disabled individuals. *Journal of Autism and Developmental Disorders, 19(3)*, 449–460.

Dunn, W. (1997). The impact of sensory processing abilities on the daily lives of young children and their families: A conceptual model. *Infants and Young Children, 9*, 23–35.

Dunn, W. (2002). *The Infant/Toddler Sensory Profile Manual.* San Antonio: The Psychological Corporation.

Dunn, W., Myles, B.S., and Orr, S. (2002). Sensory processing issues associated with Asperger syndrome: A preliminary investigation. *American Journal of Occupational Therapy, 56*, 97–102.

Dunn, W., Saiter, J., and Rinner, L. (2002). Asperger syndrome and sensory processing: A conceptual model and guidance for intervention planning. *Focus on Autism and Other Developmental Disabilities, 17(3)*, 172–185.

Gray, C.A., and Garand, J.D. (1993). Social Stories™: Improving responses of students with autism with accurate social information. *Focus on Autistic Behavior, 8*, 1–10.

Gutstein, S.E., Burgess, A.F., and Montfort, K. (2007). Evaluation of the relationship development intervention program. *Autism, 11*, 397–411.

Harper, C.B., Symon, J.B.G., and Frea, W.D. (2007). Recess is time in: Using peers to improve social skills of children with autism. *Journal of Autism and Developmental Disorders, 38*, 815–826.

Jaegermann, N., and Klein, P.S. (2010). Enhancing mothers' interactions with toddlers who have sensory-processing disorders. *Infant Mental Health Journal, 31*, 291–311.

Keane, E. (2004). Autism: The heart of the disorder? Sensory processing and social engagement— illustrations from autobiographical accounts and selected research findings. *Australian Journal of Early Childhood, 29*, 8–14.

Kern, P., and Wakeford, L. (2007). *Playground Favorites: An Interdisciplinary Approach to Outdoor Play for Young Children*. Paper presented at the Annual Conference of the American Music Therapy Association, Louisville, Kentucky.

Kern, P., Wakeford, L., and Aldridge, D. (2007). Improving the performance of a young child with autism during self-care tasks using embedded song interventions: A case study. *Music Therapy Perspectives, 25(1)*, 43–51.

Koegel, L.K., Koegel, R.L., Frea, W., and Green-Hopkins, I. (2003). Priming as a method of coordinating educational services for students with autism. *Language, Speech, and Hearing Services in Schools, 34(3)*, 228–235.

Kuoch, H., and Mirenda, P. (2003). Social story interventions for young children with autism spectrum disorders. *Focus on Autism and Other Developmental Disabilities, 18(4)*, 219–227.

Law, M., Cooper, B., Strong, S., Stewart, D., Rigby, P., and Letts, L. (1996). The Person–Environment– Occupation Model: A transactive approach to occupational performance. *Canadian Journal of Occupational Therapy, 63*, 9–23.

MacDonald, R., Clark, M., Garrigan, E., and Vangala, M. (2005). Using video modeling to teach pretend play to children with autism. *Behavioral Interventions, 20(4)*, 225–238.

Maekawa, T., Tobimatsu, S., Inada, N., Oribe, N., *et al.* (2011). Top-down and bottom-up visual information processing of non-social stimuli in high-functioning autism spectrum disorder. *Research in Autism Spectrum Disorders, 5*, 201–209.

Mahoney, G., and Perales, F. (2003). Using relationship-focused intervention to enhance the social-emotional functioning of young children with autism spectrum disorders. *Topics in Early Childhood Special Education, 23*, 77–89.

Mahoney, G., and Perales, F. (2005). Relationship-focused early intervention with children with pervasive developmental disorders and other disabilities: A comparative study. *Journal of Developmental and Behavioral Pediatrics, 26(2)*, 77–85.

* Mahoney, G., Kaiser, A., Girolametto, L., MacDonald, J., *et al.* (1999). Parent education in early intervention: A call for a renewed focus. *Topics in Early Childhood Special Education, 19*, 131–140.

Maione, L., and Mirenda, P. (2006). Effects of video modeling and video feedback on peer-directed social language skills of a child with autism. *Journal of Positive Behavior Interventions, 8(2)*, 106–118.

Marr, D., Mika, H., Miraglia, J., Roerig, M., and Sinnott, R. (2007). The effect of sensory stories on targeted behaviors in preschool children with autism. *Physical and Occupational Therapy in Pediatrics, 27*, 63–79.

McCoy, K., and Hermansen, E. (2007). Video modeling for individuals with autism: A review of model types and effects. *Education and Treatment of Children, 30*, 183–213.

Miller-Kuhaneck, H., Henry, D.A., and Glennon, T.J. (2007). *Sensory Processing Measure: Main Classroom Form and School Environments Forms*. Los Angeles: Western Psychological Services.

Olsen, L.J. (1999). Psychosocial frame of reference. In P. Kramer and J. Hinojosa (Eds.) *Frames of Reference in Pediatric Occupational Therapy (Second Edition)*. Baltimore, MD: Lippincott, Williams and Wilkins.

Paterson, C.R., and Arco, L. (2007). Using video modeling for generalizing toy play in children with autism. *Behavior Modification, 31(5)*, 660–681.

Pillay, M., Alderson-Day, B., Wright, B., Williams, C., and Urwin, B. (2011). Autism spectrum conditions—enhancing nurture and development (ASCEND): An evaluation of intervention support groups for parents. *Clinical Child Psychology and Psychiatry, 16*, 5–20.

Register, D., and Humpal, M. (2007). Using musical transitions in early childhood classrooms: Three case examples. *Music Therapy Perspectives, 25*, 25–31.

Robertson, J., Green, K., Alper, S., Schloss, P.J., and Kohler, F. (2003). Using peer-mediated intervention to facilitate children's participation in inclusive childcare activities. *Education and Treatment of Children, 26*, 182–197.

Rosenberg, N., and Boulware, G.L. (2005). Playdates for young children with autism and other disabilities. *Young Exceptional Children, 8*, 11–20.

Sawyer, L.M., Luiselli, J.K., Ricciardi, J.N., and Gower, J.L. (2005). Teaching a child with autism to share among peers in an integrated preschool classroom: Acquisition, maintenance, and social validation. *Education and Treatment of Children, 28(1)*, 1–10.

Schaaf, R.C., Miller, L.J., Seawell, D., and O'Keefe, S. (2003). Children with disturbances in sensory processing: A pilot study examining the role of the parasympathetic nervous system. *American Journal of Occupational Therapy, 57*, 442–449.

Shumway-Cook, A., and Woollacott, M. (2000). *Motor Control: Theory and Practical Applications (Second Edition)*. Hagerstown, MD: Williams and Wilkins.

Smith, I.M., Koegel, R., Koegel, L.K., Openden, D.A., Fossum, K.L., and Bryson, S.E. (2010). Effectiveness of a novel community-based early intervention model for children with autistic spectrum disorder. *American Journal on Intellectual and Developmental Disabilities, 115*, 504–523.

Sturmey, P., and Fitzer, A. (2007). (Eds.) *Autism Spectrum Disorders: Applied Behaviour Analysis, Evidence and Practice*. Austin, TX: Pro-Ed.

Smith, L.B., and Thelen, E (2003). Development as a dynamic system. *Trends in Cognitive Sciences, 7*, 343–348.

Wakeford, L. (2008). Baggie books. *Journal of Occupational Therapy, Schools, and Early Intervention, 1*, 283–288.

Wakeford, L. (2010). Sensory processing: Key points and ideas for application in music therapy. *imagine*, Volume 1, Podcast Handout, p. 4.

Wakeford, L., and Baranek, G.T. (2011). Occupational therapy. In D.G. Amaral, G. Dawson, and D.H. Gschwind (Eds.) *Autism Spectrum Disorders*. New York: Oxford University Press.

Wolery, M. (1994). Instructional strategies for teaching young children with special needs. In M. Wolery and J.S. Wilbers (Eds.) *Including Children with Special Needs in Early Childhood Programs*. Washington, DC: NAEYC.

Chapter 13

Family-Centered Practice

Integrating Music into Home Routines

Darcy Walworth, Ph.D., MT-BC
UNIVERSITY OF LOUISVILLE
LOUISVILLE, KY

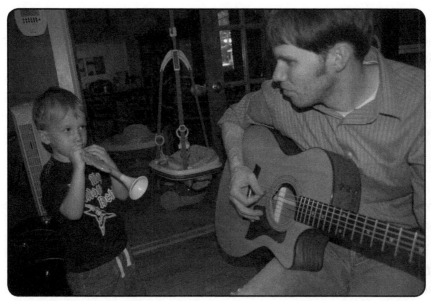

Embedding music into family routines is achievable and beneficial to improve communication, emotional regulation, and transition times for families and children with autism spectrum disorders. (Darcy Walworth)

Parents of young children with autism spectrum disorders (ASD) who attend music therapy sessions may be guided to transfer intervention strategies and techniques into their home activities and routines. This chapter explores the need for family-centered practice providing music therapy service in natural environments and addresses myths surrounding parents' hesitancy to sing or create meaningful music with their children who have ASD. Tips and comments for parents about embedding music into family routines are discussed and organized by prominent areas of needs of children with ASD. The chapter also includes considerations for music therapists to effectively involve parents within this protocol.

Guiding principles

The Division of Early Childhood (DEC) recommends focusing on five guiding principles of effective practices when working with young children with ASD and their families. These support: (1) a family-centered and strength-based approach, (2) natural and inclusive environments, (3) developmentally sound interventions, (4) functional goals that are oriented toward active child engagement, and (5) services that are provided in a coordinated and systematic manner (Sandall *et al.*, 2005).

These principles interlock to form a foundation for effective service delivery that is reflected throughout this book and within this chapter. The pages that follow will more thoroughly examine two main concepts that further strengthen this foundation: family-centered practice and providing music therapy services in children's natural home environments.

Family-centered practice

The idea of parents and professionals partnering to provide a more comprehensive and quality care for children with special needs has been developing since the 1970s (Wells, 2011). Today, families are encouraged to be involved in the therapeutic process, extending the location of where children learn from the therapeutic sessions to the child's natural environments (Gabovitch and Curtin, 2009; Schertz, 2010). However, discrepancies in the delivery of family-centered practice exist between children with ASD and those with other special needs. Families of children with ASD are less likely to receive services based on family-centered practice. Furthermore, African-American families with a child with ASD are more than two times less likely than Caucasian families of children with ASD to receive family-centered services (Montes and Halterman, 2011) even though reports verify that family-centered practice consistently yields better outcomes for children with special needs (American Academy of Pediatrics, 2003). Family-centered practice focuses on (a) incorporating family priorities, (b) supporting a strong parent–child interactive relationship, and (c) building the family's capacity to promote the child's development (Schertz, 2010, p. 13).

FAMILY NEEDS, VALUES, AND PREFERENCES

When parents and siblings of children with ASD are empowered with positive supports and strategies, they can play a vital role in the therapeutic process and development of their child's skills. Both mothers and fathers report negative effects in coping with stress, mental health, and monetary strain as a result of raising a child diagnosed with ASD, while siblings' reports are mixed between experiencing depression and being well adjusted (Gabovitch and Curtin, 2009). When questioned about family-centered practice, parents of children with ASD report a need for professionals to be open-minded, positive, and to think within the framework of the strengths their family and child possess. Open communication and respect for family system routines also are highly valued by parents. The successful incorporation of family-centered practice can alleviate anxiety and self-doubt that many families face when trying to accommodate many service providers and treatment options for their child (Gabovitch and Curtin, 2009). To be successful, service coordination has to occur within multiple systems where the family is involved and with appropriate education, advocacy, and monitoring (Lindeke et al., 2002). The ultimate goal for interventionists may be to enable families to meet their own needs (Prelock and Hutchins, 2008).

SUPPORTING FAMILY–CHILD INTERACTIONS

The first step in this process may be to provide information to families that is relevant to evidence-based practice within available treatments; this may build confidence and respect between care providers and families, and foster collaboration between all treatment team members (Abbey and Foster, 2009). Next, interventions should be planned to support the interactions between family members and the child with ASD rather than the therapist's interactions with the child (Schertz, 2010). The parent–child relationship is central for young children's development because learning occurs in the natural environments and during daily routines. Providing services in the family's home where siblings and other family members are present is therefore valuable, especially when working with infants and toddlers with ASD (Sandall et al., 2005). Carefully planned music therapy interventions may strengthen the relationships through music-making while supplying invaluable resources for future interactions and challenging situations the child with ASD may face (Walworth, 2010).

EMPOWERING PARENTS TO FOSTER THE CHILD'S DEVELOPMENT

Parents are their child's primary partner for providing stimulation, support, and motivation for learning and development. Therefore, parent-mediated interventions may enable family members to respond to daily life situations and may promote the development of their child with ASD (Schertz, 2010). The inclusion of services within the family's home may give children the skills they need to be successful during daily activities and family routines. With the support of a certified music therapist, parents and children with ASD may be guided to respond to naturally occurring changes within the home environment. Families may be empowered to learn, facilitate new social communication and emotional regulation skills, foster seamless transitions, and encourage joint engagement to possibly help the child with ASD generalize skills to the home environment.

Natural environments

Providing interventions in the natural environment of children with ASD is recommended practice (National Research Council, 2001). Natural environments are places where children regardless of their level of ability would spend time (McWilliam, 1996). So, for young children with ASD, the family home or community settings (e.g., community-based childcare programs or playgrounds) are natural environments where music therapy interventions should take place (Kern and Aldridge, 2006). Children with ASD demonstrate difficulty in transferring newly learned skills from settings where they were initially learned to new settings. Practicing these skills across different environments where they are needed may be necessary. The process of accessing previously learned responses does not occur as readily when there are environmental changes (Cowan and Allen, 2007). By conducting training for parents, music therapists may be able to provide avenues for embedding interventions that may promote the child's development through naturally occurring everyday situations.

Interventions for teaching children with ASD functional skills in the natural environment are often based on natural teaching strategies (Franzone, 2009). The National Autism Center (NAC) (2009) identifies naturalistic teaching strategies as an established treatment for individuals with ASD. Naturalistic teaching strategies vary in technique, but all share the goal of increasing the child's ability to generalize the skills learned to settings the child has yet to experience with the newly learned response; incorporating these strategies with children with ASD is gaining increasing acceptance by experts (Cowan and Allen, 2007). Examples of natural teaching strategies include focused stimulation, incidental teaching, milieu teaching, embedded teaching, responsive education, and prelinguistic milieu teaching (NAC, 2009).

Considerations for music therapists

Music therapists need to be flexible when delivering services in the context of family-based practice. Embedded music therapy interventions may be provided along the continuum of direct to consultative services in the child's natural environments (Humpal and Colwell, 2006). The collaborative consultative approach may allow for individualized interventions using music for functional skill improvement in young children with ASD while empowering parents and caregivers to embed the intervention in the family's home or community settings (Kern, 2005). Music therapists may also familiarize themselves with natural teaching strategies (especially those being used with the target child) and incorporate them into music therapy interventions when providing home and community-based services for young children with ASD and their families.

Identifying a child's communication, behavioral, and coping strengths is the first step in assessing a child within a home or community environment (Prizant *et al.*, 2006). Chapter 4 offers a detailed discussion of music therapy assessment tools for young children with ASD. Creating a plan for embedding music for the child's development into the family routines across settings and daily activities may be better achieved when the music therapist has an accurate picture of the strengths, values, and preferences of each child and family system (Walworth, 2010).

A music therapy plan might unfold as follows. Before engaging in singing or playing a song to support their child's learning, parents may prefer having the music therapist demonstrate how the music will function in the home or community environment. Parents may hesitate to sing or make music with their children due to preconceived reasons. Music therapists may help parents feel more comfortable by coaching them to use music intentionally with their children who have ASD and by dispelling common myths about their singing and music-making skills (see Table 13.1). If the focus is taken off their singing ability and instead is realigned with how their child reacts to the music intervention at home, parents may feel more comfortable implementing music techniques with their children with ASD.

During the implementation of the music therapy intervention in the family's home or a community setting, music therapists need to regularly assess the child's progress while providing continuous support to parents and caregivers (Kern and Aldridge, 2006).

Using music for specific needs in the home environment

Core areas of needs that might benefit from including music therapy interventions in the home environment of children with ASD may include: (1) verbal and non-verbal communication, (2) emotional regulation, (3) transitions, and (4) joint engagement between parent and child. This section provides a brief description of four selected core areas included in the SCERTS® Model (Prizant *et al.*, 2006). Examples and explanations are described through tips and comments under each area; these may guide parent/child music-making in the home environment.

Communication

As discussed in Chapter 11, children with ASD have deficits in social communication and speech-language development. Various facets of communication such as *Reciprocity* and *Motivation to Communicate* may possibly be supported by music-making in the family's home by parents who support the child's communication by creating natural learning opportunities through music.

Table 13.1 Common myths surrounding why parents may hesitate to sing with their children

Statements	Discussion
I will scare people away if I open my mouth and sing.	Most people can sing with enough accuracy that the tune of the song can be identified. Creating a group experience engages others in singing; once a melody is distinguishable, others can join in so not just one voice is heard. After experiencing this a few times, the person will be less intimidated by starting a song alone because the expectation of others joining in the singing will be stronger.
I can't sing as well as the CD recording.	None of us has the luxury of our voices being processed and mixed before being heard. Recordings actually have many shortfalls that live singing does not. Live singing allows for spontaneous stopping and starting, speeding up and slowing down, and repeating certain phrases. Recordings do not allow for those changes as easily, if at all. Singing to engage a child may require changing the song to preserve interest and attending to the music. Live music is consistently a more engaging method of singing for this very reason.
No one wants to hear me sing.	Many children will love the times when a parent tries to interact and engage with them through music. Initiating a positive interaction using a song that a child likes may elicit interest and usually enjoyment. This means that the child does want to hear the parent sing. Be aware of auditory sensitivity and gauge the volume of singing accordingly.
I can never remember all of the words to the song, so it is hopeless to try and sing.	Remembering song lyrics is a difficult task for many people. There is nothing wrong with using printed lyrics when singing. Many websites have printable lyrics to a large number of songs from many different genres. Be sure to look up from the lyric sheet and engage with the child to allow engagement to occur and to avoid losing the entire purpose of singing.
I can never remember any songs to sing other than "If You're Happy and You Know It."	Certain songs may get stuck in your head. There are some quick solutions: Have a song list that is kept in a high traffic area of the house as a reminder for possible songs to use, or place a label on the underside of toys or items with the name of a song that can be sung when playing with that toy.
I feel so _____ when I sing.	That blank can be filled in with many different words (e.g., uncomfortable, silly, self-conscious, embarrassed). Usually people stop using those words to describe how they feel about singing when they begin to realize the positive benefits of singing in front of children. The negative words are often replaced by positive terms (e.g. great, fun, happy). The empowering process of branching out of a comfort zone and grabbing hold of a new interaction technique can be very rewarding—for both parents and children!

RECIPROCITY

Due to the lack of social communication skills, children with ASD may need to learn the back-and-forth flow of communicative exchanges (Prizant *et al.*, 2006). When a musical instrument is shared between two people, a natural reciprocity may be established (Walworth, 2010).

MOTIVATION TO COMMUNICATE

Many children with ASD will communicate when they are motivated to express a desire (Prizant *et al.*, 2006). Music is a natural motivator for many children, including those with ASD (Kern, 2008).

TIPS AND COMMENTS FOR PARENTS

- Parents may set up the environment to encourage communication for obtaining a favored song or instrument (e.g., by playing the instrument or singing in a novel way to capture the child's attention, or enticing the child by placing the instrument out of the child's reach, thus requiring the child to communicate to get what he or she wants).

- Once the child successfully communicates and is given the instrument, a favorite song can be sung to keep the child engaged in a meaningful interaction. The song then may be anticipated when the instrument is presented; thus the song itself may become intrinsically rewarding.

- Pausing within the song and waiting until the child sings a word within the context of the song may naturally reinforce the child to sing as the song continues. For example, if a child likes the song "Twinkle, Twinkle, Little Star," the parent can sing "Twinkle, twinkle, little...," pausing and waiting for the child to sing or say "star." Once the child sings or says "star," the parent may continue with the next phrase.

Emotional regulation

Children with ASD often have difficulty with emotional regulation, demonstrating abnormal responses to events in their surroundings. They may have trouble adjusting to changes and transitions, which may result in aggression, stereotypic behaviors, self-injury, or tantrums (Prizant *et al.*, 2006). *Distracting, Focusing, Supporting,* and *Expressing,* four functions of music, can encourage emotional regulations (Walworth, 2010). Parents may assist the regulation of the child's emotions by intentionally applying the four functions of music during stressful moments.

DISTRACTING

Distracting a dysregulated child with ASD from the negative catalyst may be very useful (Laurent and Rubin, 2004). The child's emotional distress may be dispelled by attending to the stimulus of the music and actively engaging in music-making (Walworth, 2010).

TIPS AND COMMENTS FOR PARENTS

- Parents may choose music that matches the emotional state of the child, considering both familiar and completely unfamiliar music. Music that is familiar to the child and previously had elicited a positive association may grasp the child's attention and distract her from abnormal responses. Similarly, the curiosity elicited by an unfamiliar sound of a completely new song or musical piece may divert the child's attention away from the stimulus that may be causing the dysregulation.

- Once the child is successfully distracted from the negative catalyst and begins to demonstrate signs of being emotionally regulated, the next function of music may be applied.

FOCUSING

Children with ASD need to learn socially appropriate ways to express their emotional state (Laurent and Rubin, 2004). When a child is making music, the music may serve as a focus for attention and an outlet for emotional expression (Walworth, 2010).

TIPS AND COMMENTS FOR PARENTS

- Parents may need to be in tune with how the child's emotions are changing over time. The ability of a child to remain focused on music may fluctuate during the process of returning to a regulated emotional state.

- Changing the music as soon as the child shows any signs of disengagement may allow the child to remain focused on the music stimulus and be more likely to reach a regulated emotional state.

SUPPORTING

Providing emotional support to a dysregulated child with ASD may be useful for regulating emotions (Laurent and Rubin, 2004). Music serves as a support for a dysregulated child because it may elicit positive, comforting, and calming feelings (Walworth, 2010).

TIPS AND COMMENTS FOR PARENTS

- Parents may support their child's emotional state by carefully observing the child's reaction to the music and then providing different musical stimuli.

- Active music-making versus listening to selected music may elicit different levels of responses from the child.

- The intensity of positive and negative emotions triggered by music may vary from child to child and across settings and times.

EXPRESSING

Finding appropriate ways to express negative feelings can be challenging for children with ASD who have difficulty with verbal communication (Prizant *et al.*, 2006). A child with ASD may release positive and negative emotions through active music-making (Walworth, 2010).

TIPS AND COMMENTS FOR PARENTS

- Parents may guide the child to a calmer emotional state by first matching the music to the child's emotional intensity (e.g., fast and loud drumming may offer a means for releasing energy and frustration).

- After the child is engaged in active music-making, he or she may be systematically introduced to a calmer emotional state (e.g., expressed through playing the drum softly and calmly).

- When the rhythmic complexity and tempo decrease gradually over a longer period of time, the changes may be hardly noticeable to the child. Therefore, the child may be more likely to stay engaged in the drumming and will naturally calm down as the drumming becomes less intense.

Transitions

Transitions are difficult to manage for many children with ASD (Prizant *et al.*, 2006). As discussed in Chapter 9, songs and sound cues can prepare children with ASD for transitions from one activity or event to the next (Kern, 2008; Register and Humpal, 2007). Parents may play a major role in supporting transitions by establishing structure and a predictable routine through music.

TIPS AND COMMENTS FOR PARENTS

- Parents may determine which music choice is best for providing a positive transition experience by first identifying when in the transition process the child typically becomes dysregulated.

- Songs that are related to walking, running, or marching (e.g., "The Ants Go Marching") are logical choices for moving from one location to another.

- Begin the transition song before the child is finished with the prior activity (e.g., playing with a favorite toy). This may allow the child to become engaged in the song before getting upset about having to stop the activity in which she was previously occupied.

- When parents always sing the same song during each specific transition, the song itself eventually may cue the child that a transition is happening; the song relays information about what will happen next.

- Once the transition has begun, the music shifts from functioning as a cue to functioning as a structure for the completion of the transition.

Joint attention

The inability to share enjoyment, interests, and achievements with others is a core deficit in children with ASD (Prizant *et al.*, 2006). When two people sing together, a natural shared attention may occur through participating in the music-making (Walworth, 2005; Walworth, Register, and Engel, 2009). Parents may play a major role in promoting joint attention by sharing their enjoyment and interest in music with the child.

TIPS AND COMMENTS FOR PARENTS

- Parents may use several specific aspects of music-making that require attention for a joint activity to occur between them and their child. For example, if the child is going to sing or play an instrument with the parent, he or she must recognize the song's beginning or ending.

- Parents may use the natural aspect of singing to request an interaction within the song. Pausing within a song may function as a natural reinforcer for participation and interaction of the child to finish the song.

- When a child learns to sing a song or play an instrumental part, parents may celebrate the child's success and share their enjoyment and interest.

Incorporating music into the home environment to support communication, emotional regulation, and transitions may encourage parents to abandon their insecurities about singing and making live music. Parents who have successfully incorporated live music with their children realize that an important purpose of singing moves away from focusing on performing and towards addressing their child's needs and sharing pleasurable moments (Walworth, 2010).

Conclusion

Effective music therapy service delivery for young children with ASD may be guided by principles that address the needs not only of the child but also of the family. While music therapy may be provided across a continuum that ranges from direct service to collaborative consultation, treatment should represent a family-centered approach that is delivered in the natural home environment and incorporates family priorities, supports strong parent–child interactive relationships, and builds on the family's capacity to promote their child's development. Music may support core areas of verbal and non-verbal communication, emotional regulation, transitioning, and joint engagement. Music therapists can offer parents a unique avenue for empowering their children by including music in natural environments. Working together, professionals and parents may support children with ASD to more comfortably attain the paramount goal of generalizing skills across different environments.

LEARNING QUESTIONS

1. What are five principles that may guide effective practices when working with young children with ASD and their families?

2. Family-centered practice focuses on (a) _____, (b) _____, and (c) _____.

3. Why should music therapy services be delivered to children with ASD in a natural environment?

4. What should music therapists consider when providing parent training in the family's home?

5. What are some common reasons parents may hesitate to sing to their child with ASD?

6. Which core areas of needs for children with ASD may be supported by music therapy interventions in the home environment?

7. Name four ways in which music may function as a support for emotional regulation of children with ASD.

8. How may parents promote their child's development through music?

Author's note

The author would like to thank Michael and Rebecca Strickland for their continual advocacy of the music therapy profession and enthusiastic inclusion of music therapy techniques into their home environment.

References

Abbey, D., and Foster, R.L. (2009). Helping families find the best evidence: CAM therapies for autism spectrum disorders and Asperger's disorder. *Journal for Specialists in Pediatric Nursing, 14*, 200–202.

American Academy of Pediatrics (2003). Family centered care and the pediatrician's role. *Pediatrics, 112*, 691–697.

Cowan, R.J., and Allen, K.D. (2007). Using naturalistic procedures to enhance learning in individuals with autism: A focus on generalized teaching within the school setting. *Psychology in the Schools, 44*, 701–715.

Franzone, E. (2009). *Overview of Naturalistic Intervention.* Madison, WI: National Professional Development Center on Autism Spectrum Disorders, Waisman Center, University of Wisconsin.

Gabovitch, E.M., and Curtin, C. (2009). Family centered care for children with autism spectrum disorders: A review. *Marriage and Family Review, 45*, 469–498.

Humpal, M., and Colwell, C. (Eds.) (2006). *Best Practices in Music Therapy Monograph: Early Childhood and School Age*. Silver Spring, MD: The American Music Therapy Association, Inc.

Kern, P., and Aldridge, D. (2006). Using embedded music therapy interventions to support outdoor play of young children with autism in an inclusive community-based child care program. *Journal of Music Therapy, 43(4)*, 270–294.

Kern, P. (2005). Single case designs in an interactive play setting. In D. Aldridge (Ed.) *Case Study Designs in Music Therapy*. London and Philadelphia: Jessica Kingsley Publishers.

Kern, P. (2008). Singing our way through the day: Using music with young children during daily routines. *Children and Families, 22(2)*, 50–56.

Laurent, A.C., and Rubin, E. (2004). Challenges in emotional regulation in Asperger Syndrome and high-functioning autism. *Topics in Language Disorders, 24*, 286–297.

Lindeke, L.L., Leonard, B.J., Presler, B., and Garwick, A. (2002). Family-centered care coordination for children with special needs across multiple settings. *Journal of Pediatric Health Care, 16*, 290–297.

McWilliam, R.A. (Ed.) (1996). *Rethinking Pull-Out Services in Early Intervention: A Professional Resource*. Baltimore, MD: Paul H. Brookes Publishing Co.

Montes, G., and Halterman, J.S. (2011). White–black disparities in family-centered care among children with autism in the United States: Evidence from the NS-CSHCN 2005–2006. *Academic Pediatrics, 11*, 297–304.

National Autism Center (NAC) (2009). *National Standards Report*. The National Standards Project—Addressing the need for evidence-based practice guidelines for autism spectrum disorders. Randolph, MA: NAC.

National Research Council (NRC) (2001). *Educating Children with Autism*. Committee on Educational Interventions for Children with Autism. C. Lord and J. McGee (Eds.) Division of Behavioral and Social Sciences and Education. Washington, DC: National Academy Press.

Prelock, P.A., and Hutchins, T.L. (2008). The role of family-centered care in research: Supporting the social communication of children with autism spectrum disorder. *Topics in Language Disorders, 28*, 323–339.

Prizant, B.M., Wetherby, A.M., Rubin, E., Laurent, A.C., and Rydell, P.J. (2006). *The SCERTS Model: Volume I. Assessment*. Baltimore, MD: Paul H. Brookes Publishing Co.

Register, D., and Humpal, M. (2007). Using musical transitions in early childhood classrooms: Three case examples. *Music Therapy Perspectives, 25*, 25–31.

Sandall, S., Hemmeter, M.L., Smith, B., and McLean, M.E. (Eds.) (2005). *DEC Recommended Practices: A Comprehensive Guide for Practical Application in Early Intervention/Early Childhood Special Education*. Longmont, CO: Sopris West.

Schertz, H. (2010). Principles of intervention for young children: Implications for toddlers and preschoolers with autism spectrum disorders. In H. Schertz, C. Wong, and S. Odom (Eds.) *Young Exceptional Children Monograph Series 12*. Missoula, MT: DEC.

Walworth, D.D. (2005). Procedural support music therapy in the healthcare setting: A cost and effectiveness analysis. *Journal of Pediatric Nursing, 20*, 276–284.

Walworth, D.D. (2010). Incorporating music into daily routines: Family education and integration. *imagine, 1(1)*, 28–31.

Walworth, D.D., Register, D., and Engel, J.N. (2009). Using the SCERTS Model assessment tool to identify music therapy goals for clients with autism spectrum disorder. *Journal of Music Therapy, 46(3)*, 204–216.

Wells, N. (2011). Historical perspective on family centered care. *Academic Pediatrics, 11(2)*, 100–102.

Chapter 14

Parents of Children with Autism Spectrum Disorders

Personal Perspectives and Insights from Music Therapists

Marcia Humpal, M.Ed., MT-BC
OLMSTED FALLS, OH

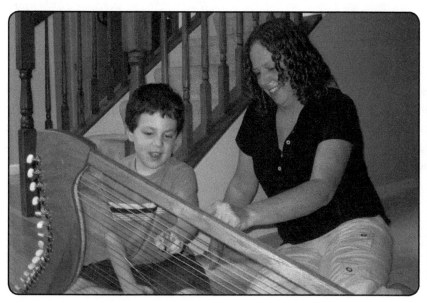

PHOTO COURTESY OF MARCIA HUMPAL

*For parents whose professional lives are dedicated to serving individuals
with disabilities, having a child with an autism spectrum disorder
may add layers of knowledge, expectations, and urgency.
(Marcia Humpal)*

Parents of children with autism spectrum disorders (ASD) are thrust into a role that invariably brings denial, frustration, and desperation, but also deep feelings of commitment, love, and joy. This chapter examines issues that generally surround families of children with ASD. Additionally, the voices of four music therapists who have both a professional and personal investment in the lives of young children with ASD are captured in interviews; no one else can speak their thoughts better than they themselves.

The impact on family life

I chose to become a parent, not an autism expert. So I have no idea how to make sense of what is out there. So it's all about trial and error, and asking lots of questions, and keeping my fingers crossed. (Parent reflecting on raising a child with ASD; in Lawsane, 2011)

The impact of having a child with ASD may permeate all aspects of family life. The child's behavior, communication, social and health issues, and unique needs in other areas may drastically alter the lives of the immediate family and interactions with the extended family, friends, and co-workers. While each family unit reacts and copes in its own way, many parents express similar perspectives about the following major areas of stress in their lives (Estes *et al.*, 2009; Hastings, 2004; Hastings *et al.*, 2005; MacNeil and Zucker, 2011; Rudy, 2010):

- their child's inappropriate behavior
- not being able to understand the child's wants and needs
- money and financial issues
- guilt and anxiety
- time commitment
- lack of leisure and recreation activities
- navigating the various systems (e.g., education, healthcare)
- too much and too little information (i.e., media reports that lack details or substantiation)
- loneliness
- effect on partner and siblings
- professionals' lack of understanding of the all-encompassing ongoing issues
- uncertainty about the child's future.

Parents

Parenting a child with ASD is a complex task. While having a child with ASD affects the family unit, some families report that they are able to work through obstacles, look to the positive experiences and personal growth that often accompany having a child with special needs, and do not always view themselves as victims, but more like people who are able to cope and accept new challenges (Fleischmann, 2004). Yet the differences in how fathers and mothers react to the diagnosis (Schertz and Odom, 2007), availability of social support (Plant and Sanders, 2007), and the accessibility of services within a reasonable distance of the home (Symon, 2005) may impact the family's life.

Parents may be trained by professionals acting as coaches to deliver intervention to their children with ASD (a method referred to as parent-mediated/parent-implemented or PM/PI). Studies of PM/PI interventions historically have focused on the characteristics of the children with ASD rather than on the characteristics of the parents who are carrying out interventions (Wakeford and Odom, 2012). However, children with ASD may come into family units that already have issues such as parental depression (Olsson and Hwang, 2001) or one or both parents may have sub-threshold characteristics of ASD (Ingersoll and Hambrick, 2011). These factors directly related to parents may influence not only the family and the child with ASD but also the experience of professionals working with that family.

Siblings

I just don't like how autism affects the family. It just—it seems like it takes up too much time, and you usually get really bored of autism, because it's in your life all the time. (Sibling's comment; in MacNeil and Zucker, 2011)

The impact of ASD on siblings is not clear-cut. Brothers and sisters of a child with ASD may experience feelings of unfairness or be expected to assume roles of protecting and advocating for their sibling. They may exhibit less intimacy or feel neglected, then experience guilt for having these feelings. Their friends may not be able or even want to try to understand why the sibling acts in certain ways. Siblings, too, worry about what the future holds in store (Bagenholm and Gillberg, 2008; Dillenburger *et al.*, 2010; Kaminsky and Dewey, 2001; MacNeil and Zucker, 2011).

A report by Hastings (2004) notes that boys with siblings with ASD, and also siblings who are younger than their sibling with ASD, had more behavior and social issues than did the normative sample. While many additional variables and larger samples need further examination, it appears that siblings of children with ASD may have more hurdles to overcome than those whose siblings have other types of disabilities. This might be because children with ASD at first glance appear normal but act in ways that are difficult for the siblings to understand or explain.

While many family members describe concerns, others express the positive effects for siblings. Those who are brothers and sisters of children with ASD may exhibit increased sensitivity to individuals who are different, the development of a helping mentality, admiration for their sibling, and good psychosocial and emotional adjustment, especially when demographic risk factors are limited (Dillenburger *et al.*, 2010; Kaminsky and Dewey, 2001; Marks and Reeve, 2007).

Grandparents

> For me, the father of four children with four other grandchildren, seeking connection with (this grandchild with ASD) is a very poignant experience. To have a grandson, who can tune me out or simply ignore me like this, make no eye contact for long stretches of time, gives me a strange and painful feeling. (Grandfather of a boy with ASD; in MacNeil and Zucker, 2011)

The extended family of the child with ASD often experiences feelings of denial, anger, and grief as do those in the immediate family. For grandparents, there is often a deeper hurt and feeling of helplessness for their own child who is the parent and whose dreams and expectations for his or her child have been shattered (MacNeil and Zucker, 2011).

The world held different views of children with disabilities when grandparents were new parents. Therefore, grandparents and the extended family need to receive information about ASD. Today, many grandparents assume active roles as caregivers when their children return to work or need additional physical or emotional support. A social worker who is the grandmother of a child with ASD offers the following suggestions to fellow grandparents (in Joshi, 2009, pp. 292–293):

1. Support your adult children without suffocating them. It takes tremendous energy to raise a difficult child.

2. Give parents some time for themselves by taking care of your grandchildren whenever possible.

3. Ask them what would help them, don't assume.

4. Be realistic about time available for you and your capacities.

5. Advocate and educate people in your grandchildren's life.

6. Enjoy little triumphs and time together with grandchildren.

7. Be equally attentive to all of your grandchildren. They need your love and nurturing.

Professionals who work with children with ASD and their families

Young children with ASD come in contact with many professionals who are called upon to assess, consult, deliver, and evaluate services. Families may need to interface with physicians and other medical personnel, developmental or early intervention specialists, psychiatrists and psychologists, social workers, speech-language pathologists, occupational and physical therapists, music therapists, adaptive physical education specialists, and others who will become part of their world. Some work as part of interdisciplinary teams; others may not. Some will seek input from the family; others will not. Some are staunch in their beliefs that a specific treatment is the best and only approach; others may be quite eclectic in their programming or handling of the child's needs. However long and tedious the road to attaining best available services may become, having multiple perspectives and ultimately an interdisciplinary team of providers is in the best interest of the child and the family (Schertz, 2010). See Chapters 1 and 10 for additional information.

Family-centered practice

In the United States, Part C of the Individuals with Disabilities Education Act (IDEA) (2004) mandates that early intervention services for infants and toddlers with disabilities be family-centered. This term refers to a systematic partnership between families and professionals that treats them with dignity and respect, honors their choices and values, and provides supports that strengthen and enhance family functioning (Dunst, 2002). Including the family in all aspects of intervention planning and implementation is paramount and supported by evidence-based practice (Sandall et al., 2005).

The National Professional Developmental Center on ASD (2008) incorporated several guiding principles from the Division of Early Childhood (DEC) in its training materials for service providers working with children with ASD and their families. Central to these principles is the importance of family-centered practice that provides effective intervention and education via a collaborative interdisciplinary approach that honors diversity and is delivered within naturalistic and least restrictive environments (Sandall et al., 2005). This model of family-centered practice has implications for professionals working with children with ASD and their families. Service delivery for intervention should (a) be family-centered and strengths-based, (b) incorporate family priorities, and (c) support the parent-child relationship, and thus enable the family to promote the child's development (Schertz, 2010). Although family-centered practice is a recommended component of effective early intervention, the relationship between providing family-centered services and achieving positive outcomes for children is complex and often misunderstood, with some professionals still harboring misconceptions and lack of understanding of the true impact ASD has on families (Dempsey and Keen, 2008; Dillenburger et al., 2004). Numerous organizations, universities, and agencies offer information exchanges, resources, and specialized training about various aspects of ASD to educate both professionals and families to increase understanding of these issues and underlying factors.

Similarities and differences in perceptions

A study by Dillenburger and colleagues (2010) examined similarities and differences of parental and professional perceptions about specific categories of issues that impacted families of children with ASD. Parents and professionals agreed on the need for effective collaboration and communication. Both acknowledged that the child's behavior was an issue of great distress. Parents were more concerned with specific deficit areas associated with ASD such as interaction, play, social skills, and communication; professionals in general were more troubled about challenging or routine behaviors, hyperactivity, or other externalizing behaviors such as erratic sleep. While both professionals and parents espoused the need for better opportunities for inclusion, advocacy, and information dissemination, and a better flow of information about available services and financial planning for obtaining these, discrepancies were evident pertaining to perceptions of family needs. Some parents felt that professionals were not open-minded or knowledgeable about various treatment options, and did not always have enough training or expertise to base interventions on scientific methods that would best meet the specific needs of their child.

Family empowerment

GROUP EXPERIENCES IN A NATURAL ENVIRONMENT

Research indicates that when parents are given opportunities to come together for group experiences with their children, they are often grateful to have a place where their children can be accepted and they feel supported. When the experience mirrors or is part of a typical recreational or enrichment opportunity, families may feel a sense of relief and even empowerment (Allgood, 2005; Humpal, 2009).

FROM THE PARENTS' VIEWPOINT

According to the literature (Drouillard et al., 2011; Lawsane, 2011; Prizant, 2008), parents report they tend to be more trusting of empathetic, knowledgeable, approachable professionals who use simple, honest language when explaining things to them. Parents want to trust not only the professional's knowledge and judgment, but also him or her as a person. Parents would like written information, not only about ASD, but about community resources and sources of support. Overall, parents yearn for their children to be evaluated and treated as individuals and not part of a "one size fits all" approach.

Assuming a dual role: Music therapists as professionals and parents

Background

Due to the statistical prevalence of ASD in the general population, it is logical to assume that some human services professionals who work with children with ASD will be or have been personally touched by the disorder. Unfortunately, there is only scant research on this topic. However, personal reflections such as the following three parental statements shed light on how both professional and personal lives are affected:

> I am a special education teacher working with three-year-old children, all of who are on the autism spectrum…a great deal of my knowledge and expertise has developed as a result of living with a child with autism…helping our students is not separate from, but contingent upon, the well being of the family. (Nagy, 2009, pp. 308–309)

> …your life is changing dramatically, and you can either be broken by that, or it can take you in another direction. And where [my son] took me was he made me into a better man. And he's really taught me that the true meaning of life is to love and to give of yourself and to be compassionate and to serve others. And I've met a lot of very impressive people in my life, but no one's taught me that more than my son, and I will be forever grateful to him. (J. Mojica, an education official who has a son with autism; in MacNeil and Zucker, 2011)

> On a personal note, it cannot be stressed enough the importance of respecting the parents…we tend to remember the negative feedback for a long time and, as a result, it places an unnecessary strain on communication between parents and school staff, to the detriment of the child involved. (Simpson, 2002, p. 6)

The following accounts and anecdotal narratives from music therapists offer personal and professional reflections and insights on being a parent of a child with ASD. Four female music therapists from various regions within the United States were selected to answer 32 questions related to (a) working with children with ASD, (b) reflections and insight about their child with ASD, and (c) personal perspectives of being a professional and parent. Three of the music therapists have one child with ASD; another has two. Of the five children, four are boys and one is a girl. Two of the children are currently adolescents, and their stories reflect how times have changed in some ways for families and young children with ASD.

In addition to giving written responses, parents spoke or corresponded with the author to offer additional comments and clarify explanations. Their personal stories that follow represent a synopsis of information delivered in their own words. Though the current ages of the children range from preschool to young adulthood, their mothers' comments (italicized in the following narratives) reflect experiences from the children's early childhood years. Each music therapist and all children have been assigned pseudonyms in the interest of preserving their anonymity and respecting their privacy.

Mary—Music crosses the spectrum and is embedded in their world

Mary has been a music therapist for 14 years. She had worked with young children with ASD, though she had no formal training in specific ASD treatment methodology. As she reflects back on those years, she now realizes her approach was a mix of techniques used by the DIR®/Floortime™ Model as well as the Hanen Program®'s *More Than Words®* (a speech program specifically designed for parents of children on the autism spectrum that demonstrates how using their child's unique strengths and preferences during everyday routines and activities can build communication skills) (The Hanen Centre®, 2011). She often worked with occupational therapists and speech/language pathologists to help children with ASD better attain their goals and objectives by using music. Mary had opportunities to work directly with parents in the home setting and also in Individual Education Program (IEP) meetings with other specialized instructional support personnel in school districts.

When Mary's first son Mark was nine months old, she expressed concerns about his development to her pediatrician. *Things I was noting at the time: No response to name, appeared deaf at times, no babbling, and later no attempt to communicate with words or sounds, no gestures.* At two years, ten months, a psychologist finally diagnosed Mark. At that time, her second son David had been born. *I didn't have a strong reaction when Mark was first diagnosed (he was diagnosed when David was one month old). I felt relieved that someone was validating my concerns... I felt like it was something I could handle. Around his third birthday, I went full force into action mode to help him as he still didn't have any language and "early intervention" didn't seem to be helping him progress.*

David, on the other hand, seemed to blossom during the next few months. He was a happy, social child. However, Mary *noticed a marked difference around 21 months when he stopped using language he had previously used...the onset of repetitive behaviors and odd ways of looking at items from the corner of his eyes.* The same psychologist diagnosed David when he was one year, ten months old. *When David was diagnosed, I had more of a reaction as I knew so much more about autism. I was also devastated that I now had two children with autism and went through more of a grieving process. I wasn't shocked when he got the diagnosis, but it was painful to see him lose skills when he had initially appeared so much more normal in development than his older brother.*

Initially, I was not aware of many supports and it took some time of research on my part to become aware of community resources... ABA, the gold standard, was not easily available because of cost. I was told by the diagnosing psychologist that Mark needed many hours a week of ABA if we wanted him to have a chance at being mainstreamed in school and becoming independent later in life. Mary decided on a home ABA program, specifically using the techniques of Applied Verbal Behavior and also began the P.L.A.Y. project (Floortime® method), offered at no cost...and delivered as a parent-training model. *Through trial and error I found the right mix for each of the boys of Verbal Behavior-based ABA and Floortime®. When we began Floortime® with Mark, David [also] was thrown into Floortime® from an early age prior to diagnosis as we didn't think of it as "sessions," rather a way of interacting and playing throughout the day. David responded well and enjoyed that way of interacting. We added a program of Verbal Behavior/Applied Behavior Analysis for him at age two years, three months. Both methods are beneficial for different reasons and I think worked well together.*

Mary's sons are both musical in their own ways. Mark initially was *extremely sensitive to sounds and music. He could not stay in the house when I taught flute students as it bothered him greatly. We did not do a lot of music with him other than soft lullabies. During his preschool years he became much more interested in live music in our home and would often request us to play or sing his favorite songs. David was highly interested in music at a young age. He would often dance, clap, and respond rhythmically in other ways. He would show a curious response if the music stopped and would resume movement when music resumed.*

Music therapy was not directly recommended for Mark; however, he did receive group music therapy as a part of services offered to his toddler classroom. Around his fifth birthday, Mary realized that this *child who I thought hated music actually had perfect pitch. His extreme sensitivity to sounds actually was a gift. It took many years of occupational therapy (OT) and me learning how to help him regulate his senses to find this out. David was involved in music therapy groups prior to his diagnosis and has always thrived in a group MT environment. He received group music therapy as part of the early intervention program for children under three and also attended a small group facilitated by the music therapist, occupational therapists, and early intervention specialists.*

Mary continues to *seek out opportunities for them to participate in music. David attends a music therapy class at a local college and Mark takes keyboard lessons, performs in recitals, and composes his own music. The family also encourages music at home. Keyboard, music software, and instruments of every kind are easily accessible to them and they utilize these tools daily.*

Mary plans to eventually resume her music therapy career. Did her previous experience working with children on the autism spectrum help her be a more effective parent to her own children with ASD? *I think of it the other way around... I think my experience as a parent of two children with ASD will make me a much stronger music therapist. I have such a deeper understanding of autism and their needs that I didn't have prior, as well as a stronger understanding of treatment models and confidence in implementing methods myself.*

Anne—Experiences empower advocacy efforts

Anne has been a music therapist for 16 years and worked with children with ASD prior to starting her family. Her music therapy training was heavily behavioral in nature, and afforded her skills that were supportive of treatments being utilized by the families and teams with which she worked. She feels that she was well equipped to write solid goals and objectives. She worked with parents within the home setting, but often those parents were glad for her to just take over and give them a short respite. In retrospect, she wishes she had gathered more input from them as to what they wanted to see accomplished through music therapy.

Dean was the second child of Anne and her husband. Anne did not suspect autism. *He was cuddly. He did not respond to his name, though; I thought he was deaf. I contacted the county department of developmental disabilities and an early intervention specialist diagnosed him with speech delay at 18 months.* When Dean was not meeting developmental milestones by age three, his family sought an evaluation with a psychologist at a major metropolitan autism center. *When we heard the diagnosis of PDD-NOS, I was shocked, saddened, yet relieved; I was heartbroken and I was determined. I had been in denial.*

Unfortunately, the family was given no referrals for services. Anne credits her previous professional experiences with helping her know where to look for help. Dean initially was part of a cross-categorical integrated preschool program, but the curriculum was not intense enough to meet his needs. Then he received more intensive home-based ABA. On the advice of another parent, Anne observed a preschool that embraced Verbal Behavior ABA techniques.

She was impressed with the way the children were engaged and actually playing. *It looked like a music therapy session! The teacher was pulling the children out of their own worlds.* Here Dean thrived and Anne was pleased. *It took the pressure off me to do everything.* Furthermore, the staff and other professionals on the team respected her experience and her knowledge of ASD, and *the level of communication was fabulous.*

Music therapy was never recommended for Dean. In fact, he did not seem to respond well to music. "Stop singing!" he will still tell his mom. Unanticipated sounds startle him. However, he likes to listen to music on his Mp3 player. Anne says he loves structured movement which is often paired with music or dramatic play.

Yet social skills are foreign to Dean, and Anne says this is very exhausting since she herself is a very social person. *Everything has had to be taught to him, nothing is intuitive. And even though he has hyperlexia and reads far above his chronological age, he's in the middle of the continuum. There are TONS of kids like him, and it is so hard to find the right fit for them.* It has also been difficult for their other son at times; recently Anne heard him confide to a friend to explain his brother: "He has 'the autism'."

Anne is not working as a music therapist now, and devotes much time to advocating for her son. She has struggled with getting the school district to provide services and had to engage an attorney at one point. *I still almost cry every time I think about how the school district treated me.* She said that assessments have not always been thorough enough to accurately reflect Dean's abilities or his needs. Anne feels that her prior experiences as a music therapist definitely helped her parent a child with ASD. They *gave me a framework for understanding and a tool for working through the process and navigating the system, and the confidence to always be an advocate.*

Anne reflects that she has learned *not to underestimate [her son's] abilities on the surface. Go observe, keep an open mind about various treatment options, and don't assume you know everything, but also don't assume you know nothing.* She advises parents to educate themselves and get their child into an intensive, targeted program early. *I found my way, but it took two years.*

Shortly after taking part in this interview, Anne and her husband decided to build a new home. They thoroughly investigated school systems before selecting a new location. Anne reports that they have moved, are happily settled into the new community, and have been successful in obtaining the services they were seeking for Dean. Ultimately, Anne's advocacy efforts paid off.

Gina—Music is what emotions sound like

Unlike the other music therapists who took part in this interview process, Gina was not a music therapist when she learned that her son Nicholas was on the autism spectrum. She was, however, a talented musician and performer; music was infused into the family's life. Not until Nicholas was 11 did Gina begin studying music therapy. *I think my professional knowledge about ASD came later; I think my experience as a musician and performer contributed more at first. In a sense, I realized after the fact that certain things I had done with my son were in keeping with MT best practices, while others I wished I could have done over!*

Nicholas had just turned three and was in a new preschool class when his family noticed he was not participating fully or responding to certain people. He also had been exhibiting some self-stimulating behaviors. A local provider of spectrum services diagnosed Nicholas with PDD-NOS. Later he was designated as having multiple disabilities, but his speech/language, gross, and fine motor skills improved significantly and the label no longer seemed appropriate. Finally in eighth grade, the school requested and provided a formal assessment. Mild Asperger's was a diagnosis upon which both the school and the family could agree.

Throughout this process, one thing always was evident: Nicholas was extremely musical.

It was obvious that he was so bright…decoding letters and numbers very early, singing (including the interior parts of Mozart symphonies and spot-on memorization of jingles and songs with perfect pitch) by about 18 months.

We did not view our son as impaired or disabled; just learning-different, perhaps needing more time. We were offered early intervention in our home, which we accepted at first…early intervention is key; not only in working with the developing mind of a child, but also in helping children with learning differences to assimilate prior to the inevitable social demands that come up later on.

Unfortunately, we had a terrible experience early on with the head of preschool special education services for the public school district…she was very negative about his potential, which frightened and disappointed us… Looking for a place that would meet their son's needs but also wanting an environment that would recognize his talents and abilities, they eventually enrolled Nicholas in a parent-supported school that placed a high value on art and music and offered some alternative therapies and enrichment opportunities. It did not offer as many traditional early intervention supports as others may have, and ultimately this placement did not meet Nicholas's need in academic areas (e.g., his high level of reading and math skills).

A chance meeting with an energetic teacher on a playground led the family back to the public school arena where Nicholas found his niche at a school that combined grade levels and had small classes taught by co-teachers. All teachers had training in special education. The family and school developed a comprehensive *Individualized Education Plan*. Nicholas attended a typical combined grade class with an in-class aide and received pull-out services for gross and fine motor and speech/ language skill training. The family was very pleased with this school: *...we wanted to kick ourselves for not finding it sooner (especially when the special education teacher said at the first meeting, "I wish I'd had him two years ago...").*

Throughout his high school years, Nicholas struggled with social and test anxiety. However, his participation in orchestra and string quartet, and the tireless support of his music teachers and friends, offered him opportunities to shine.

Gina is now a hospice music therapist and continues to share music with her son. *My son has played violin since third grade, and now plays bass as well. We play, practice, and rehearse together all the time, go to concerts and favorite shows; we attend all his performances with orchestras and small ensembles; he has participated in many of our hospice events, and has "sat in" with my band on occasion... We never treated our child differently, but rather told him that his struggles are not unique; that there is a way through them into a rich and fulfilling life. We have told Nicholas that understanding this about himself will help him learn compassion, because everyone has difficult things to face. As he matures, he seems to take this more to heart.*

Gina offers this advice: *Start early with intervention; use a strengths-based approach while also addressing areas that need work; encourage participation in music and MT, not just if your child has a talent for it, but for all the social skills it teaches; find someone you can talk to about the difficult parts and challenges of parenting and decision making; read, research, and know your options; be a tireless advocate and trust your own instincts...remember, no one knows your child better than you do! Decisions can always be changed or adjusted...better to make a choice, move on, and monitor it than to become stuck. I think the greatest challenge for me personally has been to stay strong in the face of what may or may not be possible; to gain comfort with uncertainty. It seems that with ASD certain things do not change, no matter how much support is provided... There is a real risk of expecting too much...but also, and potentially more damaging, is the trap of low expectations.*

As a post-script to Nicholas's journey, Gina reports that he received two scholarships to a local community college where he now plays in the string ensemble and college community band. Gina sums up her experiences by recounting this vignette: *My husband and I had our last annual meeting with the special education representative, psychologist, music teacher, lead teacher, and speech teacher in attendance. The speech teacher mentioned a quote that [Nicholas] had shared with her, "Music is what emotions sound like." Everyone commented that it was a great quote...where did he find it and who said it? Nicholas said, "I said that." Everyone smiled. It occurred to me that despite the not-knowing and all the years of questions, we had somehow arrived at this wonderful shared moment, another gift that [Nicholas] has given us. How cool is that?*

Brit—Music therapy works and it's worth fighting for

Brit has been a music therapist for almost 30 years. Before her children were born, she worked with children with ASD, though at that time was not aware of specific treatment methodologies. She utilized more traditional behavioral methods *because they integrated well with music therapy interventions.* Brit conducted music therapy sessions in a hospital setting; parents were not allowed on the unit during therapy times.

The second girl to arrive in her family, Kayla was not diagnosed until she was three. Brit began to notice autistic tendencies when Kayla was around 18 months old. At her two-year check-up, Brit inquired if Kayla might have ASD. *The doctor told me, "No, she wouldn't be able to nurse if she had autism." He diagnosed a speech delay and we started a full-day program complete with various therapies at age two. But it took another year and a change to another doctor to get the actual diagnosis.* A pediatric neurologist told the family that Kayla, now age three, had autism.

I was heart-broken. I remember resenting hearing about all the things my friends' and co-workers' children were doing, when my daughter had so many delays. I felt sorry for myself, questioned God, and wondered why me, why us?

Kayla received excellent early intervention in a full-day special education program with occupational, physical, and speech therapies. A case manager made regular visits to the house. Thanks to a waiver program, funding was available for sensory integration and augmentative communication equipment and also covered music therapy services.

Brit recognized that as Kayla's needs and behaviors changed, her programs would require adjustments. *Our daughter received chiropractic care and trigger point acupuncture for a few years. She has been on various nutritional supplements for several years. Speech therapy with PECS and then augmentative communication devices using PECS has been a big part of her treatment throughout her life. Occupational therapy and sensory integration was very helpful when our daughter was three to five years old. We started one-to-one ABA when she was five years old for about six months and then we moved to a school that offered Discrete Trial Training in a small classroom setting. She has also received individual music therapy at various points in her life.* Brit was not always satisfied with the quality of services offered, however. *Especially in the public school system, we have had to advocate for the right services in all three districts in which we have lived since our daughter was diagnosed.*

There were definite challenges along the way. *We had to fight for ABA access, but lucky for us, another family had just won a lawsuit against the district for ABA and so it didn't take a long time to obtain ABA. We had to seek outside legal support and evaluations to obtain music therapy, increased speech therapy, measurable IEP goals, and improved behavioral plans.* The family had to be proactive and search for expert professional help. They are grateful for *legal advice from a special education attorney, and private evaluations by a neuropsychologist, speech therapist, and an educational consultant.*

The school district never had provided music therapy, but Brit knew Kayla responded well to music. The family sought a music therapy evaluation, but the school officials claimed *the only reason we wanted music therapy for our daughter was so we could give our music therapy friends work at the school.* Those who directly participated on

Kayla's educational team had been very aware and respectful of Joan's professional expertise, and *once the music therapist started working with [them], the team started verbalizing the value of the service for our daughter.*

Now music therapy is on Kayla's IEP as a consultative service and she also receives music therapy privately. Brit today uses her music therapy skills in a position advocating for the recognition of the benefits of music therapy and the music therapy profession.

Brit offers these pieces of advice: *Although it's great to provide music in the home to assist your child with their skill development, it is important to seek outside support and treatment. Just as it never works well to be your child's piano teacher, you need someone else to be your child's music therapist.* She has learned from Kayla *that routines are comforting; organization can make your life simpler; rushing through life causes stress; rhythmic repetition is fun; we all have some autistic tendencies; maybe the rest of us have the skewed view of the world.*

She also reflects and looks to the future: *I can't imagine our daughter being "typical." Everyone that works with her loves her and the community-at-large is doing better with accepting her for who she is right now. I feel that as she gets older, there is an acceptance that we need to focus less on changing her behaviors and we need to focus more on shaping her environment to help her be successful. Reminds me of music therapy!*

Conclusion

The stories, like the people relaying them, are unique. However, there are similarities that come to the foreground of each family's experiences. All reported that they recognized indicators that sent up warning signs early on: inability to interact, no or limited speech, lack of eye contact, lack of response, or strange behaviors. Most of the children are highly musical and the parents include aspects of music in the routines and experiences provided for their children (e.g., singing, playing, listening, and moving to music). All music therapists felt that they were respected as professionals, but reported some dissatisfaction with the people and facilities that were available to serve the needs of their children with ASD. Citing an abundance of service providers that seemed to lack compassion and even expertise, plus cost issues and difficulty in finding appropriate providers, the four music therapists reported frustration with the system. They learned to become strong advocates for their children, and rated this quality as essential.

The reflections from the four music therapists mirror many of the same concerns and frustrations of all parents of children with ASD. Much useful and insightful information can be gained by examining reflections from parents, professionals, and professionals who also are parents of children with ASD. This awareness perhaps may shape the thoughts, words, and actions of those who work with families, molding them into more attuned and thereby more effective helping professionals.

> ## Learning questions
>
> 1. Name five aspects of having a child with ASD that are often sources of stress to parents.
>
> 2. How might siblings react to having a brother or sister with ASD?
>
> 3. What is family-centered practice and how does it apply to working with children with ASD?
>
> 4. Give five examples of what parents like to see in professionals who deal with their children with ASD.
>
> 5. What unique issues might professionals who are also parents of children with ASD face?
>
> 6. What are specific ways music therapists may utilize music with their children with ASD in their own home settings?
>
> 7. How might insights from music therapists who are parents of children with ASD inform your future practice?

Author's note

The author wishes to thank the music therapists who graciously shared their families' life stories, Linn Wakeford for her helpful review, and Petra Kern for the inspiration for this topic.

References

Allgood, N. (2005). Parents' perception of family-based group music therapy for children with autism spectrum disorders. *Music Therapy Perspectives, 23(2)*, 92–99.

Bagenholm, A., and Gillberg, C. (2008). Psychosocial effects on siblings of children with autism and mental retardation: A population-based study. *Journal of Intellectual Disability Research, 35*, 291–307.

Dempsey, I., and Keen, D. (2008). A review of processes and outcomes in family-centered services for children with a disability. *Topics in Early Childhood Special Education, 28(1)*, 42–52.

Dillenburger, K., Keenan, M., Doherty, A., Byrne, T., and Gallagher, S. (2010). Living with children diagnosed with autism spectrum disorder: Parental and professional views. *British Journal of Special Education, 37(1)*, 13–23.

Dillenburger, K., Keenan, M., Gallagher, S., and McElhinney, M. (2004). Parent education and home-based behaviour analytic intervention: An examination of parents' perceptions of outcome. *Journal of Intellectual and Developmental Disability, 29*, 119–130.

Drouillard, B., Gragg, M., Miceli, R., Mullins, A., Beneteau, A., and Tiede, A. (2011). Parents' advice for professionals working with autism spectrum disorders and their families. Presentation at the 2011 IMFAR Conference, San Diego, CA. Retrieved from http://imfar.confex.com/imfar/2011/webprogram/Paper7988.html.

Dunst, C. (2002). Family-centered practices: Birth through high school. *Journal of Special Education, 36(3)*, 139–147.

Estes, A., Munson, J., Dawson, G., Koehler, E., Zhou, X., and Abbott, R. (2009). Parenting stress and psychological functioning among mothers of preschool children with autism and developmental delay. *Autism: The International Journal of Research and Practice, 13(4)*, 375–387.

Fleischmann, A. (2004). Narratives published on the Internet by parents of children with autism: What do they reveal and why is it important? *Focus on Autism and Other Developmental Disabilities, 19(1)*, 35–43.

Hastings, R. (2004). Brief report: Behavioral adjustment of siblings of children with autism. *Journal of Autism and Developmental Disorders, 33*, 99–104.

Hastings, R.P., Kovshoff, H., Ward, N.J., degli Espinosa, F., Brown, T., and Remington, B. (2005). Systems analysis of stress and positive perceptions in mothers and fathers of pre-school children with autism. *Journal of Autism and Developmental Disorders, 35*, 635–644.

Humpal, M. (2009). A community music program for parents and children with and without special needs. In J. Kerchner and C. Abril (Eds.) *Musical Experience in Our Lives*. Lanham, MD: Rowman and Littlefield Education.

Ingersoll, B., and Hambrick, D. (2011). The relationship between the broader autism phenotype, child severity, and stress and depression in parents of children with autism spectrum disorders. *Research in Autism Spectrum Disorders, 5*, 337–344.

Joshi, S. (2009). Grandparents: The role they play. In S. Joshi, B. McLaughlin, and C. Riggi (Eds.) *Courage, Heart and Wisdom: Essays on Autism*. Denver, CO: Outskirts Press.

Kaminsky, L., and Dewey, D. (2001). Siblings relationships of children with autism. *Journal of Autism and Developmental Disorders, 31(4)*, 399–410.

Lawsane, J. (2011). Parent reflections on raising a child who has an ASD. *Autism Spectrum Disorders Network News, 2*, 1.

MacNeil, R., and Zucker, C. (2011). Autism now series. *PBS NewsHour*. Retrieved from www.pbs.org/newshour/news/autism.

Marks, R., and Reeve, R. (2007). The adjustment of non-disabled siblings of children with autism. *Journal of Autism and Developmental Disorders, 37*, 1060–1067.

Nagy, K. (2009). From one gift came many more. In S. Joshi, B. McLaughlin, and C. Riggi (Eds.) *Courage, Heart and Wisdom: Essays on Autism*. Denver, CO: Outskirts Press.

National Professional Developmental Center on ASD (2008). Foundations of autism spectrum disorders: An online course. Session 4: Guiding principles. In *Foundations of Autism Spectrum Disorders: An Online Course*. Chapel Hill, NC: FPG Child Development Institute, The University of North Carolina.

Olsson, M., and Hwang, C. (2001). Depression in mothers and fathers of children with intellectual disability. *Journal of Intellectual Disability Research, 45(6)*, 535–543.

Plant, K., and Sanders, M. (2007). Predictors of caregiver stress in families of preschool-aged children with developmental disabilities. *Journal of Intellectual Disability Research, 51*, 109–124.

Prizant, B.M. (2008). Parent–professional relationships: It's a matter of trust. *Autism Quarterly, Fall*, 34–37.

Rudy, L. (2010). Why is autism stressful for parents? *About.com Guide*, June 22, 2010. Retrieved from http://autism.about.com/b/2010/06/22/why-is-autism-stressful-for-parents.htm.

Sandall, S., Hemmeter, M.L., Smith, B., and McLean, M.E. (Eds.) (2005). *DEC Recommended Practices: A Comprehensive Guide for Practical Application in Early Intervention/Early Childhood Special Education*. Longmont, CO: Sopris West.

Schertz, H. (2010). Principles of intervention for young children: Implications for toddlers and pre-schoolers with autism spectrum disorders. In H. Schertz, C. Wong, and S. Odom (Eds.) *Young Exceptional Children Monograph Series 12*. Missoula, MT: DEC.

Schertz, H., and Odom, S. (2007). Promoting joint attention in toddlers with autism: A parent-mediated developmental model. *Journal of Autism and Developmental Disorders, 37,* 1562–1575.

Simpson, J. (2002). Increasing access to music therapy: The roles of parents, music therapists, and AMTA. In B. Wilson (Ed.) *Models of Music Therapy Interventions in School Settings.* Silver Spring, MD: The American Music Therapy Association.

Symon, J. (2005). Expanding interventions for children with autism: Parents as trainers. *Journal of Positive Behavioral Interventions, 7,* 159–173.

The Hanen Centre® (2011). About Hanen®. Retrieved from www.hanen.org/About-Hanen.aspx.

Wakeford, L., and Odom, S. (2012). Describing parents in intervention studies: Literature review and implications. Manuscript in preparation.

PART 5

Selected Resources

Chapter 15

Resources Within Reach

Information at Your Fingertips

Petra Kern, Ph.D., MT-DMtG, MT-BC, MTA
MUSIC THERAPY CONSULTING
SANTA BARBARA, CA

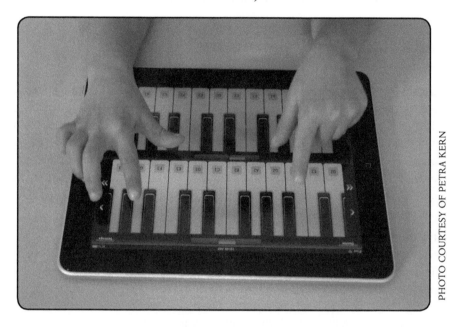

*Using high-quality online resources in our practices
and services for young children with autism spectrum
disorders and their families keeps us up-to-date.
(Petra Kern)*

Responding to the increased incidence of autism spectrum disorders (ASD), multiple organizations, institutes, companies, and individuals have developed informational resources and products for children with ASD, their parents, practitioners, researchers, policy makers, and others. However, the vast amount of information about ASD on the Internet can make it difficult to identify pertinent information. The purpose of this chapter is to present a selection of high-quality online resources related to ASD for use in professional development and clinical practice in music therapy, including informational websites, briefs, podcasts, blogs, and applications (apps). How to stay informed in this fast-paced world of technology, be aware of future implications of online resources, and applications in music therapy practice are also addressed.

Professional development sites
Websites
National Professional Development Center on Autism Spectrum Disorders
http://autismpdc.fpg.unc.edu
> This multi-university center supports the use of evidence-based practice for children and adolescents with ASD by providing free (a) information on evidence-based practices (e.g., briefs), (b) 37 Internet training modules for professional development providers and practitioners (additional modules are in preparation), (c) eight *Foundation of ASD* online course sessions, (d) conference presentation materials, and (e) links to partners, model sites, and related resources.

National Autism Center
www.nationalautismcenter.org
> This nonprofit organization is dedicated to providing leadership and evidence-based resources about ASD to families, practitioners, and communities. The center includes (a) an ASD clinic (offering diagnostic assessment services, a social development program, and parent support), (b) an onsite learning facility and distance learning lab (targeting parents and practitioners), (c) an online research center (presenting collaborative research projects, research findings, and dissemination events), and (d) an online library (offering Questions and Answers, the *National Standards Report*, resource articles and guides, and links).

Learn the Signs. Act Early.
www.cdc.gov/ncbddd/actearly/index.html
> This website of a public awareness campaign launched by the Centers for Disease Control and Prevention (CDC), National Center on Birth Defects and Developmental Disabilities (NCBDD), and other collaborators aims to educate parents about key developmental milestones (for children between the ages of three months and five years), early signs of ASD and other developmental disorders, screening, and early interventions. Free products for families, early childhood educators, and healthcare providers include an interactive milestone chart and checklist, a video on developmental milestones, talking tips for parents, fact sheets on screening and

developmental disabilities, as well as complete resource kits for different stakeholders. Some of the materials are available in multiple languages.

First Signs®: ASD Video Glossary
www.firstsigns.org/asd_video_glossary/asdvg_about.htm

This web-based tool was created by Amy M. Wetherby, PhD, Director of the Florida State University FIRST WORDS® Project, and Nancy D. Wiseman, Founder and President of First Signs®. It contains numerous video clips demonstrating typical and delayed development in young children and points out red flags and diagnostic features of ASD. The video materials are free of charge to parents and professionals. In addition to information about the nonprofit organization, the general First Signs® website discusses early signs of developmental delays, screening, diagnosis, and treatment (including music therapy). Selected articles, books, videos, and related links are available at this website, too.

MusicWorksPublications.com: Autism Workbooks and Toolbox
http://musicworkspublications.com/courses/autism

Created for beginning music therapists by MusicWorksPublications.com, these self-study courses address basic information about ASD, music therapy settings and service delivery models, and common strategies applied to music therapy demonstrated by examples. Each of the three courses comes with a workbook in pdf format and audio files discussing the content for each chapter.

Online briefs and fact sheets

Evidence-Based Practice Briefs
http://autismpdc.fpg.unc.edu/content/briefs

The National Professional Development Center on Autism Spectrum Disorders has created briefs for 24 identified evidence-based practices for children and adolescents with ASD. Brief components, which can be downloaded for each practice, include (a) a general description of the practice, (b) a list of references supporting the effectiveness, (c) step-by-step directions for implementation, (d) an implementation checklist for intervention fidelity, and (e) supplementary materials (e.g., data collection sheets) for some of the identified practices.

Facts About Autism
www.nationalautismcenter.org/pdf/nac_facts_about_autism.pdf

Facts About Autism is a two-page fact sheet updated by the National Autism Center in 2012, which includes information about the symptoms, prevalence, diagnosis, causes, and recommended treatments of ASD.

Autism Spectrum Disorders
www.nichcy.org/InformationResources/Documents/NICHCY%20PUBS/fs1.pdf

The National Dissemination Center for Children with Disabilities (NICHCY) offers a six-page ASD fact sheet, which is available in English and Spanish. This 2010 publication includes a case scenario, general information about ASD and the changing diagnostic criteria within the forthcoming *DSM-V,* as well as information on educational aspects and tips for parents and teachers.

Information Kit
www.cdc.gov/ncbddd/actearly/downloads.html
> This set of fact sheets and flyers is part of the CDC *Learn the Signs. Act Early* campaign. It includes information on developmental milestones, developmental screening tools, and condition-specific items (e.g., Asperger syndrome, attention-deficit/hyperactivity disorder, ASD, cerebral palsy, intellectual disabilities, vision loss, and hearing loss). All PDFs include English and Spanish versions as well as translation into other languages.

Podcasts and blogs

Podcasts on CDC: Autism Awareness
www2c.cdc.gov/podcasts/browse.asp
> CDC offers several podcasts related to ASD topics that can be downloaded for free.

National Institute of Mental Health (NIMH): Video and Audio about Autism
www.nimh.nih.gov/media/index-autism.shtml
> NIMH provides video/audio documentation of interviews with experts in the field.

Kennedy Krieger Institute: Focus on Autism
www.podcastdirectory.com/podcasts/archive.php?iid=9457
> *Focus on Autism* is an audio podcast series featuring scientists of the Kennedy Krieger Institute who speak about the latest research and developments in the field of ASD.

AutismPodcast: Your Audio Connection to Autism
www.autismpodcast.org
> Via interviews conducted by a father of a boy with ASD, these podcast episodes feature individuals, parents, and experts who make special contributions to the field of ASD.

University of California TV: Podcasts on Autism
www.uctv.tv/search-moreresults.aspx?catSubID=68&podcasts=yes
> Sponsored by the UC Davis M.I.N.D. Institute, University of California Television releases video podcasts of lectures on a broad range of ASD topics.

Nurse Practitioner Schools: Top 50 Autism Research Blogs
http://nursepractitionerschools.org/top-50-autism-support-and-research-blogs
> This website provides an annotated list of 50 support and research blogs about children with ASD, families, and friends.

Autism Speaks Official Blog: It's Time to Learn
www.autismspeaks.org/blog
> This organizational blog presents a variety of updated information on topics such as awareness, fundraising, science, meetings, and events related to ASD.

MT Research Blog: Bringing Current Research to Music Therapy Clinicians
www.musictherapyresearchblog.com/?cat=4
> This blog, hosted by two certified music therapists, summarizes research articles on selected topics such as ASD and/or music therapy.

FAQs: Autism.com: A Resource for Practical Ideas
http://faqautism.com

These short blog posts (also available as five-minute audio podcasts) by a certified music therapist speak to daily life situations that individuals with ASD, their families, and practitioners may face, providing practical tips and creative solutions (musical and non-musical) for addressing these issues.

Tools for clinical application
Websites

AutismShop.com™
www.autismshop.com

Hosted by the Autism Resource Network, this online shop carries numerous books (including a children's section), software, CDs and DVDs, games, toys, small instruments, visual and sensory items, jewelry, gifts, and cards related to ASD.

Do2Learn: Supporting Special Needs
www.do2learn.com

This website offers a variety of educational books, customized picture cards and schedules (available in six languages), and learning software for children with disabilities, including ASD. Free online learning games, activities for skill development, songs, and a sounds-sing-along, as well as a teacher toolbox with classroom management ideas, learning strategies, worksheets, and monitoring forms, are available.

Different Roads to Learning: Your Complete ABA and VB Resource
www.difflearn.com

This website provides a wide variety of Applied Behavior Analysis (ABA) products such as books, DVDs, software, flashcards, visual supports, assessment kits, staff training tools, timers, counters, scheduling tools, picture communication, token boards, games, toys, and academic materials. One section is dedicated specifically to early intervention/special education and ASD.

Tuned Into Learning™: Music for Special Education
www.tunedintolearning.com/store.html

Designed by an autism specialist and music therapist, this comprehensive music-assisted learning curriculum targets specific goal areas for children and teens with ASD, developmental disabilities, and neurological disorders. Each of the nine volumes includes (a) a booklet with color visuals, lesson plans, learning objectives, adaptations, and instructor guides, (b) a music CD with original songs, and (c) a CD-ROM with songs, data sheets, flash cards, and worksheets. The website also provides free tip sheets and research bibliographies for download.

Autism Technology
http://sites.google.com/site/autismtechnology

This website provides best-practice recommendations for technology use with individuals with ASD and suggests latest technology-based tools (such as apps, robots, videos, computer games, and virtual reality) to support (a) social and affective skills, (b) language development, and (c) motor, sensory, and behavioral skills. This comprehensive online source also provides hyperlinks to related websites, an annotated list of apps for autism (see https://autismapps.wikispaces.com/), research-based publications, and innovative technology initiatives.

Apps for Children with Special Needs
http://a4cwsn.com

This website demonstrates from a user perspective how selected special education apps work. Video demonstrations feature skill improvements in children with special needs (including ASD).

Apps for iPhone, iPod, and iPad
(*indicates that a free version is currently available)

AUTISM SPECTRUM DISORDERS (AGES 0–5)

*Model Me Going Places™
http://itunes.apple.com/us/app/model-me-going-places/id347813439?mt=8

This series of social skills training apps are designed to familiarize children with ASD with locations in the community (e.g., hairdresser, mall, doctor, playground, grocery store, and restaurant). Children learn by observing peer models demonstrating appropriate behaviors via photo series that include audio/text narrations and background music.

Eye Contact—Toybox
http://itunes.apple.com/us/app/eye-contact-toybox/id358972670?mt=8

Some cultures value eye contact as an important part of communication. This app (and additional apps from FizzBrain) allows children with ASD to practice eye contact by identifying numbers appearing in a person's eyes. Children earn stars for correct answers; these can be used for instance to select toys in a virtual playroom.

*TapToTalk™
http://itunes.apple.com/us/app/taptotalk/id367083194?mt=8

This Augmentative and Alternative Communication (AAC) device allows children with ASD to select from albums with different topics and corresponding pictures that have text labels (e.g., the album "hungry" includes pictures of a snack, fruit, vegetable, bowl, and a meal—each leading to another series of pictures). When the child taps the picture, a recorded voice gives the response. The library offers over 2500 pictures (including musical instruments) and allows individual picture and text uploads as well as voice recordings in any language.

iSpeech Toddler Sign Language
http://itunes.apple.com/us/app/ispeech-toddler-sign-language/id324321945?mt=8

Two computer-animated children model about 60 basic language signs that may be useful for toddlers, parents, and practitioners to communicate with each other. Each sign is labeled with a vocal output and described in a text box.

Stories2Learn
http://itunes.apple.com/us/app/stories2learn/id348576875?mt=8
> This app allows parents and practitioners to access pre-written social stories or create a personalized story for social learning (e.g., turn-taking). Photos, text, and audio messages can be uploaded and are displayed in an electronic book format. This app can also be used to create a visual schedule that guides children with ASD through the day or an activity (e.g., a music therapy session).

*See.Touch.Learn™
http://itunes.apple.com/us/app/see-touch-learn/id406826506?mt=8&ls=
> This picture learning system (with six free exercises) helps children with ASD learn new words and concepts by choosing pictures that match the question posted as text or vocal output. Correct answers are acknowledged with a specific sound cue; cheering people applaud if the lesson is successfully completed.

*AutismXpress
http://itunes.apple.com/us/app/autismxpress/id343549779?mt=8
> This app helps children with ASD learn about facial expressions that represent emotions such as happy, sad, and angry. When one of the 12 comic-like picture icons is touched, an animated facial expression with a distinguished color, sound, and text appears.

*AutismApps
http://itunes.apple.com/us/app/autism-apps/id441600681?mt=8&ign-mpt=uo%253D4
> This comprehensive list of apps for individuals with ASD and other special needs allows users to search for topic-specific apps within 30 categories (e.g., ABA, Behavior and Social Skills, and Music). Links to video demonstrations and reviews of apps as well as a "new apps" category are featured.

SPECIAL EDUCATION TOOLS
Autism News Reader
http://itunes.apple.com/us/app/autism-news-reader/id319164790?mt=8
> This app can access the latest news and reports about ASD.

*IEP Check List
http://itunes.apple.com/us/app/iep-checklist/id348702423?mt=8
> This app is a checklist for parents and professionals for developing a child's Individualized Education Plan (IEP). Items on the checklist include a list of team members; current performance; annual goals; services, supports, and aids; special factors; student placement; state and district assessments; and a transition plan among others. Besides writing notes, the user can record IEP meetings, make voice notes, prioritize items, and email the checklist to others.

Behavior Tracker Pro and Skill Tracker Pro
www.behaviortrackerpro.com/products/stp/STP-for-iPhone.aspx
> Both apps are designed to track data related to behaviors of children with ASD for comprehensive Applied Behavior Analysis (ABA)-based treatment plans.

Configuration options include tracking of individual skills and targets, number of probes, corrected responses on consecutive days, and retention checks. Member profiles, document management, video capturing, and data charting by frequency, duration, or rate are available as well.

Super Duper® Data Tracker
http://itunes.apple.com/us/app/super-duper-data-tracker/id432397161?mt=8
This app allows documenting clients' progress during sessions by tracking data (i.e., tally, correct, incorrect, approximated, and cued) on individual goals during both individual and group sessions. Session notes and graphed data can be added and emailed to parent and interdisciplinary team members.

iRewardChart
http://itunes.apple.com/us/app/irewardchart-parents-reward/id341306389?mt=8
Children can earn stars for accomplishing tasks or an award certificate for special recognition that can be printed or sent to social network pages. The app offers rewards from a default list, but also allows setting up specific rewards for each child (e.g., playing the drums).

MUSICAL INSTRUMENTS

*Virtuoso Piano Free 2 HD
http://itunes.apple.com/us/app/virtuoso-piano-free–2-hd/id304075989?mt=8
This app features a six-octave concert grand piano, which allows playing color-labeled keys (with glow touch) individually or as chords with up to five fingers. The keyboard also can be split into mirror images so that two people can play it.

PocketGuitar
http://itunes.apple.com/app/pocketguitar/id287965124?mt=8
Pressing and strumming strings like any other guitar can activate this virtual guitar. The app allows switching to an electric bass or ukulele and offers a variety of sound effects such as distortion, chorus, and reverb.

iBone
http://itunes.apple.com/us/app/ibone-the-pocket-trombone/id306629300?mt=8#
This virtual trombone responds to touch and breath for producing sounds through the iPhone or iPad. Slurring up and down with the finger will change the notes; raising and lowering the bell changes the pitch. Users can play along with six songs that come with this app.

Pocket Drums
http://itunes.apple.com/us/app/pocket-drums/id301294780?mt=8Drummer
This six-piece drum kit has four different drum layouts and offers 24 styles (i.e., Birch, Classic, Country, Delay, Electronic, Funk, Fusion, Garage, Indian, Japan Vintage, Jazz, Latin, Marching, Melodic, Natural, Pop, Punk, Reverb, Rock, Tribal, Vintage, Weird, Wood, and World). Users can utilize its additional features such as a metronome or multi-track recording capability, improvise to its drum loops, and experiment with pitch control.

Hand Drums

http://itunes.apple.com/us/app/hand-drums/id380564151?mt=8

This app features 19 hand drums (e.g., bongos, djembe, cajon) with over 50 beats and loops as well as accompaniment options from its own library or from a personal iPod. Multi-track recording, pitch control, a metronome, and drum rolls also are available.

*Voice Changer Plus

http://itunes.apple.com/us/app/voice-changer-plus/id339440515?mt=8

This app allows users to record their own voices and transform them into over 40 different sounds (e.g., echo, reverse, haunting, choir, whisper, or crowed).

*Pocket Shaker

http://itunes.apple.com/app/pocket-shaker/id313139592?mt=8

Shaking the iPhone, iPod, and iPad or tapping the screen activates the sound of percussion instruments such as a cabasas, castanets, cowbells, shakers, rattles, or gongs.

Air Harp

http://itunes.apple.com/us/app/air-harp/id364524199?mt=8

By tapping one or multiple strings this virtual harp allows users to create their own music (in G Major on 15 strings) or choose from over ten free songs available in an easy-to-read sheet music system displayed under the strings.

*Amazing Xylophone

http://itunes.apple.com/us/app/awesome-xylophone/id423063965?mt=8

This is a virtual xylophone with colored keys. Users can play single and two notes on a chromatic scale. One or two bars can be activated by tapping them with the animated xylophone mallets.

iMaracas

http://itunes.apple.com/us/app/imaracas/id287861647?mt=8

A pair of colorful maracas appears on the screen. Shaking the iPhone, iPod, or iPad activates the sound.

*Kalimba Free

http://itunes.apple.com/us/app/kalimba-free/id300802995?mt=8

This digital kalimba (or African Thumb Piano) has seven prongs, which can be tapped one or more at a time. Melodies can be created in the key of C and G Major.

Ocarina

http://itunes.apple.com/app/ocarina/id293053479?mt=8

This app is sensitive to breath, touch, and movement. It creates sounds when the user blows into the microphone of the iPhone or iPad and changes notes when the holes are covered. It does play vibrato when the device is tilted. Key and mode changes, as well as access to a social network of ocarina players worldwide, are also available.

*Kazoo

http://itunes.apple.com/us/app/kazoo/id287655381?mt=8

By tapping on letters next to a picture of a kazoo, the player can make kazoo-like sounds.

*Baby Scratch
http://itunes.apple.com/us/app/baby-scratch/id338290357?mt=8

This virtual DJ turntable allows production of scratching music from the "Baby Scratch Library" or the recording of children's voices and subsequent scratching by moving a finger over the LP.

*Soundrop
http://itunes.apple.com/us/app/soundrop/id364871590?mt=8#

By drawing lines on the screen, users can manipulate the sound of dropping dots and thereby create unique music.

*Beatwave
http://itunes.apple.com/us/app/beatwave/id363718254?mt=8#

Beatwave creates beats and unique tunes by setting dots on a squared screen. Colorful stripes moving over the dots activate the sounds and create waves.

Bloom
http://itunes.apple.com/WebObjects/MZStore.woa/wa/viewSoftware?id=29279
2586&mt=8&ign-mpt=uo%3D4#

This app functions as an instrument, composition tool, and artwork. By tapping the screen, users can create unique melodies with 12 different moods that idle and are accompanied by visualizations. Shaking the device will clear all previous music.

MadPad HD
http://itunes.apple.com/us/app/madpad-remix-your-life/id456072329?mt=8

This app allows capturing environmental sounds (e.g., car, kitchen tools, nature) and turning them into soundboard sets that can be activated by rhythmically tapping.

Moozart
http://itunes.apple.com/us/app/moozart/id405194870?mt=8

This app allows children to compose and save their own songs by dragging sound-making farm animal icons onto music stave. Children can also follow along with preloaded songs and manipulate the tune by interspersing animal sounds.

Tappy Tunes™
http://itunes.apple.com/us/app/tappytunes/id299495181?mt=8

By tapping the screen in time and rhythm, the player activates a selected song (notes and chords are preloaded in sequence) accompanied by colorful animated graphics.

MUSIC TOOL KIT FOR MUSIC THERAPISTS

*Metronome
http://itunes.apple.com/us/app/metronome/id287965434?mt=8

This virtual metronome marks 2/4, 3/4, or 4/4 time signatures by giving a regular tick sound at a selected rate from 1 to 210 beats per minute.

*Guitar Tuner
http://itunes.apple.com/us/app/guitar-tuner/id310457191?mt=8#

This electronic guitar tuner plays single notes or all six strings in a row in standard tuning (E A D G B e) and allows selecting alternative tunings (e.g., Drop D, Open C).

ClearRecord
http://itunes.apple.com/us/app/clearrecord-premium-noise/id395704227?mt=8

This voice recorder suppresses ambient noise during recording and allows controlling playback speed without modifying pitch. It also features efficient storage of recordings.

*SoundHound
http://itunes.apple.com/us/app/soundhound/id355554941?mt=8

By singing, humming, or playing ten seconds of a piece of music into the iPhone or iPad's microphone, this app searches for close matches and offers different interpretations available in iTunes. Alternatively, one can say the title of a song or artist name to receive matching results.

*SingFit
http://itunes.apple.com/us/app/singfit/id442827581?mt=8

Developed by a music therapist, this app supports users in singing along and recording songs by providing lyrics and melody guides while singing. The app also permits changing keys and sharing recordings via email, Facebook, and Twitter. Users can subscribe to the SingFit catalogue to download songs (categorized by genre, age, and level of difficulty), or make use of free sample songs.

Songwriters Pad™
http://itunes.apple.com/us/app/songwriters-pad/id380151611?mt=8

This songwriter tool will assist with organizing sections of a song (i.e., verse, chorus, bridge), find creative expressions for song lyrics (including a rhyme dictionary), record melody lines, and export the song in written or audio form.

*Virtual Sheet Music
http://itunes.apple.com/us/app/virtual-sheet-music/id322312746?mt=8

This app allows downloading classical sheet music from a virtual library with over 50 free items. The music sheet can be played from the iPad screen or printed on paper. MP3 files connected to the sheet music allow listening to the musical piece.

*Slow Down Music Player
http://itunes.apple.com/us/app/slow-down-music-player/id314296369?mt=8

This app allows slowing down the music of one's own song library without changing the pitch.

OnSong for iOS
http://itunes.apple.com/us/app/onsong-for-ios/id364493059?mt=8#

This app allows importing and storing song sheets, transposing and highlighting chords in any key, reading it on a scroll screen, listening to song recordings, and exporting or sending via different media.

*TuneWiki
http://itunes.apple.com/us/app/tunewiki-lyrics-radio/id320088832?mt=8

This app accesses one's song lists on the iPhone, iPod, or iPad, and provides the lyrics in a subtitle (which can be translated in more than 40 languages), related Internet radio stations, and music video. The TuneWiki Community feature allows searching for song lyrics by artist, title, or phrases, exploring new music from around the world, and presenting the TuneWiki users' 50 top songs.

Additional information, resources, products, and supports for ASD can be found on organizational and networking websites. A selection of prominent ASD organizations and networks are listed in Table 15.1. Most of these organizations have annual conferences, which bring together experts who provide first-hand information about the latest developments in the field.

Table 15.1 Selected examples of organizations and networks for ASD	
Organizations	Networks

• Autism Speaks
  www.autismspeaks.org
• Autism Society of America
  www.autism-society.org
• Autism Europe
  www.autismeurope.org
• International Society of Autism Research
  www.autism-insar.org
• Organization for Autism Research
  www.researchautism.org
	• Autism Network International
	  www.autreat.com
	• Autism Consortium
	  www.autismconsortium.org
	• Interactive Autism Network (IAN)
	  www.ianproject.org

Staying informed

Although the information presented in this chapter is current and accurate at the time of publication, it may become outdated, updated, or available in different formats in the near future. The constant expansion of information on ASD, and on related interventions and tools for children with ASD, requires continuous investigation to provide relevant effective services, be accountable, maintain credibility, and receive funding. Therefore, it is crucial for parents and practitioners to understand how to locate, appraise, apply, and evaluate new online resources. Figure 15.1 outlines five basic steps for identifying and applying high-quality online resources.

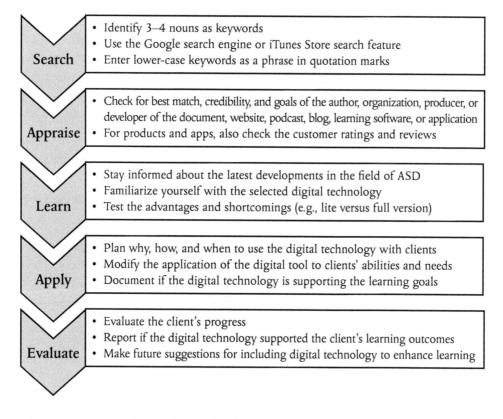

Figure 15.1: Five steps for identifying and applying high-quality online resources

Future implications

Dissemination of information on ASD is shifting from printed to online materials (e.g., websites, online journals, podcasts, blogs), and online learning has become prevalent in many professional fields serving individuals with ASD. Additionally, a growing number of instructional technology applications are currently being customized to the needs of children with ASD. These hold great promise for enhancing specific skill sets. Virtual learning environments, social networking tools, and digital devices such as the iPhone, iPod, and iPad have created new learning opportunities, allowing practitioners and researchers to explore new ways of providing effective therapy. Intentional use of the latest digital technology may motivate children with ASD to learn (e.g., by using the same devices as their peers), match their learning styles (e.g., visual learning), or compensate for specific barriers to engagement (e.g., accessibility of tools).

Music therapists and others serving young children with ASD and their families must become proficient in using digital devices and software applications that are available now, as well as those that will be developed in the future; these devices may enhance children's learning outcomes. With the music sector also undergoing a dramatic shift (e.g., to digital music, instrument apps, and online musical tools), music therapists need to actively develop, explore, and evaluate new possibilities of the digital world for the benefits of their clients. Digital technology may change the way we provide music therapy services to children with ASD and their families, far beyond what we can currently imagine.

The responses to the following two questions provide additional perspectives and predictions from three professional music therapists:

1. How do you use digital technology and devices (i.e., iPad and apps) in clinical practice for children with ASD?

2. What are your predictions about online learning and high-tech devices for children with ASD in the future?

I use music technology resources such as the iPad and client-preferred apps to facilitate the creative expression and engagement of children with ASD, especially when their fascination with and enjoyment of these resources enable a therapeutic relationship to develop through these shared technology-enhanced music experiences.

I predict that technology devices and online interaction environments will continue to become more powerful, transparent, intuitive, and easier to use by both children with ASD and those who work with them, including caregivers, teachers, and professionals such as music therapists. (Robert Krout, Ed.D., MT-BC, Professor and Director of Music Therapy, Southern Methodist University, Dallas, Texas)

I have used several apps with children with ASD. There are several music apps that have excellent sound quality. The iPad bells and xylophones are easy to activate, colorful, and have a reaction when touched (shaking/ringing or mallets moving). These are engaging to children and can be used to learn pre-academics, social skills, and creative exploration. Music can be added to academic apps (apps for learning letters, colors, etc.) in order to further motivate children to learn using the iPad. Many children that I work with now use the iPad as their primary AAC device—using simple "yes/no" or picture/word communication apps.

I think that the future will be full of online and high-tech learning opportunities and I think there will be a real place for technology in the treatment and functioning of children with ASD. As children with ASD find ways to communicate using technology, they will be able to show their parents, teachers, and communities their true personalities and abilities. (Blythe LaGasse, Ph.D., MT-BC, Assistant Professor of Music Therapy, Colorado State University, Fort Collins, Colorado)

I supervise a practicum in an elementary school where our university students work with a class of preschoolers with developmental delays and a class of young children with varying degrees of hearing loss. For both groups of children, visuals are a must, and for that, the iPad is ideal. We may not be ready to throw out the laminating machine yet, but we will be soon.

Children with ASD will always benefit socially from face-to-face interactions with others; however, for those with little to no language, the iPad can aptly facilitate their communication with others—thus, opening doors that might have otherwise been shut tight. For practicing music therapists, especially those who work with young children, the iPad will soon be as necessary as a guitar. In the near future, I believe college curricula will include survey courses in iPad applications for music therapists. (Alice-Ann Darrow, Ph.D., MT-BC, Professor of Music Therapy and Music Education, Florida State University, Tallahassee, Florida)

LEARNING QUESTIONS

1. Identify one prominent professional development, organization, and network site that focuses on issues related to ASD.

2. Where can one download evidence-based briefs and fact sheets on ASD?

3. What is your favorite ASD podcast/blog and why?

4. Describe three products/apps and how you would use them in clinical practice.

5. Why should music therapists stay informed about new products and technological advances?

6. How do you identify and apply high-quality online resources?

7. What are your predictions about future online learning and high-tech devices for children with ASD?

Chapter 16

Annotated Bibliography

Selected Research At-a-Glance

Marcia Humpal, M.Ed., MT-BC
OLMSTED FALLS, OH

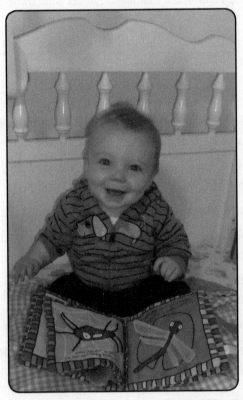

We are never too young or too old to learn from research and literature.
(Marcia Humpal)

Research both from within and outside the music therapy profession informs evidence-based practice. This chapter provides a brief overview of selected studies found throughout this book. Because of the rapidly evolving discoveries surrounding autism spectrum disorders (ASD), it is essential for music therapists to keep abreast of peer-reviewed publications that offer rigorous information for effective interventions and supports for young children with ASD and their families. Science is not static, but an ongoing search for explanations and predictions. While the selected studies reflect current knowledge in music therapy, readers are encouraged to look beyond these examples and to be vigilant seekers of ongoing research-based information to inform clinical practice.

Treatment studies supporting the effectiveness of using music with young children with ASD

- Brownell, M. (2002). Musically adapted social stories to modify behaviors in students with autism: Four case studies. *Journal of Music Therapy, 39(2)*, 117–144.

  This single case experimental design study evaluated the effect of using musical social stories with four first and second graders with ASD to modify targeted behaviors. The behaviors were selected by each child's classroom teacher and were those most interfering with the child's successful social or academic development (e.g., dealing with echolalia, following directions, and using a quiet voice). The musical-social story condition was equally effective to reading of social stories in three of four cases, and more effective in one of the cases.

- Buday, E.M. (1995). The effects of signed and spoken words taught with music on sign and speech imitation by children with autism. *Journal of Music Therapy, 32(3)*, 189–202.

  This investigation used a within-subjects design to examine the use of music as a strategy to teach manual signs to ten children with ASD between ages four and nine. The imitation of sign and speech in conjunction with music or rhythm favored use of music over rhythm training.

- Finnigan, E., and Starr, E. (2010). Increasing social responsiveness in a child with autism: A comparison of music and non-music interventions. *Autism, 14(4)*, 321–348.

  This single case experimental design study with a three-year-old child with ASD demonstrated that music play sessions employing a variety of instruments, toys, and "piggyback" songs with guitar increased the child's social responsive behaviors (i.e., eye contact, imitation, and turn-taking skills). In addition, the child exhibited no avoidance behaviors (e.g., looking away, walking away, or pushing away a toy or adult) during music therapy sessions.

- Kern, P., and Aldridge, D. (2006). Using embedded music therapy interventions to support outdoor play of young children with autism in an inclusive community-based childcare program. *Journal of Music Therapy, 43(4)*, 270–294.

This multiple baseline design study, conducted with four boys with ASD, ages three through four, sought to determine if embedded music therapy interventions can improve children's peer interaction on a university-based inclusive playground. While the musical adaptation of the playground itself did not greatly improve social interactions of children with ASD, it did facilitate their play by attracting them to the sound source. Playground songs composed by the first author and embedded through a teacher and peer-mediated intervention resulted in increased peer interactions and meaningful play for the target children with ASD.

- Kern, P., Wakeford, L., and Aldridge, D. (2007). Improving the performance of a young child with autism during self-care tasks using embedded song interventions: A case study. *Music Therapy Perspectives, 25(1)*, 43–51.

This alternating treatment design study investigated the effectiveness of embedding information within songs to prompt multiple-step self-care tasks for a three-year-old child with ASD enrolled in an inclusive classroom. Musical versus verbal presentations of the task sequence were compared across three self-help tasks. The song intervention was more effective than lyric/spoken intervention for hand-washing and cleaning-up while lyrics/spoken words appeared more successful for toileting.

- Kern, P., Wolery, M., and Aldridge, D. (2007). Use of songs to promote independence in morning greeting routines for young children with autism. *Journal of Autism and Developmental Disorders, 37(7)*, 1264–1271.

Using an ABAB withdrawal design, this study evaluated how songs composed specifically for two three-year-old boys with ASD could assist them during the morning greeting routine of their inclusive classrooms. The songs, composed by the music therapist, delineated each step of the morning greeting routine. Classroom teachers were taught to sing these songs, embedding them into the routine. Results indicated that the songs supported the children's independence in entering the classroom, greeting the teachers and/or peers, and engaging in play.

- Kim, J., Wigram, T., and Gold, C. (2008). The effects of improvisational music therapy on joint attention behaviors in autistic children: A randomized controlled study. *Journal of Autism and Developmental Disorders, 38,* 1758–1766.

  Ten boys between the ages of three and five took part in this randomized controlled trial single subject design comparing improvisational music therapy and play sessions with toys. Upon analysis of sessions, improvisational music therapy yielded significantly more and longer eye contact and turn-taking than did play sessions.

- Kim, J., Wigram, T., and Gold, C. (2009). Emotional, motivational, and interpersonal responsiveness of children with autism in improvisational music therapy. *Autism, 13(4),* 389–409.

  This article described emotional, motivational, and interpersonal responsiveness of ten young children with ASD between the ages of three and five during improvisational music therapy. Results of this repeated measures within subjects comparison design indicated that improvisational music therapy produced significantly more and longer events of joyful facial expressions, emotional synchronicity, and initiation of engagement than did toy play conditions.

  Note: Though based on the same study as Kim, Wigram, and Gold (2008), this entry includes different outcome descriptions.

- Lim, H.A. (2010). Effect of "Developmental Speech and Language Training Through Music" on speech production in children with autism spectrum disorders. *Journal of Music Therapy, 47(1),* 2–26.

  Fifty children between the ages of three and five took part in this experimental design study that compared the use of music training, speech training, and no-training to aid verbal production with young children with ASD. Music training was given to the children via a music video that contained songs and pictures of targeted words, using a music therapy developmental speech and language training through music technique. Results of pre- and post-testing indicated that both music and speech training are significantly effective for improving acquisition of functional vocabulary words and speech production in young children with ASD. Low-functioning participants in particular showed a greater improvement after the music training as compared with speech training. The study also suggests that children with ASD may gain important linguistic information by perceiving patterns embedded in musical stimuli.

- Lim, H.A., and Draper, E. (2011). The effects of music therapy incorporated with Applied Behavior Analysis Verbal Behavior approach for children with autism spectrum disorders. *Journal of Music Therapy, 48(4),* 532–550.

In this within subjects experimental design study, 22 children with ASD, between the ages of three and five, took part in a comparison of developmental speech-language training, using an Applied Behavior Analysis Verbal Behavior (ABA VB) approach and music incorporated with this method. A single group intervention with three training conditions and four verbal operant conditions was utilized. Results showed that both music and speech training are effective in ABA VB training, with music being more useful in areas of echoic production.

- Simpson, K., and Keen, D. (2010). Teaching young children with autism graphic symbols embedded within an interactive song. *Journal of Developmental and Physical Disabilities, 20,* 165–177.

This study investigated the use of music to teach communication skills. In this single case design study, three children with ASD, ages three to four, were taught a song about animal names while the animal symbols were simultaneously shown in a PowerPoint presentation on an Interactive Whiteboard (IWB). Children were asked to touch the symbol on the IWB that corresponded to the animal named in the song. Using the IWB facilitated correct receptive labeling by all the study participants,. However, there was little generalization of these results to other contexts.

- Wimpory, D., Chadwick, P., and Nash, S. (1995). Brief report. Musical interaction therapy for children with autism: An evaluative case study with two-year follow-up. *Journal of Autism and Developmental Disorders, 25(5),* 541–552.

This single case experimental design study described how Musical Interaction Therapy (MIT) was employed with a three-year-old child with ASD to improve non-communicative behavior. Musical accompaniment depicting the child's mood or type of activity was provided during times of mother–child play. Results indicated that MIT aided playful joint action that generalized beyond therapy and was sustained over time.

Literature reviews supporting the effectiveness of using music with young children with ASD

- Gold, C., Wigram, T., and Elefant, C. (2006). Music therapy for autistic spectrum disorder. *Cochrane Database of Systematic Reviews, Issue 2.* Art. No.: CD004381. doi:10.1002/14651858.CD004381.pub2.

In this Cochrane review, the authors identified three small randomized controlled or controlled clinical trial studies ($N = 24$) that met the criteria for inclusion in their systematic review for comparing music therapy to "placebo" therapy, no treatment, or standard care. The outcomes resulted in small to medium effect sizes indicating that music therapy was significantly more effective than the non-music therapy conditions for addressing verbal and gestural communicative skills, but did not have a significant effect on behavioral issues. The authors concluded that the studies did not offer great applicability to clinical situations because the music therapy treatment (though presented daily) was conducted for only one one week and resulted in only short-term effects.

- Reschke-Hernandez, A.E. (2011). History of music therapy treatment interventions for children with autism. *Journal of Music Therapy, 48(2)*, 169–207.

  This historical overview examines music therapy and treatment of children with ASD from 1940 to 2009. The author presented a history of autism diagnosis, reviewed the historical strengths and limitations of music therapy practice with children with ASD (1940–1989), appraised strengths and limitations of music therapy practice with children with ASD (1990–2009), and discussed future directions for music therapy research and clinical practice with this population.

- Whipple, J. (2004). Music in intervention for children and adolescents with autism: Meta-analysis. *Journal of Music Therapy, 41(2)*, 90–106.

  This meta-analysis examined 12 dependent variables from nine quantitative studies, revealing that using music yields significant treatment benefits (overall effect size of $d = 0.77$) in interventions with children and adolescents with ASD. The areas of social (challenging, self-stimulatory, mealtime out-of-seat behaviors), communication (eye contact, verbalization, spontaneous speech, social acknowledgment, and communicative acts), and cognitive skill enhancement (gross motor task completion, computer task response accuracy, shape identification, vocabulary comprehension, and point and look at stimulus) appear to be particularly benefical.

Descriptions of music therapy practice supporting the effectiveness of using music with young children with ASD

- Allgood, N. (2005). Parents' perception of family-based group music therapy for children with autism spectrum disorders. *Music Therapy Perspectives, 23(2)*, 92–99.

  This qualitative treatment case study investigated parents' perceptions of family-based music therapy services for their children with ASD who were between the ages of four and six. Data were gathered via pre-interview sessions and in post-interview focus groups with parents from four families. Parents responded positively to a seven-week family-based group music therapy intervention, articulating new insights about themselves and their children.

- Gadberry, A. (2011). A survey of the use of aided Augmentative and Alternative Communication during music therapy sessions with persons with autism spectrum disorders. *Journal of Music Therapy, 48(1),* 74–89.

This cross-sectional survey study was conducted with 187 certified music therapists who work with clients with ASD in the United States. Only 14.6 percent used aided Augmentative and Alternative Communication (AAC) with their clients who utilized them outside of music therapy. Picture schedules were the most commonly employed. Furthermore, 40 percent of music therapists report having been trained in the use of AAC.

- Kaplan, R.S., and Steele, A.L. (2005). An analysis of music therapy program goals and outcomes for clients with diagnoses on the autism spectrum. *Journal of Music Therapy, 42(1),* 2–19.

This program evaluation report tracked data pertaining to music therapy service delivery in a community-based music school over two program years for 40 clients with ASD ranging in age from 2 to 49 years. Areas examined and information tracked about each (listed in rank order herein) included music therapy interventions (interactive instrument playing, musical instrument instruction, interactive singing, and making instrument or song choices), session types (individual was most often conducted), formats most frequently used (activity-based, lesson-based, client-led/shadow, ensemble), goals most frequently addressed (language/communications skills followed by behavioral/psychosocial skills), assessed level of difficulty of clients and their situations (levels of difficulty did not seem to affect attainment of objectives), and generalization of skills to other settings (positive generalization to non-music areas).

- Lim, H.A. (2010). Use of music in the Applied Behavior Analysis Verbal Behavior approach for children with autism spectrum disorders. *Music Therapy Perspectives, 28(2),* 95–105.

This article discussed how music may be used to treat young children with ASD within the Applied Behavior Analysis Verbal Behavior approach and also described a music therapy language training session protocol. The author concludes that pairing targeted verbal behavior with musical experiences might establish effective automatic reinforcement and increase the frequency of communicative behaviors and social interactions.

- Walworth, D.D. (2007). The use of music therapy within the SCERTS® Model for children with autism spectrum disorder. *Journal of Music Therapy, 44(1),* 2–22.

This paper described the SCERTS® Model, a comprehensive curriculum designed to assess and identify treatment goals and objectives for children with ASD. A national survey of music therapists who serve clients with ASD revealed that they are working on various treatment goals listed in the SCERTS® Model, but may not have identified or are unaware of the many additional goals that they actually are addressing. The author explains that music therapy may be aligned with the multidisciplinary treatment goals and objectives of the SCERTS® Model and also suggests that it could be used as an assessment tool to measure clients' progress.

- Walworth, D.D., Register, D., and Engel, J.N. (2009). Using the SCERTS® Model Assessment tool to identify music therapy goals for clients with autism spectrum disorder. *Journal of Music Therapy, 46(3)*, 204–216.

A post hoc descriptive analysis of videotaped sessions submitted by 33 music therapists sought to identify the areas of the SCERTS® Model that the music therapists focused on within their sessions for young children with ASD. The frequency of SCERTS® domains and goals that were addressed were compared following coding of the sessions by four independent observers. Results indicated that music therapists worked on all three SCERTS® domains (i.e., social communication, emotional regulation, and transactional support). Furthermore, 58 of the 320 possible sub-goals in the social partner and language partner stages were addressed with at least a 90 percent frequency. The authors noted that the SCERTS® Model Assessment may yield a substantial number of additional untapped goals and sub-goals appropriate for music therapy intervention.

- Wigram, T., and Gold, C. (2006). Music therapy in the assessment and treatment of autistic spectrum disorder: Clinical application and research evidence. *Child: Care, Health and Development, 32(5)*, 535–542.

This report examined the potential effects of utilizing improvisational music therapy with children with ASD. Designated case studies and controlled trials appear to demonstrate that improvisational music therapy may help improve communicative behavior, language, emotional responsiveness, attention span, and behavior control.

LEARNING QUESTIONS

1. Which studies support social skill improvements in children with ASD through music therapy interventions?

2. Which studies support using music therapy interventions to improve communication for young children with ASD?

3. What additional goal areas for young children with ASD may be effectively supported by music therapy interventions? Cite at least one research article that substantiates each.

4. How might studies inform and influence your clinical practice?

Author's note

The author wishes to thank Talia Morales and Michelle Lazar of Coast Music Therapy, Inc. for sharing resources for the development of this chapter.

The Editors

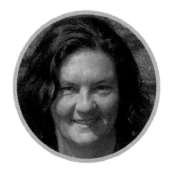

Petra Kern, Ph.D., MT-DMtG, MT-BC, MTA is a certified music therapist in the United States, Canada, and Germany and earned her doctoral degree from the School of Medicine at the University of Witten-Herdecke. She is the owner of the California-based company *Music Therapy Consulting* and Adjunct Professor at Marylhurst University and the University of Louisville. Previously she taught at the State University of New York at New Paltz and the University of Windsor, and continues to guest lecture and conduct workshops at universities worldwide.

Dr. Kern has worked in several clinical settings, serving the youngest to the oldest with various disabilities and health issues. In 2008, she received the Research/Publications Award of the American Music Therapy Association (AMTA) for her studies with young children with autism spectrum disorders, which she conducted at the Frank Porter Graham Child Development Institute at the University of North Carolina at Chapel Hill. Her work has been published in *Young Exceptional Children, Young Children, Children and Families, Teaching Young Children,* the *Journal of Autism and Developmental Disorders,* the *Journal of Music Therapy, Music Therapy Perspectives, Music Therapy Today,* and *imagine.*

Dr. Kern is a frequent international speaker and serves as the immediate Past President of the World Federation of Music Therapy (WFMT). She is on the editorial boards of *Music Therapy Perspectives,* the *Canadian Journal of Music Therapy,* and *Music and Medicine.* She is also the founder and editor of *imagine,* an early childhood online magazine published by AMTA, and the co-chair of AMTA's Early Childhood Network. For more details, please visit her website at www.musictherapy.biz.

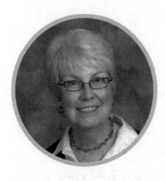

Marcia Humpal, M.Ed., MT-BC operates a small private practice following her retirement after a long career with the Cuyahoga County Board of Developmental Disabilities in Cleveland, Ohio, United States. She is a music therapist for the Toddler Rock program at the Rock and Roll Hall of Fame, and sees early intervention parent/child groups through the Outreach Department of Baldwin-Wallace College, and the West Shore YMCA.

A past Vice-President of the American Music Therapy Association (AMTA), the co-founder of its Early Childhood Network, and former member of the editorial board of *Music Therapy Perspectives*, she currently co-chairs AMTA's Strategic Priority on Music Therapy and ASD Workgroup and serves on the editorial team of *imagine*. Marcia is a frequent presenter at national and international conferences, and has numerous publication credits, including co-editing *Effective Clinical Practice in Music Therapy: Early Childhood and School Age Educational Settings*. She was the recipient of the AMTA Award of Merit in 2004 and was honored by her alma mater Baldwin-Wallace College as an Outstanding Educator in 2006.

The Contributors

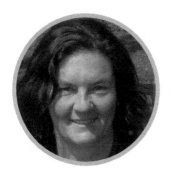

Petra Kern, Ph.D., MT-DMtG, MT-BC, MTA, owner of *Music Therapy Consulting*, has a clinical and research focus on young children with autism spectrum disorders, inclusion, and staff training. She is recipient of the AMTA 2008 Research/Publications Award, editor of *imagine*, and author of numerous publications. A former scholar at UNC at Chapel Hill, Dr. Kern taught at the University of Windsor, SUNY New Paltz, and currently at Marylhurst University and the University of Louisville. She serves as the immediate Past President of WFMT, on various editorial boards, and is a frequent international speaker and guest university lecturer.

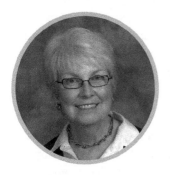

Marcia Humpal, M.Ed., MT-BC maintains a small private practice in the Cleveland, Ohio area. Her clinical work focuses on early intervention, autism spectrum disorders, music in educational settings, and inclusion. She was a member of the advisory panel for Sesame Street's *Music Works Wonders* project, and has several publication credits. A frequent national and international presenter, she also guest lectures at college and universities and continues to work on numerous committees and assignments for AMTA.

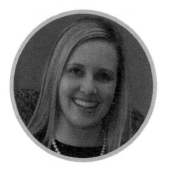

Jennifer Whipple, Ph.D., MT-BC, Professor and Director of Music Therapy at Charleston Southern University, is a Fellow of the National Institute for Infant and Child Medical Music Therapy. Author of the 2004 published meta-analysis on music intervention for children and adolescents with autism spectrum disorders, Dr. Whipple's primary research interests are developmental intervention with preterm infants and teacher training for successful inclusion of students with special needs.

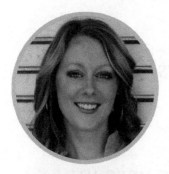

Linda K. Martin, MME, MT-BC has been working with children with autism spectrum disorders since 1998 in early intervention and school settings. She specializes in assessments, behavioral intervention, and supporting families through diagnosis. An international presenter, she focuses on the use of music-assisted curriculum as well as evidence-based practices in autism spectrum disorders intervention.

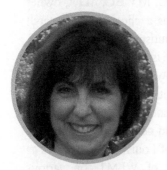

Angela M. Snell, M.S., MT-BC is an experienced school music therapist specializing in autism spectrum disorders, early childhood, behavior disorders, assessment, and inclusive education. A contributing author in two books on early childhood and school age music therapy, she has a Master's of Science in Educational Leadership and is currently earning a Specialist of Arts in Special Education Administration.

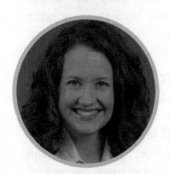

Darcy Walworth, PhD, MT-BC is the Director of Music Therapy at the University of Louisville. Co-chair of AMTA's Strategic Priority on Music Therapy and ASD Workgroup, Dr. Walworth has published in the *Journal of Music Therapy, Journal of Pediatric Nursing, Pediatric Nursing Journal,* and *Journal of Neonatal Nursing.* Her research focus areas include neonatal and early childhood developmental music therapy interventions.

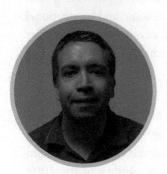

Mike D. Brownell, MME, MT-BC is owner and director of *Music Therapy Services of Ann Arbor,* Michigan where he provides services to children with developmental, physical, learning, and emotional disabilities. He has served on the editorial board of *Music Therapy Perspectives* and as a guest reviewer for *Autism: The International Journal of Research and Practice.*

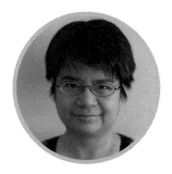

Nina Guerrero, M.A., MT-BC, LCAT, Research Coordinator at the Nordoff-Robbins Center for Music Therapy, New York University, oversees projects investigating effects of Nordoff-Robbins music therapy on communication, social interaction, and creative expression in young children with autism spectrum disorders; music perception and speech perception in children with cochlear implants; and physical, psychological, and social well-being in stroke patients.

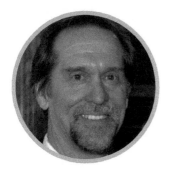

Alan Turry, D.A., MT-BC, NRMT, LCAT is Managing Director of the Nordoff-Robbins Center for Music Therapy at New York University. The first music therapist formally certified to run a Nordoff-Robbins training course, he is responsible for the overall administration, research, clinical services, and the training program at the Center. An international lecturer, Dr. Turry also teaches clinical improvisation in the New York University Master's program.

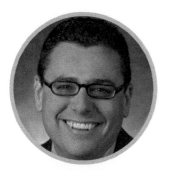

John A. Carpente, Ph.D., MT-BC, LCAT is Assistant Professor of Music Therapy at Molloy College where he founded the Center for Autism and Child Development. Also the Founder and Executive Director of the Rebecca Center for Music Therapy, Dr. Carpente participated in supervision and case conferences with Dr. Stanley I. Greenspan from 2005 to 2010 while creating the Rebecca School's DIR®-based Music Therapy Program.

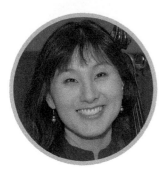

Hayoung A. Lim, Ph.D., MT-BC, Neurologic Music Therapist, is Director of Graduate Studies in Music Therapy at Sam Houston State University. Her published research focuses on music's effect on children with autism spectrum disorders, and music's influences on cognition, speech/language, and physical rehabilitation. She is the author of *Developmental Speech-Language Training through Music for Children with Autism Spectrum Disorders* published by Jessica Kingsley Publishers.

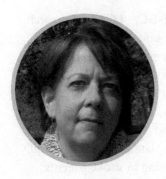

Linn Wakeford, M.S., OTR/L is an Associate Professor in the Division of Occupational Science and Occupational Therapy at the University of North Carolina at Chapel Hill. Author of several publications on sensory processing issues related to children with autism spectrum disorders, she serves as the Intervention Coordinator for the Early Development Project, an early intervention research project targeting very young children at risk for autism spectrum disorders.

Subject Index

Author Index

CPI Antony Rowe
Chippenham, UK
2017-10-29 20:03